The Psychopharmacology Sourcebook

THE PSYCHOPHARMACOLOGY SOURCEBOOK

Mark Zetin, M.D.

Deborah Tate, M.S.W.

LOWELL HOUSE

LOS ANGELES

NTC/Contemporary Publishing Group

The Psychopharmacology Sourcebook is intended solely for educational and informational purposes and not as medical advice. Please consult a medical or health professional if you have any questions about your health.

Library of Congress Cataloging-in-Publication Data

Zetin, Mark.
    The psychopharmacology sourcebook / Mark Zetin, Deborah Tate.
        p. ; cm.
    Includes bibliographical references and index.
    ISBN: 0-7373-0266-6 (alk. paper)
        Mental illness—chemotherapy. 2. Psychopharmacology. I. Tate,
        Deborah. II. Title.
        [DNLM: 1. Mental Disorders—drug therapy.
        2. Psychopharmacology. 3. Psychopharmacology—methods.
        4. Psychotropic Drugs—therapeutic use.
        WM 402 Z61p 1999]
    RC483.Z48 1999
    616.89'18—dc21
                                                                                                99-051478

Published by Lowell House
A division of NTC/Contemporary Publishing Group, Inc.
4255 West Touhy Avenue, Lincolnwood, Illinois 60646-1975 U.S.A.

Copyright © 1999 by NTC/Contemporary Publishing Group, Inc.

All rights reserved. No part of this work may be reproduced, stored in a retrieval system, or transmitted in any form or by any means electronic, mechanical, photocopying, recording, or otherwise, without the prior permission of NTC/Contemporary Publishing Group, Inc.

Printed in the United States of America

International Standard Book Number: 0-7373-0266-6

99 00 01 02 03 04 RRD 18 17 16 15 14 13 12 11 10 9 8 7 6 5 4 3 2 1

CONTENTS

INTRODUCTION — IX

CHAPTER 1 PSYCHIATRIC DIAGNOSIS — 1
- What is Diagnosis? — 1
- History of Present Illness — 5
- Evaluating an Illness (Symptom Description) — 5
- Past Psychiatric Treatment — 6
- Medical History — 7
- Family History — 7
- Habits — 8
- Developmental History — 8
- Current Life Situation — 8
- Review of Systems — 9
- Mental Status Exam — 9
- Physical Exam — 9
- Laboratory Examinations — 10
- How to Help Your Doctor — 11
- Defining Target Symptoms — 12

CHAPTER 2 ANXIETY DISORDERS: PANIC AND PHOBIAS — 17
- Medical Causes of Anxiety — 19
- Epidemiology — 19
- Panic Attacks — 20
- Medical Treatment of Panic Disorder — 23
- Psychotherapeutic Treatment of Panic Disorder — 29
- Specific Phobias — 30
- Social Phobia — 30
- Family Issues in Panic Disorder and Anxiety Disorders — 57

Chapter 3 Obsessive-Compulsive Disorder — 61
- Multiple Disorders — 64
- Drug Treatments for OCD — 66
- Family Issues with OCD — 91

Chapter 4 Post-Traumatic Stress Disorder — 99
- How PTSD Affects Families — 104
- Education About PTSD and Its Effects — 105
- Anger Plays a Key Role in Family Disruption — 106
- Triggers — 107
- Family History Is Important — 109
- Substance Abuse and the Alcoholic Family — 110
- Codependency — 111

Chapter 5 Generalized Anxiety Disorder — 113
- Benzodiazepine — 114
- BuSpar — 116
- Other Anxiety Disorders — 122
- Drugs to Avoid When Treating Anxiety Disorders — 122

Chapter 6 Insomnia and Minor Tranquilizers — 123
- Family Issues with Insomnia — 129
- Benzodiazepine Treatment Issues — 132

Chapter 7 Depression — 137
- How a Psychiatrist Diagnoses Depression — 137
- Drugs That Cause Depression — 138
- Unipolar and Bipolar Mood Disorders — 139
- Subtypes of Depression — 140
- Illness and Depression — 142
- Depressions Unresponsive to Drugs — 143
- Psychotherapy or Medications? — 144
- Suicide — 146
- Laboratory Evaluation of Depression — 147

Choosing the Proper Medication for Treatment
  of Depression 148
The New Generation of Antidepressants 153
Safety and Overdose Risk 154
How to Best Utilize Medication Trials 154
What Happens When the Medicine Does Not Work? 155
Response Lag 158
Duration of Treatment 159
Drug Dosing 160
MAO Inhibitors 163
BuSpar 164
Seasonal Affective Disorder 165
Refractory Depression 165
Electroconvulsive Therapy (ECT) 168
Family Issues in Depression 230

CHAPTER 8 BIPOLAR AFFECTIVE DISORDER (MANIC DEPRESSIVE ILLNESS) 243

Acute Mania 245
Acute Bipolar Depression 247
Long-Term Maintenance Treatment 248
Family Dynamics in Bipolar Disorder 271
Enmeshment in Families with Bipolar Affective Disorder 271
Denial of the Illness 274
Realistic Expectations Are Important 274

CHAPTER 9 SCHIZOPHRENIA 279

Schizophrenia 280
Family Issues in Schizophrenia 308
Communication 309
Negative Effects of Criticism 311
Emotional Aloofness Requires Patience 312
Helpful Hints 313

A Behavioral Contract for the Schizophrenic Family
Member Living at Home   314

Chapter 10 Alcohol and Drug Abuse   317
Alcoholism   317
Tranquilizer Abuse   320
Stimulant Abuse   321
Opiate Abuse   322
Nicotine Addiction   323
Family Issues of Substance Abuse   325
Interventions Can Help   326
Secondary Gain and Enmeshment Play Roles in Issues of
    Substance Abuse   327
Substance Abuse Leads to Chaos in Relationships   329

Summary and Conclusions   323
Diagnosis   323
Goal Setting   334
Medicines, Psychotherapy, and Self-Help   336
Self-Observation   337
Medication Trials   337
Duration of Treatment   338

Appendix 1
Common Drugs: Their Uses, Advantages, and Side Effects   339

Appendix 2
Drugs Categorized by Brand and Generic Names   347

Glossary   349

Suggested Reading   357

Index   359

INTRODUCTION

WHO SHOULD READ THIS BOOK?

Many people today are taking advantage of the benefits available to them through the field of psychiatry and psychiatric medications; yet, unless someone has worked with a psychiatrist before, it is unlikely that he will know what to expect, or how to adequately prepare all of the medical and personal information a psychiatrist needs to give an accurate diagnosis and to prescribe proper medications for successful treatment. This book attempts to demystify psychiatry, giving readers the tools they need to collaborate with the psychiatric practitioner.

We have written this book for the person who is considering taking a psychiatric medication, or who has been taking one and has questions about it. Some readers are planning to go to a psychiatrist or primary care physician to request a psychiatric medication evaluation. Others may have already gone and been given one or more medications. Still others might be considering seeing a psychiatrist because a psychotherapist says they may have a "chemical imbalance," and they wish to know what this term really means. No matter which of these apply to you, as an informed consumer, you can work better with your doctor toward getting well if you understand the process of psychiatric diagnosis and treatment.

ASSUMPTIONS ABOUT THOSE WHO ARE SEEKING PSYCHIATRIC HELP

When someone comes to a psychiatrist for a consultation, there are several assumptions the practitioner will make about him or her. If the patient does not follow these ground rules, no psychiatrist can do a really comprehensive evaluation and arrive at a treatment plan that makes sense.

1. *The doctor will assume that you have a problem.* By coming to him or her, you are acknowledging that you have difficulties that cause you some real pain, and symptoms that interfere with your quality of life, not just complaints from someone else. Your symptoms might include depression, anxiety, ritualistic behavior, hallucinations, or binge eating. A psychiatrist would hope that you are willing to acknowledge that something is a problem for you and that you want to overcome this problem.
2. *You are clean and sober, or you are willing to get counseling to become so.* Alcohol and drug abuse can cause psychiatric symptoms for which the treatment is often simply abstinence. If you are currently drinking heavily, frequently using cocaine or amphetamines ("speed"), smoking marijuana on a daily basis, or using diet pills or barbiturates ("downers"), then it makes little sense for a psychiatrist to prescribe psychiatric medication for you. All these abusable drugs can cause depression, anxiety, hallucinations, and numerous other symptoms. When the drugs are stopped, the symptoms typically clear up over a period of a month or so. If you are using any

of these addictive substances, it would be well worth attending a twelve-step program such as Alcoholics Anonymous or Cocaine Anonymous to begin the process of recovery.
3. *You are willing to be honest with your doctor about your problems and collaborate with him or her regarding your treatment.* Although there are some limits to doctor-patient confidentiality, such as requirements to report symptoms to managed care and insurance organizations, and to report child and dependent elder abuse to social service agencies, a psychiatrist will assume that your evaluation is based on honest disclosure of your problems. Of course, if you have been ordered into treatment by a court with the understanding that your doctor will have to give a report to a judge, or if you are coming to treatment to avoid legal problems, you will be less likely to be fully honest. Be aware, however, that this choice can get in the way of your treatment and recovery. Many of the symptoms we will be talking about, such as depression and anxiety, don't carry a moral connotation or the sense of embarrassment that addiction, shoplifting, gambling, or other compulsive or abusive behaviors do.
4. *You are willing to take medicines on a daily basis, even if the symptoms you experience come and go.* Psychiatric treatment is often based on three stages: using medications to stabilize the acute symptoms of an illness, continuing to take the drugs for several months beyond that point, and, for many people, long-term maintenance treatment. The goal is to both eliminate your symptoms and to prevent them from coming back. One important point to be aware of is that many illnesses are intermittent. For example, panic attacks may occur only one to five times a week, and yet the medication used to prevent them has to be taken every day. Depression or mania may come in episodes lasting for a few weeks or months, but with several years between occurrences; yet for some people suffering from these disorders, long-term maintenance treatment to prevent recurrence is fully justified.

5. *You are willing to tolerate a few side effects.* The focus of modern psychiatry has evolved from simple symptom suppression to the major goals of long-term prevention of recurrences and restoration of quality of life. For some people, this will mean six to twelve months of treatment; for many others, this means lifelong medication. In this way, psychiatric medications are similar to those taken for other illnesses, such as hypertension, diabetes, and arthritis. Because of this long-term commitment, however, it is very important that side effects be minimized or at least kept tolerable. Although you must be willing to put up with minor side effects, if those you experience are more than a nuisance, you must complain about them assertively to your doctor and ask for a change of dosage or medicine.

The unfortunate but common alternative to this scenario can be seen in the person who takes the medicine until her symptoms get a little better, at which point the side effects seem to outweigh the benefits of continuing the drug. Usually, the patient may stop the medication, only to see symptoms rapidly return within a few months. Then she will start another medication trial that lasts only until the side effects again become overwhelming. This cycle of going on and off medications every few months or years is counterproductive because, in some cases, the response to the original medication may be lost over time. Careful dosage adjustment or selection of alternative medications can minimize most side effects.

ABOUT THE AUTHORS

You are probably wondering about our qualifications to teach you about psychiatric medications. If you are not, you should be. It's only fair to ask that anyone who treats you or consults on your treatment should be a specialist in this area. Mark Zetin, M.D., is a board-certified psychiatrist and has been a full-time member of the faculty at the University of California, Irvine, for fifteen years. Throughout that period, he has had a small private practice that has now become his full-time occupation. In his practice he sees patients referred by psychotherapists for medication evaluation, and some patients referred by other doctors for a second opinion or for a medication management plan that these doctors are not comfortable performing.

Most typically, he will initially see a new patient for a fifty-minute appointment. Then he will ask for past treatment records, laboratory data, and information from the psychotherapist, using this information to formulate a diagnostic and medication treatment plan. Whenever possible, he likes to see a patient with a family member to get a broader perspective on the problems.

Most of his professional life is spent working with patients who are taking psychiatric medication. This book is the result of innumerable conversations about these medicines with his patients.

Deborah Tate is a licensed clinical social worker who has been in private practice for the last ten years. Debbie sees a wide variety of people and families on an outpatient basis and is also involved in various teaching projects, including her work as a volunteer faculty member at the University of California, Irvine, teaching family therapy. She has also spent several years in hospital psychiatry working with the families of severely disturbed adolescents and adults, as well as veterans and others with severe post-traumatic stress disorder. As a clinical social worker, she has worked extensively in a team approach with psychiatrists and other mental health professionals.

ABOUT THIS BOOK

This book covers the major problems seen by an adult psychopharmacologist and clinical social worker. We have made no attempt to include rare and esoteric problems or up-to-date journal article references. In each chapter we give an overview of diagnosis and treatment and then include the details of illustrative cases. These have been edited to delete irrelevant information or potential identifiers, but otherwise are accurate case histories taken when the patient was evaluated. At the end of each chapter, we also include a section offering pertinent information to family members who are trying to help a loved one suffering from a particular disorder.

Each chapter contains case studies from Dr. Zetin's practice. Hopefully, they will serve as examples for doing your own case report to bring to your psychiatrist. They illustrate many of the points discussed in the text, as well as raise many questions about the ins and outs of the treatment process. We really don't claim to know it all, but we hope by including this human dimension to the psychiatric illnesses, and their impact on people's lives, we may provide lessons for the reader in how to manage, or not to manage, important treatment issues. The unfolding of the individual cases often serves as a caution about the impact of illness on individuals and their families, and demonstrates how medications, individual and family therapy, and lifestyle changes (or the absence of these) may all interact in a person's life in important ways. These cases are part of the reality of dealing with psychiatric problems; they are not fictionalized and we haven't selected only the patients with the best outcomes.

A WORD OF CAUTION ABOUT PSYCHIATRISTS

The field of psychiatry is still evolving, as is the professional identity of its practitioners. Psychiatrists subspecialize in numerous areas including:

- pharmacotherapy, also called psychopharmacology (drug treatment)
- psychotherapy
- psychoanalysis (intensive long-term psychotherapy)
- behavior therapy
- child and adolescent therapy

- medical-legal evaluations (for example, those concerning child custody or criminal responsibility)
- treating the medically ill with psychiatric problems (also known as consultation-liaison psychiatry)

Not all psychiatrists are especially interested in psychopharmacology; some do mostly psychotherapy. It is most important to ask your doctor what his or her major areas of interest and expertise are in order to see if there is a good match with your needs and expectations.

Your relationship with a psychiatrist may be lifelong. Choose carefully by interviewing him or her. Ask about hospital affiliation (if you have needed or feel you might need hospitalization), advanced fellowship training, publications, and recent continuing education activities. Ask about hours, fees, insurance arrangements, and other details that will make a difference to you.

If you need help finding a psychiatrist, consider the following ideas.

- Go to a patient support group and ask for the names of the best specialists in your area.
- Call the nearest university medical center and request a list of its faculty or recent graduates with a special interest in the kind of problem you have.
- Phone several psychotherapists (psychologists or social workers) and your family doctor and ask them for their top choices of referrals. If the same name keeps coming up from several of these sources, that doctor is probably well respected and kind to his patients. Consider that person as a potential choice.

In some circumstances, when an individual's symptoms are unrelenting and do not respond to psychotherapy alone, it is beneficial for a psychotherapist to work together with a psychiatrist to help find a medication that will alleviate or stabilize the patient's symptoms enough for emotional healing to occur. Jim is such a case.

Jim: A case of psychiatric medication assisting therapy

Every time Jim was involved in a social situation, he would find himself so overwhelmed that he would turn away rather than face speaking to anyone. He had a hard time going to school and was unable to work, and felt depressed and very angry at himself as he watched others who could do these tasks with ease. At times, he would go on binges of smoking marijuana to ease the pain of what he perceived as his failed social encounters. At one point, Jim used so much cocaine that he almost died. This wasn't a conscious attempt to kill himself, but it certainly demonstrated a desperate attempt to resolve his social phobia.

In therapy, Jim painfully recounted memories of his father's social phobia and his mother's lifelong depression, and his fears that he would end up like them. He also recounted numerous occasions when, as a child, he was the brunt of cruel jokes by both peers and adults when he awkwardly stammered in social situations, unable to speak or even to know what to say.

Jim worked hard in therapy, learning social skills and working through his poor self-image and traumatic childhood. In spite of his efforts, his depression seemed relentless. Finally, Jim's therapist referred him to a psychiatrist for medication. Jim tried Prozac, which proved useful in the first year. At that point, something else was needed to further release him from his depression and social phobia. When his psychiatrist finally had him stop Prozac and then placed him on Nardil, Jim soon found his efforts at being social more fruitful. The more successes he was able to have, the more his social skills grew and the more free he became. His therapy was able to progress more quickly as a result of the Nardil, since it took the edge off his fear and reduced his depression.

Emily: Finding relief from debilitating major depression

Emily is another excellent example of how psychotherapy and psychiatry can work together. The first time Emily came to Deborah Tate for psychotherapy was after her sixteen-year-old daughter Melanie had attempted suicide. During a brief hospitalization, Melanie revealed that her now twenty-year-old brother Mitch had molested her throughout her childhood. Mitch denied participating in this behavior, but estranged himself from the family. This situation left Emily feeling empty, depressed, remorseful, and worthless as a parent, and caused her to have problems with concentration. Despite many personal achievements, both socially and in her work, Emily lost her ability to see herself as a viable parent, wife, and professional. She utilized her therapy very productively and was soon able to resolve her symptoms of depression, especially in the areas of working through her grief and beginning to communicate more effectively with her husband and two daughters.

Two years into treatment, however, Emily again presented with symptoms of major depression coupled with obsessive thoughts about death. These symptoms had started to develop when repressed memories of being molested by her stepfather began flooding her mind. Her guilt became unrelenting as she began to believe that not working through her own history of earlier abuse had somehow placed her daughter and son into a similar taboo relationship. Emily also revealed that throughout her life she had experienced routine morbid thoughts about being murdered or falling prey to a terminal illness. These thoughts became unbearable at times, as if a voice were speaking to her saying things such as, "You're going to die because you've been a bad person," "You should take a gun to your head and shoot yourself before someone else does,"

"You're going to get AIDS because of that blood transfusion you had . . . it doesn't matter that it was twenty years ago . . . what do doctors know about when AIDS began?" Since she was very bright and knew that these were only obsessive thoughts, Emily was able to brush them away as quickly as they came. She had even neglected to report them to me during her two years of treatment. Nevertheless, they continually tormented her.

It was at this point that I referred Emily to a psychiatrist for a medication evaluation because I realized that therapy alone was not going to alleviate her symptoms. Although therapy was able to help Emily work through many of the issues she had around being molested as a child, cope with much of the loss of relationship with her son, and become a more effective communicator within her family, it was ineffective in relieving her obsessive thoughts about death. In fact, as Emily delved further into her heavy issues, her obsessive thoughts worsened for awhile. This created a dilemma: She needed to work through these old unresolved issues in order to feel psychologically whole, but dealing with them temporarily made her symptoms worse. Her baseline symptoms were becoming intolerable. At this point, I sent her to a psychiatrist who did a thorough evaluation of her condition and placed her on Anafranil. Within a few weeks, Emily's obsessive thoughts of death and major depressive symptoms ceased.

Use of medication did not deter Emily from experiencing her feelings; it actually enhanced her ability to utilize her therapy more productively. On the other hand, her obsessive thoughts had only led her to a dead end. Once these thoughts ceased through the use of medication, there were no more dead ends, but only openings for Emily to grow.

Parts of this story may ring a bell for you, or perhaps you may have quite a different story from your childhood or adult life. The point we wish to make, however, is that when psychiatric symptoms are unrelenting, they may require a team approach, as well as a variety of therapeutic techniques. In Emily's case, ongoing individual and family therapy coupled with psychotropic medication created a winning combination, leading her toward psychological growth and a sense of well-being.

CHAPTER 1

PSYCHIATRIC DIAGNOSIS

WHAT IS DIAGNOSIS?

Psychiatric diagnosis begins with the collection of information in the context of the doctor-patient relationship. This is followed by a synthesis of that information that involves looking for known patterns, formulating a series of diagnostic possibilities, gathering more information, then reaching a conclusion, which means labeling the illness and finally formulating a logical treatment plan. This process is performed differently by different professionals, but it can be broadly divided into two general approaches to diagnoses: the *nonmedical model* and the *medical model*.

In either case, the information gathered by the mental health professional will ultimately be used for a *DSM-IV* diagnosis. Used by all American mental health professionals as the defining rule book for making a diagnosis, the American Psychiatric Association's *Diagnostic and Statistical Manual,* fourth edition (*DSM-IV*), requires diagnosis of acute psychiatric problems (Axis I), personality traits or disorders (Axis II), listing of medical problems (Axis III), psychosocial stressors (Axis IV), and overall level of function (Axis V).

Nonmedical Diagnosis

The nonmedical diagnostic process employed by many psychologists, social workers, and psychoanalytic therapists involves obtaining a *developmental history*, looking carefully at the patient's transference and relationship issues, and examining the patient's behaviors and thoughts.

A developmental history is the narrative story of an individual's life. This history is assumed to be important because early childhood experiences, attachment to parenting figures, traumas, and relationships within the family of origin and within the school system have a long-lasting impact. By learning about the individual's growth-promoting experiences, role models, and ideals, as well as his losses and disappointments, his current problems can be placed within a lifetime perspective. This makes it possible for the counselor and the client to discuss the patient's repetitive behaviors in relationships with others, and his flexible, adaptive coping abilities.

Telling the narrative of one's life story to an interested, concerned listener is in itself often a therapeutic experience. If that listener is capable of being quiet, empathetic, and reflective, and does not impose her own agenda on the process, the development of transference often occurs. *Transference* is the projection of feelings from early relationships onto a person in a current relationship.

We are seeing transference in action when a patient comes to the therapist's office after a few sessions, experiences strange feelings, and then "realizes" that she is having these feelings because the therapist is in some way acting like a parent or some other significant figure in her life. When a patient can combine transference with the healthy ability to observe it, she will often make a statement such as, "The way you said that reminded me of the way my father scolded me." If a patient does not have the ability to step back and observe the process, she will experience a much more direct reaction, which might involve "button pushing" and responses similar to those she remembers from her childhood interactions with her father.

The combination of telling one's life story and developing transference is central to the process of psychodynamic or psychoanalytic psychotherapy. Utilizing these techniques, recurrent themes and unconscious driving forces become manifest in transference and can be interpreted and brought into conscious awareness by the therapist.

An alternative therapeutic approach, one that is much more structured and focused on the here and now, is to look at the occurrence of symptoms and the thoughts and feelings that immediately preceded them. Often a very careful look at the situations, interpersonal interactions, and thoughts that led up to the occurrence of a particular symptom will make it much more understandable. By keeping a diary of the patient's thoughts and apparent underlying assumptions, inferring the scripts imprinted the patient from childhood, and looking at the connections between these scripts and the development of a client's symptoms, a cognitive behavioral therapist can assist a patient in realizing the distortions, catastrophizing, and overgeneralizations that contribute to anxiety and depression. By challenging these old assumptions, the person can learn to change for the better the way that he reacts to difficult situations, learning to cope in much more adaptive ways.

It is important to realize that the psychodynamic approach looks for a person's symbolic internal meanings and the long-term conflicts that led to the development of his symptoms, while the cognitive behavioral approach is more focused on the here-and-now thoughts that lead to uncomfortable feelings. Neither of these approaches is as highly focused on examining the symptoms and their time course as is the medical model.

Medical Diagnosis

The medical model, as taught to medical students, is applicable across every specialty. With this system, diagnosis of an illness follows the process of taking a clinical history, performing a physical examination, reviewing clinical records of past treatment, and obtaining laboratory data. The medical model provides the basis for a very systematic and highly structured approach to all medical problems, as well as a generalizable attitude to new problems. In this book, we will focus primarily on the patient's clinical history rather than on his or her physical and lab data because it is in the history taking that most psychiatric diagnoses can be made. This is the time during which the patient has the greatest opportunity to contribute meaningful information to aid his or her diagnosis.

In the following pages, we will review the parts of the clinical history and provide a simple outline for them. It is important to understand how this procedure works because if you know the parts of the clinical history and how to organize it, you may very well be able to write your own history and provide it to your doctor at the time of your medication evaluation, giving him or her your most important information in a very concise and organized way.

IDENTIFYING DATA

The identifying data is your basic background information (sometimes called demographics), including your age, gender, education, occupation, marital status, and employment situation. This information is important because there are certain demographic risk factors associated with psychiatric illnesses. For example, schizophrenia and manic-depressive illness usually have their onset in the late teens and twenties, while Alzheimer's dementia typically begins in the sixties and seventies.

CHIEF COMPLAINT

This is the main symptom or problem for which you are seeking help. Your chief complaint might be described as simply "panic attacks" or "I don't feel like doing anything—nothing is fun." Perhaps an individual might complain that his or her spouse demands changes and can't tolerate the patient's fears, lethargy, social isolation, or extreme overactivity. Another individual with a long treatment history might come to the psychiatrist's office saying, "I've tried everything. No medicine works for me. They all just give me side effects." Whatever the complaint, the rest of the interview will attempt to put the problem into long-term perspective and make sense of it in terms of diagnostic possibilities.

HISTORY OF PRESENT ILLNESS

This is the long-term history of the patient's problems. At what age did they begin? Is the long-term course of the complaint episodic or continuous? Does the patient experience times of getting better, either spontaneously or with treatment? If the symptoms disappear periodically, for how long are they gone? Do they completely disappear or are they just less intense for awhile? Are there things in the patient's life that tend to trigger the problems or make them worse? Is this the first time the patient has experienced this problem, or is it a recurrence of a long-standing pattern? Do episodes of the illness tend to begin when triggered by definite precipitating events, or do they come on "out of the blue"? Frequent triggers for psychiatric illnesses include stressful life events, especially separations and losses, substance abuse, medical illnesses, and discontinuing effective maintenance medication.

EVALUATING AN ILLNESS (SYMPTOM DESCRIPTION)

As part of evaluating an illness, it is important to look at many dimensions of the symptoms. Since no one can possibly remember the full range of all the symptoms that can occur in a psychiatric illness, a psychiatrist will ask the patient to think about and list all the changes she can recall in the way she thinks, feels, behaves, and functions physically in relation to her illness. Thinking, for example, may be altered by poor concentration, unusual pessimism or optimism, the inability to focus and concentrate, the inability to make decisions, or by an unusual sharpness and clarity. Feeling may be characterized by states of anxiety, sadness, elation, worry, or anger. A patient's behavior may be changed in terms of sociability, such as becoming very withdrawn from friends, being unwilling to answer the telephone or the doorbell, and going home immediately after work; or behavior may go in the opposite direction as the patient actively seeks out more people and experiences increased laughing, talking, joking, and tremendous energy. Behavioral symptoms or changes may involve rituals such as washing, counting, checking, calorie-counting during food preparation, compulsive exercise, or compulsive, ritualistic self-care and hygiene.

Biologic functioning refers to the very basic activities of life, such as eating, sleeping, and sexuality. Changes in these core functions are very common in someone with a major psychiatric illness. Appetite, sleep, and/or sexual desire may be increased or decreased, and all of these changes fit into common patterns in mood and anxiety disorders.

Another important question that a psychiatrist will explore with a patient is, "How well do you get?" Wellness is often defined in terms of global functioning in work, social, and play areas. Chronic illness may carry a burden of residual long-term symptoms, including demoralization and loss of effectiveness in life leading to unemployment, social isolation, and a lack of recreational outlets. On the other hand, these symptoms may be temporary disabilities, occurring only during the worst episodes of an illness.

PAST PSYCHIATRIC TREATMENT

By asking about past psychiatric treatment, a clinician will try to discover what worked in the past and what did not work. For example, the psychiatrist will ask the patient what medications were tried, at what dose and blood level, for how long, and with what benefits and side effects. If a patient can provide a simple list of past medications and his responses to them, this can be a huge help to the practicing psychopharmacologist in deciding what drugs to avoid because of patterns of intolerable side effects and which ones to consider because of the patient's partial or full response to them in the past. Similarly, it is worth discussing the psychotherapy approaches that have been helpful or not helpful, in terms of what might be useful now. It is also important to discuss the patient's past experiences with hospitalization or day treatment (partial hospitalization), and her feelings about using such avenues of help in the future.

MEDICAL HISTORY

A patient's medical illnesses, operations, hospitalizations, current medications, and allergies to medications are all important in helping a psychopharmacologist assess what medications might be acceptable. A physical condition or the medications taken for the treatment of such a condition may affect the selection of psychiatric drugs because of possible drug interactions or side effects.

FAMILY HISTORY

Because our appreciation of the genetic component of many psychiatric illnesses is continually growing, the importance of knowing family psychiatric and medical history cannot be overestimated. A family history of medical illnesses may indicate that the patient is at risk for problems such as thyroid disease, diabetes, hypertension, or cancer. A family history of drug or alcohol problems may be a clue to untreated psychiatric illness in the patient's relatives, and a history of suicide is certainly an important indicator of suicide risk. Most important, a family history that uncovers members with problems very similar to the patient's, and their subsequent treatment with psychiatric medications, can be a gold mine of information in deciding what drugs to try. I am often quite amazed at the number of patients who know that a parent or sibling has a similar psychiatric problem and has sought treatment for it, but have never explored the medications taken by that relative. Often, the family member has been doing extremely well on a specific medication, which then becomes a potential drug of choice for the patient.

HABITS

Health-promoting or health-injuring habits are an important part of assessing a patient. Substance abuse, alcoholism, and cigarette smoking are all factors that may make it more difficult to treat the patient with psychiatric medicines, or may require special dosage adjustments. Dramatic drops in cholesterol level or dieting may sometimes worsen depression. Conversely, a healthy diet and exercise may make a psychiatric illness easier to treat.

DEVELOPMENTAL HISTORY

The most important issues in development are the patient's early relationships with his or her parents, siblings, and extended family; a history of any major psychological, physical, or sexual traumas; relationships with peers and teachers while growing up; and relationships with friends or lovers, teachers, and employers as an adult.

CURRENT LIFE SITUATION

It is quite important to know who is living in the patient's home, what the relationships with those individuals are like, and about the patient's work situation. When these environments are abusive and emotionally intolerable for a person, this potentially creates a condition we refer to as chronic stress. There is no medication that will make a highly critical and emotionally abusive boss or spouse any more tolerable, or decrease the patient's sense of distress in having to deal with such an individual. If family burnout is present or the family is hostile, safety of the ill patient sometimes demands hospitalization until all the patient's symptoms are controlled. At other times, the availability of a support system can help to avoid the hospitalization of the patient.

REVIEW OF SYSTEMS

This is a simple inquiry into whether there are any physical symptoms that are bothering the patient. Common problems such as headaches, palpitations, indigestion, cough, fever, weight change, change in bowel or bladder habits, or physical pains may be the functional manifestations of psychiatric problems; or they may represent an undiagnosed physical illness for which lab evaluation and a consultation with an internist may be very useful.

MENTAL STATUS EXAM

This is the psychiatrist's equivalent of a physical exam. The mental status examination is done largely as part of the preceding interview and includes an evaluation of how the person is thinking, feeling, and behaving during the interview. Also included are certain formal tests of a patient's cognitive abilities, such as asking the date and the location of the interview, who the president of the United States is, the interpretation of proverbs, how certain objects are similar to one another, and testing a person's memory for digits and words.

PHYSICAL EXAM

Some psychiatrists are comfortable performing a full physical exam, while others prefer to refer this part of an evaluation to a family physician or internist. Often a psychiatrist with a full year of medical internship, or with some time spent practicing in primary care as an internist or general practitioner before training to be a psychiatrist, will be much more confident in his or her diagnostic abilities than a psychiatrist without this experience. Generally, however, a psychiatrist will not have personnel and equipment for performing a breast exam, pelvic and rectal exam, or an electrocardiogram, and will refer these tests to a colleague.

LABORATORY EXAMINATIONS

Unfortunately, despite decades of searching for the biologic markers of schizophrenia, depression, mania, panic attacks, and numerous other conditions, there are no good biological markers for a psychiatric illness. You can't go to the lab and have a blood sample taken for a test to diagnose any of these illnesses. Even though some indicators of these illnesses exist, these are mostly employed in research and are not typically used in a clinical setting.

A psychiatrist more commonly makes use of a clinical laboratory to rule out (eliminate from consideration) common medical problems in the patient, problems that might be masquerading as psychiatric symptoms. What tests are done depends largely on the patient's age and risk factors; for example, an intravenous drug user or prostitute would be at a much higher risk for hepatitis, syphilis, or AIDS than would an individual who had never injected drugs. On the other hand, an older person who was a smoker would be at greater risk for lung problems than a young individual who had never smoked.

A typical screening laboratory panel might consist of a complete blood count (to check for anemia or chronic infection), a chemistry panel (to check liver, kidney, and bone metabolism), lipids (cholesterol and triglycerides to evaluate risk of heart disease), thyroid functions, a urinalysis (to check for kidney disease and bladder infections), a stool for occult blood (a screening for stomach and intestinal cancer), a prostate specific antigen in older males (to screen for prostate cancer), a chest x-ray (especially in smokers), an electrocardiogram, and a mammogram for women over forty years of age or so. These sorts of tests are essentially the ones that would be ordered by an internist or psychiatrist, with slight variations based on the patient's health history and age, the practitioner's available resources, or external cost factors, such as the patient's insurance coverage.

HOW TO HELP YOUR DOCTOR

Prior to going for a psychiatric diagnostic evaluation, there are many things you can do that will be extremely helpful to your psychiatrist and make the process far more efficient. The first thing is to gather your records. If you have had psychological testing, psychiatric hospitalization, laboratory blood tests, medical hospitalizations, or seen other doctors for similar problems in the past, it is well worth gathering together these records . My suggestion is then to photocopy them all, giving one set to your new doctor and keeping another set at home as part of your own personal records. If you do not remember the psychiatric medicines you have taken over the years, but usually go to the same pharmacy, you can make a visit to the pharmacy to request a computerized printout of your past drug prescriptions. If you can compile a list of the medications you have tried, including the duration of use, dose, response, and side effects, this will be very useful in helping your psychiatrist choose what drug to try next.

The next step is to call any relatives who might know details of your family history. If you believe that a relative has been treated for any kind of psychiatric problem, try to find out what treatment worked best for him or her and what did not work. Sometimes, the secrets of the family history only come out when you call a parent and specifically ask him or her about them. In these cases, the family secrets of a generation ago, such as someone having a nervous breakdown, committing or attempting suicide, or suffering from alcoholism may be very important clues as to what illness runs in your family. Sometimes a family member may not have been labeled as psychiatrically ill but their behavior pattern suggests that they were. Perhaps such an individual is remembered as being eccentric, afraid to leave the house, prone to crying spells, or having had episodes of tremendous energy in which the family fortune was spent in a grandiose burst of optimism for a get-rich-quick scheme.

If you are working with a psychotherapist, asking him or her to provide a summary of your diagnostic evaluation, type of therapy provided, and treatment response would be very helpful. Often your therapist has spent many hours getting to know a lot about you. Since your psychiatrist will be asked to make a medication decision based on a relatively brief period of assessing you, the therapist's perspective will be very valuable.

If you are willing to take the time and effort to do this, write up a clinical history of yourself using the outline provided in this chapter. You will see numerous examples throughout this book; they are real evaluations of real patients seen in Dr. Zetin's practice.

Most psychiatrists appreciate an organized presentation of the information and will take a few minutes to read it at the beginning of an evaluation. With this information in hand, they will be able to inquire in great detail and in a very focused way into those areas that seem to be problems for you.

DEFINING TARGET SYMPTOMS

I will often ask a patient, "What would an ideal medication do for you?" The purpose of this question is to try to define a few of the most bothersome symptoms that drug treatment might help. These symptoms may include depression or anxiety, insomnia, low energy, obsessive thoughts, compulsive rituals, uncontrolled eating, suicidal thoughts, or even hallucinations. If you can define a few target symptoms, it becomes possible to graph the severity of these symptoms over time. The easiest method is to keep a journal of medications and results. If the medication you are trying is unsuccessful, your symptoms will continue to fluctuate at about the same intensity. If the medication is successful, the symptoms should be relieved within about a month or two. In cases where a series of different medication trials are necessary to treat a very difficult problem, this method allows the tracking of the patient's symptoms to determine which medications were helpful and which were not. Daily self-observation is of central importance in almost every form of psychotherapy, and is a valuable habit that can lead to better decisions about which medications are working.

Figures 1.1 and 1.2 provide worksheets to complete before your first psychiatric consultation.

PSYCHIATRIC HISTORY

Identifying Data (Age, gender, marital status, occupation)

Chief Complaint (The main problem)

History of Present Illness (Long-term patterns, treatments, helpful/harmful events)

Evaluating an Illness (Changes in thinking, feeling, behaving, biologic functioning when ill; target symptoms that treatment should help control)

Past Psychiatric Treatment (For each medication tried):
Drug   Dose   How long   Response   Side effects

Medical History (Illnesses, operations, hospitalizations, medications, allergies)

Family History (Psychiatric problems, drug/alcohol problems, suicide, nervous breakdown, shock treatment)

Habits (Cigarettes, alcohol, caffeine, street drugs, diet, exercise)

Developmental History (Family of origin, growing up, school, major relationships)

Current Life Situation (Home and work or school)

Review of Systems (Physical symptoms that are problems now)

Figure 1.1   Pyschiatric History

RECORDS TO OBTAIN AND BRING TO THE PSYCHIATRIC EVALUATION

For each indicate:
R = requested   **O** = obtained   **N/A** = not applicable

____ Past psychiatrists' diagnostic/treatment summaries

____ Psychotherapist's diagnostic/treatment summary (current therapist)

____ Psychotherapists' diagnostic/treatment summary (past therapists)

____ Psychiatric hospital discharge summaries

____ Medical/surgical hospital discharge summaries

____ Psychological testing reports

____ Pharmacy records of medications prescribed

____ Recent history and physical report

____ Lab tests obtained during the last year

____ List of psychiatric medications tried by close (blood) relatives and responses

____ List of all current medications with dose, purpose, blood levels (if obtained), and response

Figure 1.2   Records to Obtain and Bring to the Psychiatric Evaluation

CHAPTER 2

ANXIETY DISORDERS: PANIC AND PHOBIAS

▪ *DRUGS DISCUSSED:*
Prozac, Zoloft, Paxil, Tofranil, Xanax, Klonopin, Nardil

The Psychopharmacology Sourcebook was written to help the reader develop a comprehensive understanding of the major psychiatric diagnoses and their treatment. We purposefully wrote this sourcebook as a team since it is commonplace for a psychiatrist and psychotherapist to work in tandem, with each mental health professional bringing a unique aspect to the treatment team. First, we explain the various aspects of each disorder, including major discussions about the choices of medications appropriate for treatment. Second, we include real case histories that demonstrate the different variables that come into play in individuals with the disorder as well as with variations of the malady. We have included a section on the family dynamics and issues that are often associated with the disorder, a very important aspect of psychiatric illness. This is a crucial area to review because often it will be family members reading this book to gain insight into how to help a loved one. Not only will those concerned be able to understand the behavior of the individual presenting with the disorder, but they will also be able to understand how their behavior impacts the problems.

Anxiety in response to truly dangerous situations is a very normal response and has important survival value in dealing with environmental hazards. Anxiety that is persistent, that interferes with everyday life, and that is grossly out of proportion to the stimulus evoking it is part of an anxiety disorder and deserves treatment.

Anxiety accompanies almost every major psychiatric and many medical disorders. Deciding when the anxiety is a primary psychiatric illness rather than due to something else can be difficult. For example, anxiety is very characteristic of individuals who are using stimulants, including cocaine. Anxiety is also typical of those withdrawing from sedative-hypnotic drugs, including barbiturates, minor tranquilizers, and alcohol. Anxiety can be an early part of a developing manic episode or decompensation into schizophrenia. Some individuals who have anxiety disorders are exquisitely sensitive to anxiety induced by drugs that stimulate the sympathetic nervous system. Typically, these are available as over-the-counter decongestants, cold preparations, and diet pills. A similar sensitivity to caffeine-triggered anxiety from coffee, tea, and cola drinks is often found in people with anxiety disorders.

Anxiety disorders comprise several more specific disorders. These include generalized anxiety disorder, obsessive-compulsive disorder, panic disorder, and phobias. Post-traumatic stress disorder is also included in this category but is discussed in a separate chapter. Not everyone who has a panic attack has panic disorder; it is only if these attacks are recurrent, sometimes come out of the blue, and leave the person worrying about the next one or changing behavior in anticipation of it that a diagnosis of panic disorder is justified.

Most anxiety is due to psychiatric problems, but occasionally medical problems may present themselves with anxiety symptoms. For this reason, review of medical causes is essential in evaluation of anxiety disorder diagnosis.

MEDICAL CAUSES OF ANXIETY

Medical causes of anxiety can include irregular heart rhythm, congestive heart failure in which the heart's output of blood is not enough to keep fluid from accumulating in the lungs, asthma, chronic obstructive pulmonary disease (especially in individuals who have smoked cigarettes for a very long time), and Cushing's disease (overactive adrenal glands). Anxiety may also occur when the parathyroid glands cause problems with calcium metabolism. Other medical causes include hypoglycemia in individuals whose blood sugar falls dangerously low between meals, epilepsy, tumors, autoimmune diseases, ulcers, and many others. Frequently, cardiologists see individuals who have panic attacks, and an ultrasound examination of the heart shows mitral valve prolapse. This does not have any real significance in how their panic attacks are treated, and no one really knows if this is a cause, a consequence, or just a coincidence of having panic disorder.

Thyroid disease may also be a factor behind anxiety; it is easy to screen for with a simple blood test. Heat intolerance, frequent bowel movements, weight loss, eyes and sometimes neck bulging, and anxiety characterize hyperthyroidism. Hypothyroidism often presents with cold intolerance, weight gain, low energy, irregular menstrual periods, repeated infections, and depression.

EPIDEMIOLOGY

The percentage of the adult population who have experienced symptoms of panic disorder in any six-month period is 0.4 percent to 1 percent; of generalized anxiety, 2.5 percent; of obsessive-compulsive disorders, about 1 percent to 3 percent. The onset of anxiety disorders typically is from about age fifteen to thirty-five years. Obsessive-compulsive disorder (discussed in chapter 3) affects males and females equally, but the other anxiety disorders affect one male for every two females. The most typical long-term course is to have the anxiety fluctuate and recur throughout the individual's life, with some periods free of symptoms and other periods of severe symptoms.

Diagnosis of the anxiety disorder is complicated by a variety of factors. Often people with these disorders are prone to self-medication with alcohol, sedatives, and other drugs. Also, depression may accompany the disorder, since the individual may have a loss of personal effectiveness that accompanies chronic illness. These symptoms also tend to generate family problems; they are often debilitating and may take away from the attention being paid to other issues in the family.

PANIC ATTACKS

Panic attacks occur in the context of many of the anxiety disorders and are the primary diagnostic feature in panic disorder. They are characterized by a very abrupt onset of intense fear that reaches a peak intensity within ten minutes with four or more of these symptoms: palpitations, sweating, trembling, shortness of breath, feelings of choking, chest pain, nausea, dizziness or faintness, feeling unreal or detached, fear of losing control or going crazy, fear of dying, numbness or tingling, and chills or hot flashes. Panic attacks typically go from initial twinges of discomfort to full-blown intensity in only a few minutes. For many individuals, the attack resolves very quickly when they are able to leave the situation that triggered the attack. These triggers can be as simple as being on the freeway, in an elevator, in a meeting room, or in a line at the grocery store. In some, the attack spontaneously resolves within a couple of minutes. Others report that they feel the residual anxiety, tiredness, and fear of having the next one for hours afterward.

Panic attacks may be situational or unexpected. Situational attacks occur in predictable circumstances. For example, some people develop stage fright when asked to talk before a group of co-workers. Others panic when asked to step into a crowded elevator or to get on an airplane. Many individuals who have panic attacks will experience an attack when faced with events related to the typically feared situation. A different kind of panic attack occurs spontaneously. Instead of having a trigger bring on the panic attack, the attack comes "out of the blue." Panic may come when the person is relaxed at home watching TV or lying in bed. Sometimes panic attacks even awaken a person from a sound sleep.

Panic attacks may occur as part of social phobia, simple phobia, or panic disorder. Agoraphobia (fearful avoidance) may or may not accompany them. The context in which the panic attacks occur determines the actual diagnosis. The symptoms of a panic attack are the same in an individual suffering from panic disorder, simple phobia, or social phobia.

People who have panic disorder often find that some attacks are full-blown while others are small attacks or partial-symptom attacks. The attacks, even those only lasting a few minutes, have a long-lasting impact on a person's life because of generalization that occurs. The person usually develops anticipatory anxiety in which he may spend a great deal of time worrying about when and if he will have the next one. The anticipatory anxiety can lead to all kinds of attempts to prevent another attack and avoid any kind of situation that might trigger one.

AGORAPHOBIA

Agoraphobia is another potential consequence of panic attacks. With agoraphobia, an individual worries about being in a place from which escape would be difficult or where help would be unavailable. Such situations are usually avoided or only endured with distress or with a "safe," helpful, and trusted companion. Agoraphobia usually follows the onset of panic attacks. The person experiencing agoraphobia finds it very difficult to separate from her source of security, most commonly her home, and so goes from being a fairly independent individual to being dependent and clinging to her loved ones. The geographic range of comfortable travel typically shrinks to a small area around home and work. Unlike the person with severe depression, the agoraphobic would like to be able to be active. In fact, she may long to go to a concert or movie, to be able to fly on an airplane, to have dinner in a restaurant, but is so afraid of having an attack or having to leave the situation and be embarrassed by this that she will avoid putting herself into such a difficult situation. This is in contrast to a depressed person who could participate in these activities but often feels, "Why bother? It won't be fun or worth the effort."

In short, panic disorder with agoraphobia involves the panic attacks just described, worry about having further attacks, and the behavioral change of avoiding places.

Panic Disorder

The onset of panic disorder frequently occurs during or after a major illness, an accident, a loss, a separation, or a period of drug abuse. People with panic attacks cannot discriminate between real and imagined danger. In fact, they often fear that the symptoms are life threatening and will visit an emergency room or call the paramedics. I had one patient who had to travel for business and checked out the location of the hospital emergency room nearest to where he was working in every major city. Another patient canceled her vacation to Puerto Rico with her husband at the last minute out of fear of having an attack on the airplane.

Panic sufferers will often get major medical workups from a cardiologist, an ear-nose-and-throat doctor, or a pulmonary doctor. The number of doctors who tell them they are physically healthy and that there is nothing wrong with them accumulates and they become progressively more frustrated, disenchanted, or angry with doctors. Sometimes ineffective medication trials (for example, with BuSpar or Inderal) lead to the false conclusion that nothing will help.

Often people who have panic disorder remember childhood difficulties separating from their parents as part of school phobia or refusal. They may also remember exactly when the panic attacks started because they caused such a dramatic change in lifestyle. The unfortunate complication of panic disorder is an increased risk of death from suicide or cardiovascular causes.

MEDICAL TREATMENT OF PANIC DISORDER

Treatment of panic disorder involves multiple medication choices. The goal is prevention of panic attacks, both the spontaneously occurring ones and those that occur in specific situations, so that the individual may resume a normal lifestyle. Typically, the individual taking medication for panic disorder finds that once he is on an adequate dose of medication, the drug will block the panic attacks. There is a sudden realization that there have not been any attacks over an unusually long time. An individual seeking treatment may have four or five attacks per week at the beginning of treatment, and after a month or two of taking an effective medication, this is down to one mild attack or less per week. As improvement occurs, the necessary behavioral changes follow relatively easily. The person stops avoiding the situations he perceived as scary; he will stop worrying about having the next attack; and he will resume living a normal life.

The first step in treating panic disorder pharmacologically or with specific psychotherapies is to educate. The patient must realize that panic disorder involves oversensitivity to monitoring of internal states, that panic attacks are uncomfortable but not dangerous, and that panic attacks can be precipitated by caffeine or other drugs, including cold pills or decongestants. It is equally important to learn that daily monitoring of the attacks is important in understanding them. A typical diary of panic attacks will include a checklist of which symptoms occurred, how many attacks occurred during the day, whether these attacks were situational or unanticipated, and a rating of how important anticipatory anxiety was during the day. The triggering events and thoughts may be important clues to understanding psychotherapy issues.

There are several different classes of drugs that have been proven highly effective in panic disorder. They may be broadly divided into antidepressants and high-potency benzodiazepine anxiolytics.

ANTIDEPRESSANTS

The antidepressants that are useful in treating panic disorder include the *tricyclic antidepressants,* such as imipramine and desipramine; the *selective serotonin reuptake inhibitors (SSRIs),* including Prozac (fluoxetine), Zoloft (sertraline), and Paxil (paroxetine); and the *monoamine oxidase inhibitors* (MAOIs), such as Nardil (phenelzine). The MAOIs are highly effective but generally are reserved for only the most difficult and unresponsive cases. It is equally important to realize that some antidepressants rarely, if ever, work for panic disorder and, generally, should not be used. These include Desyrel (trazodone), Ludiomil (maprotiline), and Wellbutrin (bupropion). The anti-anxiety drug BuSpar (buspirone) is also ineffective in panic disorder. Serzone (nefazodone), Remeron (mirtazepine), and Effexor (venlafaxine) may work for panic disorder, but the data from controlled studies is not yet adequate to recommend them as first-line treatments.

Antidepressant treatment of panic disorder seems to be a painfully slow process during the first month. Imipramine or desipramine may be started at a daily dose of 10 mg with instructions to increase the dose by 10 mg every couple of days until bothersome side effects begin to occur or the panic attacks are gone. Typical doses of these tricyclic antidepressants are between 50 mg and 300 mg daily with tremendous individual variation in the amount required to get rid of the panic attacks. A higher dose may be required to treat agoraphobic symptoms than that required to block the panic attacks. Panic disorder patients have exquisite sensitivity to side effects of these drugs and the jittery, insomniac, "speedy" feeling of having had too much coffee is commonly reported if the dose escalation is too fast in the first few weeks. The tricyclic antidepressants may cause carbohydrate craving, which shows up in an individual making statements such as "I never wanted dessert before and now I want two scoops of ice cream and seconds on pie." Anticholinergic effects include dry mouth, blurred vision, difficulty urinating, and constipation. Increased appetite and weight gain are not unusual with the tricyclic antidepressants. Typically, imipramine is slightly more sedating and has more of the anticholinergic effects, while desipramine is slightly more activating and energizing and causes a bit more nervousness.

The tricyclic antidepressants are available as generic drugs and, because of this, they are very inexpensive. These drugs are not "happy pills" and are not abusable, addicting, or difficult to stop using. Until the recent development of the selective serotonin reuptake inhibitors (SSRIs), most experts in the field considered them the first-choice treatment for panic disorder.

The SSRIs began to be available in the United States in 1988 and since that time, Prozac, Zoloft, Paxil, and Celexa have all been marketed with FDA approval for depression. Most of these drugs also appear to be very effective in treating panic disorder. Only Zoloft and Paxil are FDA approved for this use. The strategy of starting at a very low dose and gradually working the dose upward until panic attacks are gone or side effects become bothersome is critically important. Many patients with panic disorder have taken a 20-mg capsule of Prozac for a day or two and sworn that they would never again try the drug because of the extreme anxiety and insomnia that it provoked. Those same individuals, when given Prozac liquid, said they could take a very tiny dose beginning at 2 mg/day, increased by 2 mg each week until symptoms were controlled, and have taken the drug and found it extremely tolerable with almost no side effects. This illustrates the point that very low doses are typically used in panic disorder patients, especially in the first few weeks of treatment until the individual has gotten used to the drug. The major goal in treating an individual with antidepressants is to encourage them to stay on the drug long enough for it to work and to minimize the side effects to allow this to happen. This is the reason for starting at very tiny doses and increasing the dose very gradually. Typically, an antidepressant takes about a month to obliterate panic attacks.

For those who fail to respond to imipramine, desipramine, or a serotonin reuptake inhibitor, the alternatives are the use of an MAO inhibitor or a benzodiazepine minor tranquilizer. Most experts consider the MAO inhibitors to be the most potent drugs in blocking panic attacks; yet they are the most difficult to tolerate because of restrictions on diet and drug interactions. The most frequently used drug is Nardil (phenelzine), with a dose gradually increased up to about 1 mg per kg daily. While on this drug, foods that are made by aging or fermentation and that are sharp and tangy are forbidden because of their tyramine content. There is a long list of foods including beer, wine, cheese, sour cream, liver, fava beans, and so on that must be avoided. Similarly, the sympathicomimetic (stimulant family) drugs, such as cold pills and appetite suppressants, must be avoided because they can raise blood pressure dramatically. High-potency narcotics such as Demerol, and selective serotonin reuptake inhibitors such as Prozac, Paxil, and Zoloft must also be avoided because of very dangerous drug interactions. (The switch from SSRI to MAO inhibitor requires a washout period of two to five weeks, depending on which SSRI was used.)

BENZODIAZEPINE ANXIOLYTICS

The alternative treatment for panic disorder is use of a high-potency benzodiazepine tranquilizer. The best-known drug in this class is Xanax (alprazolam) and this is the only tranquilizer that is FDA approved for the treatment of panic disorder. Klonopin (clonazepam) is similar and has been submitted for FDA review. Xanax doses range from 2 to 10 mg/day in the treatment of panic disorder and has to be highly individualized so that the dose is enough to prevent panic attacks and yet not enough to leave the individual feeling tired, forgetful, uncoordinated, or drunk. The tremendous advantage of Xanax in the treatment of panic disorder is that it may be used on an as-needed basis. Most individuals with panic attacks carry a few tablets with them in a pocket or purse as a "security blanket," knowing that if they do have a panic attack, they have something they can take that will help to shorten its duration. Similarly, if they have to go into a difficult situation, they have an as-needed medicine they can use shortly beforehand to decrease the likelihood of having a panic attack.

Daily regular dosing studies tell an important story. Double-blind studies comparing drugs to placebo (sugar pills) have shown that Xanax has the advantage over the antidepressants and placebo early in treatment. Xanax is significantly better than placebo in the first week. The antidepressant drugs typically take three or four weeks to be truly effective. By the end of one month of treatment, Xanax and antidepressants (such as imipramine) are comparably effective.

Some individuals taking Xanax become clock-watchers and feel the effect of each dose wearing off four to eight hours after they take it. These individuals find that they are taking the drug every four to eight hours around the clock, and they are quite aware of an increase in anxiety and a kind of mini-withdrawal if they miss a dose. The situation is highly analogous to a cigarette smoker whose nicotine level rises and falls with each cigarette and who finds himself craving the next cigarette an hour or two after the last one. Xanax is a highly addicting drug and most individuals who have taken it for more than a few months find it very difficult to stop using. If it is to be discontinued, a gradual tapering off over one to three months is far safer and more tolerable than abrupt discontinuation. Nonetheless, it is a very well-tolerated drug. The side effects occasionally reported with chronic use include stiffness, pain, eyes tearing, visual clouding, chest tightness, labored respiration, sweating, and mood swings in some individuals.

Klonopin (clonazepam) is the alternative high-potency benzodiazepine tranquilizer for the treatment of panic. It has a much longer half-life, typically one to three days, so that it can be taken on a once-daily basis. This eliminates clock-watching. It is easier to taper off of when an individual has been stable long-term because very gradually falling levels of a drug cause less withdrawal than rapidly falling blood levels. In placebo-controlled studies, an average dose of Xanax is about 5 mg/day; of Klonopin, about 2½ mg/day. When these drugs are compared, they are generally equivalent in their effectiveness. Klonopin may create a slightly higher risk of depression emerging during long-term use than Xanax; one study reported 5.5 percent of patients on Klonopin versus 0.7 percent of patients on Xanax having depression during the course of treatment of panic disorder.

Dosages

Do people have to use higher and higher doses of tranquilizers over time? In some panic disorder studies using Xanax or Klonopin, patients are first stabilized on the medicine over one or two months, then given the option to continue treatment for an additional six months with ongoing monitoring. Interestingly, the effective treatment dose decreases slightly over time. This is reassuring because substance abusers often escalate the dose of these drugs; therefore, most psychiatrists prefer to avoid prescribing minor tranquilizers to individuals with any history of substance abuse or dependence. The recovering alcoholic is often painfully aware of his risk of getting "hooked" on tranquilizers and his Alcoholics Anonymous friends have warned him to beware of this risk many times.

A meta-analysis looking across many different studies to determine whether drugs are comparably effective was performed by Janicak. He reported that the selective serotonin reuptake inhibitors are equally effective as the tricyclic antidepressants. He determined that alprazolam is equally effective as the tricyclic antidepressants. In his analysis, the percentage of people responding to each class of drugs is as follows: tricyclic antidepressants, 63 to 72 percent; selective serotonin reuptake inhibitor, 73 to 80 percent;

and MAOI, 90 percent; with a placebo response rate ranging from 30 to 51 percent.

New treatments that may be helpful in difficult cases of panic disorder include Depakote (divalproex) and Neurontin (gabapentin), both of which are used primarily as anticonvulsants but have a growing range of applications in psychiatry and neurology.

PSYCHOTHERAPEUTIC TREATMENT OF PANIC DISORDER

No discussion of panic disorder pharmacology would be complete without mention of the psychotherapy approach that is most effective; namely, *cognitive behavioral therapy*. In this therapy, the patient is taught that oversensitivity to monitoring bodily sensation with catastrophic misinterpretation of normal body signals leads to the fear response and an exaggeration of the significance of body signals. The person is taught to reproduce the physical symptoms of a panic attack by hyperventilating, spinning around, or exercising and then is desensitized to these sensations by being taught that they are not dangerous and can easily be tolerated. Another important technique in treating panic disorder is *hypnosis* or *relaxation training* to assist the patient in gaining a sense of self-control.

Whether the first-choice treatment of panic disorder should be medications, cognitive behavioral therapy, and relaxation training, or some combination of all is currently controversial, since the goal of pharmacotherapy is to eliminate the attacks and the goal of cognitive behavioral therapy is to induce attacks and desensitize the individual to the symptoms. The goal of relaxation training is to provide an alternative physiologic response to panic.

The choice of treatment modality will often be a matter of patient preference, motivation to practice behavioral techniques or tolerate medication side effects, availability of a specially trained therapist, attitude toward medication, and many other factors.

SPECIFIC PHOBIAS

Specific phobias are characterized by excessive, unreasonable, and persistent fear of an object or situation. The person avoids the object or situation completely, or endures it only with great distress. Exposure to the object provokes situationally bound or predisposed panic attacks. By definition, such a phobia interferes with a person's life and has at least a six-month chronicity. Specific phobias have generally been ignored by psychopharmacologists and considered the realm of behavior therapists because exposure therapies appear to be very effective, while drugs merely suppress symptoms in a way that does not last or generalize to other situations.

SOCIAL PHOBIA

Until recently, social phobia was very underrecognized. It is characterized by a fear of social performance situations in which the person is exposed to unfamiliar people or possible scrutiny by others. He fears he will act in a way that will reveal his anxiety or that will be humiliating or embarrassing. The person either avoids such social situations or endures them with great distress; or he has a situational panic attack. Usually the individual recognizes on an intellectual basis that the fear is excessive or unreasonable and that it interferes with normal social and work performance. For many, the fears apply to most social situations such as social conversations, small group participation, dating, speaking to authority figures, going to a party, or even going into a store and interacting with a clerk. Social phobia may be accompanied by a long-term avoidant personality disorder in which the person chronically feels socially inhibited, inadequate, sensitive to rejection, and is unwilling to get involved with people unless given reassurances of being liked. Often such a person is afraid of being criticized or rejected or feeling inadequate, socially inept, unappealing, and inferior. Social phobia has peak initial onset in the age range from eleven to fifteen years, with more that 80 percent of cases developing prior to age twenty-five; 69.5 percent of sufferers are female. The disorder affects about 2.8 percent of the population. Social phobia may be underdiagnosed for various reasons: lack of appreciation of how much impairment it causes in the person's life, viewing it as part of a personality trait (shyness) or disorder, considering it as part of some other disorder, or not realizing that drugs are effective in treating it.

For a specific social phobia such as *performance anxiety* related to public speaking, acting, or performing at a musical recital, the beta-blocking antihypertensive drugs are very effective. A dose of Inderal (propranolol) of 20 to 40 mg an hour before a performance can dramatically decrease the physiologic arousal symptoms experienced by a musician or public speaker and may even improve the quality of the performance. For the person who has generalized social phobia, cutting across most social situations, the SSRI antidepressants such as Paxil (paroxetine) or the MAO inhibitors such as Nardil (phenelzine) appear to be the most effective drugs. High-potency benzodiazepines such as Xanax 3 mg/day or Klonopin 1.5 mg/day are also very effective.

Since depression often accompanies social phobia (due to the debilitating effects on one's life), it is necessary to first treat the depression with medication. Often SSRI antidepressants will also reduce anxiety symptoms over a period of one to three months. Then behavioral therapy is essential, to teach the basic social skills of carrying on a conversation and expose the individual to social situations to practice relaxing and learn that the fear, for example, of public speaking, is a very common one. *Assertiveness training* is central to basic self-expression; simply recognizing that one has an opinion or wants something and that it's okay to speak up and say so is a major life lesson. Often individuals with social phobia will begin treatment on their own by going to groups such as Toastmasters or taking a public speaking or acting class in college, since they recognize their need to overcome the symptoms. Unfortunately, the most readily available and rapidly acting drug to decrease anxiety in social situations is alcohol; therefore, alcohol abuse is a risk for individuals with social phobia.

Here are some actual case histories of people with panic disorder and phobias. Though their identities have been disguised for reasons of confidentiality, they are all very real people.

Rick: Panic disorder with agoraphobia

Rick is a forty-two-year-old Caucasian male who is married and has a fifteen-year-old stepdaughter. He has completed one year of college and works in the communication field. Initially, he was complaining of panic attacks.

When I first met with Rick, he recounted a long and difficult ordeal of attempted medication trials with only modest results. Rick has had panic attacks since the late 1960s and was first treated with imipramine alone at a dose up to 120 mg. He experienced dry mouth and no positive benefit. He was later treated with imipramine, combined with the MAO inhibitor Nardil in 1978 by another psychiatrist, with a very questionable response. He was further treated with Pamelor for four years at a dose up to 150 mg daily, and reported feeling lethargic with a questionable response. When he went off the Pamelor, he felt unusually good for three days. He reported later being treated with Anafranil (clomipramine) at an unknown dose for several weeks a few years ago. He was tried very briefly on Prozac and felt slight nausea and no real benefit. At that time he had never been treated with Zoloft or Paxil. He was also given Valium in the 1970s and hated the tired feeling at 5 mg/day; later he was given Xanax 0.25 mg three times daily, which was slightly helpful. He tried biofeedback in 1978 without benefit. Rick reported that his maternal uncle probably had panic attacks.

Rick painfully described his symptoms. He said that at times he has the sense of going crazy, that everything is falling out from under him, and that he might lose control. He reported feeling like he had heat cramps, that he wanted to curl into a fetal ball. When he panics he feels his palms sweating, numbness in his fingertips, faint, lightheaded, and dizzy, with symptoms lasting up to sixty minutes. He stated that he has major panic attacks twice a month and minor ones daily.

Because of these attacks Rick has avoided airplanes, open spaces, and going out to the desert. He has also avoided boats, places were he feels isolated or trapped, elevators, and tunnels. This leaves him unable to enjoy activities with his friends and family. Just spending an hour with Rick made it clear that he was suffering from panic disorder with agoraphobia.

Diagnostic and Treatment Plan: On his next visit, Rick came in asking questions about emergency treatment of panic attacks, requesting an injector for a barbiturate, and stating that in the past a doctor had given him this. He was overwhelmed by the potential for suffering more panic attacks. I very strongly discouraged him from seeking barbiturate medication in Mexico and told him that my plan and hope was to prevent recurrence of attacks by using an appropriate antidepressant medication. I also told him that use of Xanax or Ativan as needed would be a reasonable approach.

In just six months, Rick was ready to challenge himself to begin flying in an airplane. After Rick learned to finely adjust the dose of Xanax based on his level of anxiety by taking doses of 0.5 mg every thirty minutes beginning two hours before getting on an airplane (to a total of 2–2.5 mg), and having gradually reached a dose of Prozac of 20 mg/day, Rick was able to take his first airplane ride in twenty years. I went along with him on this trial airplane ride and brought along injectable Ativan at his request to reassure him. His psychologist, who had been teaching him relaxation techniques, also went along, as did his wife. He was pleased to surprise his parents by flying from Southern California to San Francisco to visit them. On board the plane, he was able to walk around and feel relaxed and even commented that flying was fun. Prior to this, his parents had always come to visit him.

Two months later, Rick had flown to Dallas for a weekend with his wife, to Modesto for a work-related training meeting, and planned to practice flying somewhere at least once a month. (It would be awhile before he would be ready to take a long flight over water, so he was not planning a Hawaii vacation yet.)

Conclusion: The intense fear of having a panic attack is debilitating. I'll describe a scenario that might occur for someone like Rick: You are about to leave your house to go to work. Suddenly your heart begins to pound as you fear you might have a panic attack today. As the fear compounds itself your palms begin to sweat, you feel faint and lightheaded, you *know* you are going crazy. For one hour you sit there stricken with fear and unable to force yourself out the door. Adding to your distress, you begin to ruminate about the phone calls that are mounting on your voice mail, the paperwork piling up on your desk, and what your coworkers are thinking of you. You feel certain your family is angry with you because you are an inadequate father. Finally, the panic subsides and then you become terrified of going through this tomorrow.

Rick was so desperate to break this cycle that he was willing to go to Mexico to buy barbiturates and syringes. With an appropriate combination of daily Prozac and as-needed Xanax as well as intensive relaxation training, however, he was able to relieve the panic attacks and begin to build confidence so he could perform daily tasks. The recovery process from panic attacks almost always includes eliminating them medically as well as positive exposure to the phobic stimuli that has been avoided.

Darlene: Panic disorder with limited avoidance

Darlene is a twenty-year-old, single female student who was about to start her junior year of college. She lives with three female roommates and has been going to summer school and working part-time. Darlene came in with complaints of stress, anxiety, many physical symptoms, and debilitating panic attacks.

Darlene began having panic or anxiety symptoms at around age fifteen, which she thought were signs of asthma. She repeatedly went to doctors and was told that she had absolutely no wheezing and, therefore, no asthma. These symptoms were not debilitating or frequent until about one and a half months ago. She indicated she had numerous stressors, including developing mononucleosis, cold sores, and impetigo; financial stressors from being unable to work for the last five weeks because of the physical problems (her father had just changed jobs and was also experiencing some financial pressures); she'd been in a relationship with a boyfriend for the last seven months whom she perceived as not giving her needed time or emotional support. Additional stressors were the deaths of her boyfriend's father and her great-grandmother.

Darlene reported that panic attacks have been occurring two or three times a day for the last one and a half months. She described numerous symptoms spontaneously, including arm and face numbness and feeling that she can't breathe. She had been trying to lie down or be by herself and use relaxation and breathing techniques to get rid of these symptoms, but without significant benefit. She reported difficulty concentrating on reading and watching television. She stated that she is aware of her breathing all of the time, except when she is asleep. During the attacks she reports a myriad of symptoms. She has dry throat and feels numbness or tingling in her hands and feet, as well as her abdomen, kneecaps, back, and lips. Her back and neck muscles tense up. She feels that it is hard to breathe and her chest is tight. Her hands are cold, she feels out of breath, and she feels she needs to cough, although there is nothing to cough up. She feels light-headed, like her nose is swollen, like her lungs don't want to breathe; and after the attacks she feels exhausted. During the attacks she feels an urge to urinate or defecate. She feels like she is going crazy. She is convinced that there is something physical causing the attacks. She describes a feeling that she will "zone out" and lose track of what she is doing at the time. She is overwhelmed when she has attacks; she thinks of going to the nearby hospital, wants to sleep until the attacks are over, and knows she must pull over if she is driving. Fortunately, she has never considered suicide during or after the attacks.

Her panic attacks typically go from onset to peak intensity within a half hour and sometimes instantaneously. They typically last about two hours but can range from one-half hour up to five hours. Triggers can be anything from going out of the house or into the car to feeling stressed. The attacks even occur spontaneously when she is feeling happy and having fun with friends.

On meeting with Darlene, I learned that she occasionally took Proventil for asthma and found that this worsened her problems. She takes Seldane occasionally for allergies but cannot tolerate decongestants.

Darlene was told by a cardiologist that she has mitral valve prolapse, based on ultrasound, but there is no significance other than the need for antibiotics before dental procedures. She recently had mononucleosis and she can't exercise due to enlargement of the spleen. She has experienced excercise intolerance; for example, developing panic attacks when bicycle riding.

Darlene's father is alive and physically healthy. He also has a history of anxiety attacks, which resolve spontaneously. Her paternal aunt has manic depressive illness and panic attacks; she got worse with neurologic symptoms while on trazodone, and it is unknown what medications she might be on now.

Darlene avoids shopping, being a passenger in the car, going out to dinner, and crowds since she has had the panic attacks. This often leaves her feeling very lonely.

She described her long-term personality as "too nice," happy, funny, motherly, caring for others, being a good student, and having a perfect life with a college sorority and a house on the beach.

Diagnostic and Treatment Plan: My diagnostic impression was panic disorder with limited avoidance. I wanted her to be educated about panic disorder so I asked her to read Sheehan's book, *The Anxiety Disease*. I prescribed Klonopin 1 mg one to four times daily, and asked her to call me in three days. At that point, if she was beginning to notice improvement of the panic attacks, she could start imipramine 10 mg and gradually increase from one to ten at bedtime as tolerated. It was very important that she continue in outpatient psychotherapy.

Two years later, Darlene was taking imipramine up to 220 mg/day, Klonopin up to 2 mg/day, and doing well. We tried switching imipramine to desipramine due to her desire to minimize tiredness, dry mouth, and constipation. She was attending classes regularly, and is with a new, very supportive boyfriend. Over the long-term, she was able to cut the medication down to just imipramine 50 mg/day and occasional as-needed Klonopin. She was about to graduate college and go to Europe for the summer.

The following winter, Darlene came in after just returning from Europe. Some panic attacks were returning so we decided to switch her medicine to Zoloft rather than endure imipramine's side effects.

The summer of that same year, she was on Zoloft at 25 mg/day for a month and pleased not to have the old side effects of constipation or tiredness, or need any of the minor tranquilizers. She will be leaving in ten weeks for graduate school.

Conclusion: For a moment, put yourself into Darlene's life. She is a bright, attractive woman who experienced panic attacks for a long time before seeking treatment. She was accustomed to seeing her father's struggle; she was overwhelmed that panic attacks were interfering in her life, unable to do tasks that most people take for granted such as shopping, going out with friends, and riding in the car with her boyfriend because of a fear of having yet another attack. She was motivated to resolve these panic attacks so she began taking medications. Unfortunately, there were side effects that were annoying, but this annoyance was tolerated because being able to go on with her life outweighed the negative factors. Her admirable persistence in her work with me led to our finding for her the best medicine with the least side effects. A few years after she was treated, her sister presented for treatment with remarkably similar symptoms, demonstrating the potential for a genetic-familial component to this disorder.

Marilyn: Panic disorder with minimal avoidance

Marilyn was first seen when she was twenty-nine years old. She is a high school graduate and has taken a few college classes. She works as a regional manager for a department store. She has been living with her boyfriend for one month. She was referred by her psychotherapist. Her chief complaint is anxiety.

Marilyn had some very difficult times in her childhood. Her mother was forty-four when Marilyn was born, was very religious, and wasn't emotionally supportive when Marilyn's father died of cancer when she was only ten years old.

At age seventeen Marilyn began having "dizzy things" with anxiety and went to the emergency room for them. She thought she was dying. Her pediatrician prescribed Valium, which she didn't take, and then Tofranil (imipramine) and various other medications. She did well for awhile and then began having the panic attacks again, including some during the night. At age twenty-three she accepted a very good job, which involved moving to Utah. To her dismay, she had a very severe panic attack, which led to her going to the emergency room. She felt forced to quit her job after only two months because of panic attacks. She feared she was going crazy. She felt dizzy and disoriented, and she returned to her mother's home. She saw a doctor, who diagnosed depression and panic disorder and hospitalized her.

A few years ago she went to her general practitioner and was given Prozac 20 mg, one or two pills a day. She found that this worked for her panic and depression, but she began having weird thoughts about using a knife or scissors to hurt herself; this was very out of character for her. She also found that the Prozac blocked sexual responsiveness. Very recently she was put on Zoloft 50 mg/day for three weeks. She felt more anxious and fidgety and insomniac while taking it, so she stopped it about five days ago.

Her attacks, though rare, could last for one to five hours, and a severe one recently led to an emergency room visit.

Symptoms include palpitations, pounding and accelerated heartbeat, sweating, trembling, shaking, shortness of breath, chest pain and tightness or pressure, nausea, abdominal distress, dizziness, unsteadiness, light-headedness, faintness, feelings of unreality and detachment, fear of losing control or going crazy, fear of dying, and hot flashes.

There were several triggers to her panic attacks including taking cold pills, going to movie theaters, and getting on airplanes. She indicated that she typically has panic attacks when her stress level decreases and that her last very severe one was during a week of vacation after working very hard. When asked what relieves her panic attacks, she described some inner dialogue work she learned from books and tapes but states that she can't do relaxation tapes because when she tries to relax she becomes more anxious. It helps her to go for a walk.

Marilyn indicated that as a regional sales manager she covers Arizona, New Mexico, and California. Though she dislikes flying, she does not avoid planes because of her panic attacks, and she occasionally has to fly for her work.

Marilyn told me that beginning around age twenty-two or twenty-three she was depressed for periods up to two months at a time. She is sure that the panic disorder started by age seventeen and was there before the depression. When depressed, she doesn't want to do anything except sit around and read. She feels tired and has insomnia and is asocial. She has no change in appetite. She has had decreased sexual interest and response both with depression and then with Prozac treatment. Her concentration is poor. She does not have suicidal ideation during the depressive episodes.

There is a family history of panic and anxiety: Marilyn's maternal grandmother had depression and anxiety and used a lot of sleeping pills and wine. She died in her fifties of cirrhosis of the liver. The patient's cousin, now age forty-three, has had panic attacks since her teenage years but has never been on medication.

Over the long-term, Marilyn describes herself as happy, a "go-getter," very reactive, and oversensitive. Her boyfriend would describe her as loving, sweet but stubborn, sticking to her morals and values, and also as being anxious.

Ideally, Marilyn would like a medicine that would help her keep even, to sleep, and to not feel at all medicated during the day.

Diagnosis and Treatment Plan: My diagnostic impression was panic disorder with very minimal avoidance.

Initially, she decided to briefly participate in an experimental medication study, but didn't get much benefit. This led to her dropping out of treatment for awhile. Less than a year later, she presented with a depression that had been gradually worsening over a period of six months. She was preparing for her wedding in two months and felt that she had let her fiancé down by not telling him of her history of depression and panic disorder. She was awakening in the middle of the night and experiencing decreased concentration, loss of interest in usual activities, low sex drive, and fatigue. She was then treated with Serzone.

Conclusion: This is one of the few patients I have met who described self-injurious thoughts while on Prozac. This very rare side effect is overreported in the public media. When it occurs, it usually requires a change of medication. Fortunately, Marilyn had the good sense not to act on these thoughts and reported them immediately. One can see the interaction of panic disorder and depression in her case; often it is hard to tell which came first. Fortunately, the antidepressants used to treat panic disorder usually treat the depression, too.

Denise: Panic disorder with agoraphobia

Denise is a forty-three-year-old married female, currently in her fourth marriage of seven years. She has two children, ages twenty-three and twenty-five. She works as a musician. She was accompanied to the interview by her husband. Her chief complaint is panic.

Denise described feeling fearful and unable to stop crying during intense panic attacks. She had an embarrassing fear of falling through transparent stairs at a large stadium two years ago while at a concert. She had a terrified feeling driving home with her husband four years ago. She had anxiety about being in the center of a room in a restaurant in 1979. She describes being afraid to go out in the world at times without being accompanied by her husband or her mother. She has recently seen a cardiologist and was diagnosed as having atrial premature beats and mitral valve prolapse. She was also recently given a prescription for Xanax .25 mg, which she very rarely uses even if she feels she is going to have an anxiety attack.

Denise described feeling fearful, tearful, dizzy, and lightheaded; has numbness in her right arm, hand, and right side of her face; and difficulty breathing. She described feeling her heart skip a beat. After the attacks, she feels tired and confused. On her better days, she tries to go to the bank or grocery store on her own but often backs out of doing so. She is usually able to go to work, but at times has to distance herself from coworkers when feeling anxious.

Other symptoms included shortness of breath, a sense of smothering, unsteadiness, palpitations, racing heart, sweating, nausea, depersonalization, derealization, chills, fear of dying, and fear of going crazy or doing something uncontrolled. She has ten of the thirteen panic symptoms described in the *DSM-IV* (with four being required for diagnosis). She described only two or three attacks occurring in the last two and a half months, but a very chronic anticipatory anxiety was present about two-thirds of the time. She described onset to peak intensity lasting about one hour, and she can't really say how long the total duration of the attacks is. She denies any loss of consciousness during the attacks, and she denies hallucinations during the attacks, but her mental clarity goes down.

She states that she has been hearing and seeing things since she was eleven years old and described a "smell of death" before a relative's death, as well as premonitions of things to come.

Denise has a family history of psychiatric illness: On her maternal side, her great-grandmother was psychiatrically hospitalized after her hysterectomy and stayed home "ill" and became a recluse. Her maternal grandmother had a difficult menopause and required Haldol. Her maternal aunt was on Vivactil for depression, had suicidal ideation, and had thoughts of killing her children while in her forties. On her paternal side, her great-grandmother was housebound since her thirties or forties, was a poet and musician like the patient, and had difficulty raising her children because of being housebound. Her father has multiple sclerosis and has been a drinker for years.

When I asked Denise how she views herself overall, she described having a lot of love for people, communicating with music and art, and trying to please people. Her husband describes her as loving, compassionate, strong, and caring as well as ambitious.

Diagnostic impressions were panic disorder with agoraphobia.

Treatment Plan: I discussed medication dose adjustment and gave Denise a prescription for imipramine 10 mg to gradually increase from one to ten daily as tolerated. I also gave her a prescription for Xanax 0.25 mg to take as needed for anxiety with an explanation that this is a highly addicting drug and should be used only for the most stressful times. I asked her to return in approximately three weeks for medication follow-up and evaluation to the response of the imipramine titration.

A year later, Denise required a few modifications to her medication regimen. She has tried imipramine (which caused sweets craving and dry mouth) and desipramine in various combinations totaling about 150 mg/day along with Klonopin 0.5 mg daily. This enabled her to go shopping on her own, get four of her songs published, and to drive places alone. She no longer wants to die, and is now feeling like her old self.

Eventually, Denise requested to try an SSRI in hopes of fewer side effects, and was prescribed Paxil 20 mg/day for the last four months. She likes it better than imipramine or desipramine because she feels calmer on the Paxil. She is still using Klonopin 0.5 mg daily.

Conclusion: Denise has a long family history of psychiatric problems, leaving her well aware of how overwhelming it can seem as you begin the process of carefully selecting the correct medication. Though tricyclics as well as SSRIs are effective in treating panic, many people choose to take the benzodiazepine minor tranquilizers such as Klonopin or Xanax, either on a regular or an as-needed basis. If these are helpful, they can be difficult to give up; it should be noted that they are addictive. However, medically appropriate use involves doses that are stable long-term and are adequate to control panic attacks. This is in contrast to abuse, which involves very sporadic use of extremely high doses with the goal of getting intoxicated.

Sam: Panic disorder with severe avoidant behavior

Sam is a thirty-year-old male who is in his first marriage for eight years. He and his wife have one child. He is a shift manager in charge of schedules for about 250 people in a manufacturing plant. He has been at his job for twelve years and was selected for a promotion, although he was unable to accept due to his psychiatric symptoms. He has a bachelor's degree in general studies. Sam's chief complaint is anxiety attacks.

I asked about the history of the anxiety attacks. Sam describes a history going back to childhood with problems being away from his mother at school, coupled with fear of being alone after school at age five. He also remembers experiencing anxiety going to a movie and getting anxious when with his father at age eleven. At that time, he also recalled having a sensation of panic and inability to swallow. At age fifteen, he converted from his Jewish background to being a born-again Christian, which led to a feeling of dizziness and lightheadedness. He felt like he listed while he was walking. He began being concerned there was something physically wrong with him. In his late teen years he would stay home to avoid the anxiety that would occur when he went out. At age eighteen he began avoiding airplane flights, being far away from home, going on camping trips, and participating in other recreational activities that he used to enjoy. In college he took a first-aid course, which included gory scenes, and feared that he would pass out and began breathing hard. At nineteen he had his first panic attack. He was on the freeway with a friend and suddenly felt that there was great danger in being in a smoggy area. He became very anxious and uptight, and then this passed. At age twenty-two he got married. Five months later he had his first, full-blown, debilitating panic attack, from which he feels he never fully recovered. He describes a gradual worsening trend from age nineteen to thirty. Sam indicated that he had been in various psychotherapies since age eight. He saw a social worker in high school and then numerous psychologists; he tried behavior modification techniques and hierarchical desensitization. He had never been tried on a tricyclic antidepressant or MAO inhibitor. He has read numerous books about anxiety disorders, but despite his reading and psychotherapy he could not escape a very restricted lifestyle in which he could not bring himself to go to the grocery store, a movie, or out to a restaurant for dinner, or get on an airplane.

Sam's medical history included mitral valve prolapse, diagnosed by echocardiogram, occasional ectopic beats on Holter monitoring with some sinus tachycardia, and mild hypertension but no dietary or medication treatment recommendations for this from his doctor.

Sam described the panic attacks as a sensation of a rush from his groin to his trunk to his head with a feeling of flushing. He felt himself gasping or breathing deeply, and felt restless. He began looking for a way out or an escape. Furthermore, he experienced tingling in his nose, facial numbness, arm numbness, a feeling of going crazy, feeling that his genitals were withdrawing into his body, and fear of passing out or dying or having a heart attack or stroke. He has experienced his heart beating hard, his body swaying, sweating, dry mouth, problems swallowing, occasional diarrhea, and fullness in his ears. The time between initial warning and full intensity of the attack ranges from two seconds to a minute, and the bad attacks last from a few minutes to an hour. He has had less than one bad attack per month because he avoids all difficult situations in which he has previously had them. He states that he has mild attacks every two days. When asked what he would be able to do if the panic attacks were adequately treated, he indicated he would have a new job, new residence, take vacations, take his daughter different places, travel with his wife, go into high-rise buildings, go out on a boat, go places with friends, go to stores and shopping malls, go visit his father and his father's new girlfriend, go to the dentist more frequently, exercise more regularly, and do things and go places by himself. Conversely, these are all things that he avoids. He feels that his marriage and his life are run by his phobias and that it's like "a monkey on my back."

Like others, he has a significant family history. His mother could not drive very far, could not take a freeway, disliked flying, and disliked elevators. He described his father as a nervous person prone to hysterics who is also obese. One half brother, age forty, has a history of experimenting with drugs. His mother was in good health until she developed breast cancer and died of metastases. There is no family history of suicide, psychiatric hospitalization, severe depression, or alcoholism.

Since the onset of severe phobias eight years ago, his illness has been controlling, with Sam having to decide everything, especially travel arrangements. He became overly introspective in addition to compulsively focusing on thoughts, abusive, obsessive, and manipulative, and began using compulsive masturbation as a release.

Obviously, his marriage is not going well; his wife is "sick and tired" of Sam's phobias controlling her life and feels angry that she has to go to social functions alone. His daughter, age four, is described as being a happy, sweet child with no behavior problems in preschool but is sometimes cranky and frustrated. Sam was also unable to continue training for a position in management because he could not travel for business meetings, could not take elevators, and was so afraid of heights.

Diagnostic impressions were panic disorder with severe avoidant behavior.

Treatment recommendations were made right away. I suggested that Sam begin a reducing diet, exercise regularly, and decrease salt intake for the first-line control of his hypertension. I discussed with him the option of using Xanax, though I warned him that it would probably not be satisfactory because of the great chronicity of his problem and the high addiction risk. I recommended and gave him a prescription for imipramine 25 mg with instructions on titrating the dose up from one to ten each evening as tolerated and a description of potential side effects. I indicated to him that if this was not successful, an MAO inhibitor such as Nardil was called for. I also indicated to him that with such a chronic history he should expect to be on medication over several years.

This treatment plan was explained to Sam in the presence of his wife and he was agreeable to it, although he had numerous questions.

We discovered over the next couple of months that the imipramine trial with documentation of a blood level that would be therapeutic in treating depression (dose of 225 mg/day, level of imipramine plus desipramine 254 mg/ml; therapeutic levels in panic were not known at the time) was a complete failure when combined with Xanax about 2 mg/day. We planned to taper off it and begin Nardil (an MAO inhibitor) after a washout period.

It took another two months to raise the Nardil up to 120 mg/day. This helped him to feel much calmer, to be able to drive the freeway easily, and get along better with his wife. He's been able to decrease his compulsive eating.

Two years later, he is still on Nardil, down to 90 mg/day, and Tenormin, 25 mg/day, for blood pressure. He is transferring jobs with the same employer and looking forward to a change. He is beginning to address long-term marital problems in which he complains that the relationship is boring, nonsupportive, and no fun; each partner resents the other for the problems that have occurred because of the life restrictions that the panic disorder had caused in the past.

Conclusion: Sam's case represents the common childhood history of school phobia and separation anxiety that came into his life long before the actual panic attacks.

As previously mentioned, some people do not respond to the tricyclic antidepressants or minor tranquilizers and then the MAO inhibitors are lifesaving. Sam's situation illustrates how any disabling psychiatric illness can impact a job and marriage. You can imagine how easily his wife might become bitter and resentful of Sam's disabilities since she naturally had her own needs and issues. These led to her pushing him away as she may have felt abandoned by him. He was left feeling distant, alone, angry, and resentful, and felt all passion had died within the marriage. We'll never know if much earlier and more aggressive biologic and marital treatment might have prevented the problem from growing to such a degree.

Paul: Panic disorder with moderate avoidance

Paul is a thirty-year-old male employed as a department manager, trainer, and sales representative. He has been married for five years and has no children. He completed college in 1974 and has one year of graduate school in English. Paul's chief complaint is panic disorder.

Paul developed panic disorder at around age twenty, while in college, along with severe anxiety and depression. He went to a psychiatrist for about a year who he reports gave him no input, and prescribed the old tranquilizer Equanil, which was largely ineffective. He indicated that the disorder continued, and by the time he was twenty-five, he had a crisis when he got on an airplane. He had a panic attack and bolted off the plane and had to drive a rental car home from Washington to California. He felt worried about doing this because he has to fly around the country for a living. This led him to see a psychologist for one year of behavioral therapy, which wasn't very helpful. He saw another psychologist for biofeedback and to treat tinnitus (ringing in the ear), for twelve sessions. This did not help the tinnitus or get rid of the panic attacks; however, it did allow him to stop using clonidine patches to control his high blood pressure.

Paul had multiple phobias including freeway driving, airplanes, elevators, dentist chairs, and sitting in the back seat of a car with no door, and sometimes with a nonopening window. He was afraid of being in situations where he would feel trapped or out of control. At one point, he went into a glass elevator and saw a sign that read "Please remain calm, there is no danger of running out of air" in case the elevator malfunctioned. He describes this as a mantra that he would say to himself when he was getting anxious.

Paul states that from the onset to peak intensity of his panic attacks is a very rapid escalation of only a few seconds. From onset to resolution typically takes from about half a minute to two minutes. Current frequency is about three attacks per week, and at worst he had them up to about four times a week, plus waking up with them at times.

Paul described symptoms typical of panic disorder. He experiences his heart pounding, a hunger for air, feeling shaky, dizziness, and feeling that he is going to go crazy or lose control. He feels tightness in his chest. He has a sensation of his hands and legs shaking, feeling light-headed, and feeling that his motions are jerky. After the attack, he experiences exhaustion and depression. He does not have urinary or bowel urgency, numbness, or tingling. He has no history of emergency room visits. He does, however, state that he keeps very close track on where the closest hospital is in all of the cities he visits on his business travels.

Paul attempts to avoid airplanes, elevators, back seats of cars, and driving in the fast lane on freeways, and states that he dislikes standing in line at the bank because he has the feeling that he might fall over.

Paul's mother saw a psychiatrist for anxiety. One uncle is a recovering alcoholic. There is no other known family history.

Paul has a very successful work history. He has been with his present company for ten years and was rapidly promoted; he works well under pressure. He enjoys training sessions where he is speaking in front of as many as two hundred people at a time.

Paul feels happy in his first marriage of five years and describes it as a great relationship, and though he feels his wife is very supportive, he has never told her of his panic disorder, due to shame about having it. They have several pets, but no children.

Paul says that he is a "people person" and well liked, despite being perceived by others as "hyper" and unable to relax. Sometimes the anxiety preoccupies him, so that he can't give his total attention to people he is with. He has some difficulty sitting still in meetings as an audience member.

Paul drinks two cups of regular coffee in the morning and I suggested that he try switching to decaffeinated coffee. He also drinks two beers a night and a glass of wine with dinner. He sometimes tries strenuous exercise, although he has found this to precipitate panic attacks at times.

The diagnostic impression is panic disorder with moderate avoidance.

Paul was very motivated to try imipramine, 10 mg, gradually increased from one to ten daily as tolerated, in an attempt to control the panic attacks. I explained to him the side effects of feeling "wired" or sedated, dry mouth, blurred vision, constipation, and weight gain. I indicated that this should be taken daily. I also gave him a prescription for Xanax 0.5 mg to use one to four tablets as needed prior to stressful events, such as getting onto an airplane, and asked him to experiment with this prior to the time he might need to use it. Three weeks later, Paul reported that the panic was much milder while on imipramine 50 mg/day, with slight constipation and dry mouth, and he was using Xanax as needed for long flights. Paul was changed early in treatment from imipramine to desipramine due to the constipation and blurred vision, and he responded by feeling more energy with desipramine. By his four-year follow-up appointment Paul had been on desipramine 125 mg/day long-term, taking Calan SR 180 mg/day for blood pressure and migraine prevention, and had been flying around the country free of panic attacks for several years. He expresses ongoing gratitude for the relief that medication has given.

Conclusion: Please note that Equanil (Miltown, meprobamate) is now obsolete; it is very similar to the barbiturates in that it is potentially lethal in overdose, habit forming, and associated with withdrawal seizures.

Paul had actually hidden his illness from his wife due to embarrassment. It is not unusual for the person with panic disorder to feel ashamed of his illness since it is difficult for others to understand. He has been highly motivated to overcome his panic attacks because he needs to fly in order to do his job. He rapidly appreciated the potency of antidepressant medications in suppressing his panic attacks and wished that he had started them long before he did, saying that he should have done this before his behavioral therapy. In fact, in severe cases, behavioral therapy is greatly enhanced when used in conjunction with medication.

Brian: Recurrent major depression with social phobia

Brian is a thirty-two-year-old, gay, single male physician who came to me complaining of depression and anxiety when dealing with people he does not know well or in group settings.

Brian was in psychotherapy for about three years. He indicates that on his own he has tried imipramine and felt anxious and dissociated and that things around him were unreal with about 75 mg/day. He next tried Nardil because he felt he had atypical depression and was rejection sensitive. He found that at a dose of 45 to 60 mg/day for three months it was quite helpful for him both in terms of the depression and of his social phobia. He found that he could raise his hand and participate more when in group or class discussions. While on Nardil, however, he felt he could not reach orgasm and he never had a restful night's sleep. He subsequently tried Prozac about a year ago for three or four weeks with no benefit and again was unable to reach orgasm, and he was insomniac and tired all the time at a dose of 20 mg/day. He later tried desipramine beginning at low doses of 10 mg, then 20 mg, then 25 mg over three weeks. While taking this he felt slightly better, but he had marked worsening of irritability, which was also a significant symptom for him.

Brian indicates that one of his major symptoms is that he feels he can't handle any stress when he is depressed. He finds himself questioning whether his improvement on weekends (when he is not working) is because he is extremely stress intolerant or the work is very stressful.

Brian indicates depression began as early as college. He had a hard time in medical school because of it. He has been depressed about 60 percent of the time over the last two or three years. He has always been able to fool people and fake it even when depressed. He indicates that dealing with being gay was a major issue, but psychotherapy helped him learn to accept this. He was able to end a seven-year relationship about two years ago, which he felt was for the best. His partner was unfaithful and Brian did not want to risk any sexually transmitted diseases. He has a support group including gay friends who were recently pushing him to get help for his depression. He is very concerned that he may be alone for the rest of his life.

Brian has clear social phobia symptoms in addition to the depression. He indicates that it was difficult for him to speak up in public or in front of a group. He occasionally takes low-dose Inderal with benefit. He also feels that people criticize him, and he is very sensitive about this. He is self-critical, especially when depressed. He relates improvement of the social phobia to becoming comfortable with being gay.

Brian was embarrassed to be coming to me for help with his depression because a doctor is supposed to be strong. He also wanted to do it himself. Also, his therapist in the past had discouraged his using medicines.

Diagnostic Impressions: Major depression, which is recurrent, and social phobia.

Conclusion: Yes, doctors have psychiatric problems, too! In Brian's case, the hazard of being a health care professional was that of self-treatment. Although Brian had found some effective medications for himself, he had gone through a lot of unmonitored medication trials. He was very aware of the difference that an MAOI antidepressant (Nardil) made on his shyness; it allowed him to participate far more fully in classroom interactions and to feel less scared of criticism or rejection. He subsequently did even better on the MAOI Parnate combined with very low dose Elavil (amitriptyline), which allowed him to experience a similar benefit with fewer side effects.

Katy: Social phobia and single episode of major depression

Katy is a thirty-seven-year-old single female with no children. She has not had a major relationship since age twenty-four and has no interest in getting married. Katy describes herself as a nice person with low self-esteem. Her friends view her as a good friend and nice, loyal, and easy to get along with. She has a master's degree and works for an advertising agency. Katy's chief complaint is that she is always nervous.

Katy was tearful as she recounted the numerous work problems she has had due to difficulty concentrating and high levels of anxiety. She has never been on any form of psychiatric medication other than one unknown anticonvulsant which she took for only a couple of days because it caused headaches.

She has been in psychotherapy for three months due to problems at work and a fear of becoming even more overwhelmed by stress, anxiety, and depression.

Katy is able to relax when she is away from work, but even on a recent vacation she had insomnia related to worry about what would happen at work.

Just two years ago Katy felt energetic, but couldn't relax well when in a situation where she had to speak in front of people. Katy says that when she has to give a public speech, her heart pounds and her throat gets tight. She feels hot and sweaty. She feels very anxious and like she is not really there. She experiences shortness of breath, and feelings of "butterflies" in her stomach, but not urgency to void. She feels shaky, her voice quivers, and she wishes she could escape. Occasionally, when she starts giving her talk, if she has a good beginning, she can focus and become calm, but other times she remains quite anxious. She found that a small amount of alcohol before speaking helped a lot. She knew this was not a good practice. She declines giving talks whenever possible even though there is about one request a month at work. She also has to go to thirty-person staff meetings at her office and she shudders if she gets called on. She indicated that these severe anxiety episodes are purely situational and never spontaneous panic attacks. She thus appears to have true social phobia and not panic disorder because of the lack of any spontaneous attacks and the predictability of these occurring only in public speaking situations.

Moreover, Katy feels she has been depressed forever. She worries a lot about things at work and puts too much importance on them. When depressed, she doesn't want to eat and she can't sleep. She says she has always been quite a worrier, but not really depressed to the point of needing help. When asked about depression symptoms, she indicated that for the last eight months she has experienced eating and sleeping problems, but that the social phobia symptoms have existed for many years. She denies previous depressions lasting for months and states that previous depressions have always been situational and have been for only two weeks or less.

In order to determine how depressed she was, I gave her a standardized, brief depression scale interview called the Seventeen-item Hamilton Depression Rating Scale. She reported feeling anxious and depressed 50 percent of the time; feeling self-reproach, letting people down, and guilt; and blaming herself and asking, "Why is this happening to me?" She has had thoughts of her own death but has never made a suicide plan or attempt. It takes her one to four hours to fall asleep at night, and she often wakes during the night and watches TV for one to three hours. She has terminal insomnia, typically waking up thirty to forty-five minutes before the alarm. She has felt less effective at her work and felt nervous dealing with people, and has decreased her actual time at work. When asked how much time she was actually working two years ago, she stated about forty-five hours a week. Now, she estimates she puts in twenty-five hours a week that is actually productive, even though she might be in the office daydreaming. There was no psychomotor agitation or retardation, but she did describe tension, irritability, and worrying a lot about what people will think about her and why people might avoid her. She described loss of appetite and eating because she is hypoglycemic rather than because she gets hungry. Her energy is about 50 percent of normal and she has neck tension and headaches that are described as diffuse and tight-band, as well as shooting. Her sex drive has decreased to 50 percent of normal although she is not currently in a relationship. She has been concerned that she could not gain weight and recently had full thyroid function tests that were normal. She has gone down from a usual weight range of 95 to 98 pounds to her current weight of 93 pounds over the last six months. She acknowledges being depressed. There was no diurnal variation in mood, no depersonalization, no paranoia, and no obsessive or compulsive symptoms. She denied menstrual variation or seasonal variation and she can be cheered up. Her concentration is okay but her decision making is not as good as it used to be. The Seventeen-item Hamilton-D score was 28. Most antidepressant drug treatment studies have an entrance criterion of 18 or more to demonstrate the necessity for antidepressant treatment.

Diagnostic impressions were social phobia and major depression, single episode.

Treatment Recommendations: I indicated to Katy that the selective serotonin antidepressants can be effective in blocking the anxiety symptoms of social phobia, but these typically take several weeks to be effective. Among the SSRIs, Paxil (paroxetine) is the most sedating, and so I started her on Paxil 20 mg/day. I also indicated to her that prior to going into very difficult situations she could use the beta blocker Inderal (propranolol) 10 mg one or two, three times daily as needed and Xanax 0.25 mg one or two, three times daily as needed short term. I encouraged her to experiment with these. Later, she was taken off the Paxil because it was not effective enough and she got a better response on Nardil in a low dose long term.

Conclusion: You can see Katy's situation is such that social phobia and depression coexist with a very difficult job situation. The social phobia complicates the job performance tremendously. When she combined psychotherapy to deal with her life stressors along with medications to cut the anxiety and depression, they were adequate to deal with her symptoms. Social phobia can also interfere with dating; in this case, Katy has adapted to her illness by making work a very high priority and finding a mate a very low one.

FAMILY ISSUES IN PANIC DISORDER AND ANXIETY DISORDERS

Like other psychiatric disorders, panic disorder in one person also affects the entire family. Working on family issues related to panic disorder can help bring greater relief of symptoms for the ailing one. Often these people had a great deal of anxiety at times of being separated from the primary caregiver or parent when they were children. This separation may have occurred for a variety of reasons, such as one parent having a major illness, the death of a parent, divorce, or military service far from home. With panic disorder and anxiety, the child develops an overdependency on trusted others and is fearful of going outside of her "safe" circle around home and work. Through this, clinging behavior develops. Growing up, there may have been a great deal of worry in the home about real or imagined dangers that further made the child fearful of venturing out into the world. Panic attacks often develop in adolescence. In some sense, panic attacks may be a more grown-up way of expressing the clinging behavior that in children may be expressed in crying, begging, pleading, or fits of rage. One person I worked with described her mother as so wrapped up in her father that she had no time for the children, who felt so needy they were fearful of leaving mother's side. Another person described her mother as afraid of dying from her renal failure, leading to the child's fear about going to school.

In addition to panic disorder expressing separation anxiety, it may be the result of enmeshment (described in detail in chapter 8 on bipolar disorder). There may be a history of one family member having a psychologically unresolved trauma that becomes "acted out" through panic attack in another. The family member with the unresolved trauma may be the parent or child of the one with panic disorder, or even a more distant relative with an issue somehow connected to the issues of the one with panic disorder. I will provide a few examples to illustrate: When Misty was eight years old, she was molested by a stranger who coerced her into his car when she was walking home from school; she was left unconscious in a nearby park. After being rescued and somewhat settled down after the trauma, Misty continued to go about her days with seemingly little problem; however, her mother Sara developed panic attacks every morning when her daughter was getting ready to go to school. In essence, Sara was acting out her own fear of separation from the child as well as the child's fear. Note that Misty, however, has a high probability of developing panic attacks at some point in her life as she naturally begins to pull away from her mother in adolescence and finds herself experiencing her own fears as well as her mother's.

Rich is yet another example. After going on a heavy drinking binge, Rich developed panic disorder and became obsessed with a fear that he would die. This led to Rich drinking more and more often, which only led to more episodes. Rich's father was a chronic alcoholic who had died just one year earlier of cancer. It was as if Rich was playing out his father's role. The complicating factor was that Rich had experienced the emotional loss of his father early in life due to his alcoholism, and that wound was further opened when his father physically died. Rich was unconsciously determined to live out the father's role and repeat history. Indeed, Rich became so toxic on alcohol that he did almost die. It was at that point that Rich sought treatment for both the alcohol problem and panic disorder.

The quicksand that can lead to anxiety and panic is apparent in the relationship between Diane and Les. They separated after many months of fighting and inability to resolve their long-standing problems of communication and intimacy. Diane took their newborn baby and left home for a week. Les began to develop panic attacks almost immediately. On further looking into Les's background, it became clear that his mother had developed panic disorder at the time Les's father left her for another woman. It wasn't surprising that Les was an infant at the time. Hence, the separation from Diane triggered an old trauma when Les was abandoned by his father and Les was now acting out his fears in the same manner as his mother. Diane also developed anxiety disorder, which can be traced back to her early separation issues with her alcoholic father and mother. It is not unusual to find that others in the same extended or immediate family present with panic disorder.

Panic attacks cause a problem in relationships, as can be seen in the many case examples presented in this chapter. Frequently, the spouse in a marital relationship is needed for the person with panic attacks to feel safe to go outside a small range of travel. This can result in the healthy partner becoming resentful of being the caregiver. The couple may grow apart or become a sick one/healthy one dyad; or the healthy one can be gratified through the power trip of being so all-important to the safety of the other. When the person with agoraphobia won't go beyond the place she considers safe without the spouse, the spouse may grow to view the person as no fun, as someone who clings, is unavailable to take trips, and too dependent. Here, too, resentment may develop as the relationship becomes one of filling needs and without pleasure; the team approach to life is lost through the dependency. As described with other disorders, secondary gain issues become important in relationships, such as when one person sends the message, "you must love me" and the other partner returns the message, "I'm wanted and needed." This allows one to be the child and the other to be the power boss. This *power boss* role can be taken to an extreme where he or she may sabotage correct use of medication to keep the power. Much like with insomnia and other psychiatric disorders, the family can unconsciously encourage one person to remain ill simply by prescribing that role for them— "you are sick; let me take care of you"—which makes it hard for the sick one to say, "I will get well." It is almost as if the sick one has to remain in that role to satisfy everyone else.

Managing panic disorder requires working from a variety of angles, including removing caffeine, diet or cold pills, or other stimulants (especially cocaine) from the ill person's life. Treatment is important and includes medication, relaxation skills, and family therapy. Aside from addressing the issues described above, family members can be instrumental in weaning the patient from being so clingy and dependent on others. An example of this weaning process is as follows: The spouse learns to identify the rising anxiety and avoidance in the ill person; he provides emotional support as he gradually pulls back from being the chauffeur and caregiver; he encourages the one who is out of sorts to express directly when she *really* needs him to assist her versus him automatically taking over the role of being always available. This may require creating a new style of communication that is more open and direct about needs as well as addressing old unresolved dependency issues from childhood. When both partners and the entire family learn to communicate more efficiently and seeking independence and growth is encouraged, all members greatly benefit.

CHAPTER **3**

OBSESSIVE-COMPULSIVE DISORDER

■ *DRUGS DISCUSSED:*
Anafranil, Prozac, Zoloft, Paxil, Luvox, BuSpar

A person is said to have *obsessive-compulsive disorder (OCD)* when he or she engages in obsessive thoughts or compulsive ritualistic behaviors that are distressing or consume more than an hour of time each day. An obsession is defined as an intrusive or recurrent thought, image, or impulse that a person attempts to ignore or suppress because it seems senseless or repugnant to him or her. A compulsion is the need to perform a task or ritual in a repetitive, seemingly purposeful way. Most compulsive behaviors are designed to prevent some future event or situation the person finds threatening or frightening. These compulsions, however, are not realistically connected to the feared event or situation. Usually, compulsive behaviors temporarily reduce anxiety. At some point during the illness, the sufferer will view his behavior as excessive, senseless, and not pleasurable despite its tension-relieving properties. At other times, this insight may be lost.

Among children and adolescents, the most common symptoms of obsessive behavior are an undue preoccupation with dirt, germs, or toxins, and the worry that something terrible will happen to them if they do not keep these things at bay. Their most common compulsions are excessive washing, tooth brushing, and grooming, as well as rituals in which they repeat actions, such as having to open and close a door three times, and checking rituals, such as needing to make sure that appliances are turned off, windows closed, and doors locked five times before leaving the house or going to sleep. The most common symptoms among adults include obsessions about contamination, pathologic doubt, and bodily concerns, such as a fear that one might have a disease, an infection, or cancer; a disproportional need for symmetry, as in having to place things in exactly the right position on the desk or table; and worry about uncontrollable aggressive or sexual impulses. Adult compulsions include such activities as asking forgiveness six times for accidentally touching someone while standing in line, confessing an illegal or immoral act done in the remote past hundreds of times, setting the dinner table several times until the utensils are exactly the same distance from the plates, washing one's hands until they are raw and cracked, taking showers until there is no more hot water, counting objects in the environment, and asking senseless questions. Hoarding is an unusual and difficult compulsion in which a person allows his house to become progressively more cluttered with what others would consider valueless junk, such as old newspapers, cans, or boxes. The "pack rat" cannot bear to part with these things because he believes they might someday have value or be useful.

The boundaries of the obsessive-compulsive spectrum of disorders are not yet well defined because many of the impulse control disorders share features with OCD. For example, *body dysmorphic disorder,* also popularly known as the "the distress of imagined ugliness," has overtones of compulsive behavior. Typically, someone suffering from this condition is overly preoccupied with what she imagines to be her body's defects. These individuals invest a disproportionate amount of time trying to camouflage the "defect" with makeup or clothes, attempting to find doctors to diagnose and surgically correct it, or simply spending prolonged periods of time staring at the "imperfection" in the mirror.

Another illness with obsessive-compulsive features is *trichotillomania*, compulsive hair pulling that often leads to large bald spots on the scalp and pulling out other hair, such as eyebrows and eyelashes. This condition typically affects females at the beginning of puberty and can become chronic. Other disorders that may share part of the OCD spectrum include obsessions about urination, compulsive facial picking (initially to remove blemishes such as pimples but ultimately leading to infections and scarring), paraphilias (unusual sexual arousal patterns), and excessive involvement in religious practices and rituals. Anorexia nervosa, in which a person displays a tremendous preoccupation with food, weight, and body image, also shares features with OCD.

Obsessive-compulsive disorder is often a very secret, controlling, and socially debilitating disease. Since symptoms often manifest mostly at home, many sufferers seek treatment only when they can no longer hide these behaviors in public, or when their families insist that the rituals have become intolerable. Sometimes loss of self-esteem, loss of the sense of self-control, withdrawal from friendships because a person is embarrassed to be around others, and decreased effectiveness on the job (for example, due to long bathroom breaks to wash) are the factors that motivate an individual to seek treatment. Often an adult suffering from OCD has experienced lesser symptoms earlier in life. These symptoms may have included separation anxiety, resistance to change or novelty, avoiding risk, ambivalent feelings about people or things, excessive devotion to work, magical thinking (unrealistic connections of cause and effect), hypermorality, and perfectionism. Conditions that commonly accompany OCD include depression, phobias, anxiety, eating disorders, substance abuse, panic, and Tourette's disorder. Tourette's, with its chronic motor and vocal tics and vocalization of profanities, is often inherited in families where OCD is present, and both conditions may manifest in these instances.

MULTIPLE DISORDERS

Sometimes simple phobias coexist with OCD. The difference between these two conditions, however, is that individuals suffering from simple phobias typically *avoid* situations or things that provoke anxiety, while the person with OCD will get stuck in a prolonged ritual response to the anxiety-provoking situation.

A person may engage in some behaviors of OCD without actually having this illness, as can be seen in those who exhibit what is called "obsessive-compulsive personality disorder." The latter is characterized by long-standing perfectionism, inflexibility, and need for control, leading to undue focus on the details of a situation while remaining ignorant of the "big picture." These individuals are controlling, stingy, conscientious, restricted in their ability to express their emotions, devoted to work which they have a hard time delegating, miserly, and stubborn, and often hoard things. A person with obsessive-compulsive personality disorder, however, does not suffer discomfort or internal conflict about her behaviors, but believes others should share her outlook and values. This individual is not likely to benefit from the medications specific to OCD, but might profit from a course of psychotherapy focused on trying to help her understand and perhaps alter her personality style and behaviors. The advantage to developing some flexibility is that the person may learn to relax, play, and have some fun in life.

A national survey involving interviews with a careful sampling of adults in the United States found that 1 to 3 percent have obsessive-compulsive disorder, and that the average age of onset of this condition is around twenty-three years of age. OCD may begin in childhood or early adulthood. For half the patients, the illness is chronic and unremitting, while in others it fluctuates over time, with episodes of illness typically lasting less than a year. Often patients struggle with OCD for several years before finally seeking psychiatric treatment. The long-term follow-up studies we have reviewed show a highly variable percentage of patients improving versus those who remain unchanged. The natural history, or untreated long-term course of the illness, is fairly unpredictable. Some people spontaneously recover, while others remain chronically ill or have symptoms that come and go throughout their lives.

Before individuals suffering from OCD can begin treatment, they must acknowledge several things to themselves. The first is that they have been fighting a long-term battle with thoughts or impulses prior to seeking treatment. They need to admit to themselves that they are suffering from a sense of demoralization because they feel powerless to control their symptoms, and that the struggle to keep their disease a secret has only resulted in guilt, helplessness, and loss of self-esteem. They may even be experiencing a fear of giving up their symptoms because these are "safe" and familiar ways of doing things. Many people find themselves demoralized by the social ramifications of OCD, which may have resulted in unwanted celibacy, broken marriages, or chronic family struggles. Once an individual has reached this state of self-awareness, admitting to himself that he is out of control and in need of help, his chances of benefiting from treatment are greatly increased because he is willing to do behavioral homework and to tolerate drug side effects.

In the treatment of OCD, psychodynamic, psychoanalytic psychotherapy, and simple relaxation techniques are ineffective. The most effective form of psychotherapy is one that exposes the patient to a series of stimuli, each successively more anxiety provoking than the last, while at the same time helping her to curb her compulsive ritualistic responses. An example of this approach might be having the patient touch a doorknob without engaging in hand washing, then touch a toilet seat, then use the toilet in a public rest room while limiting hand washing to under one minute. Individuals undergoing this therapy show long-term gains in winning control over their illness. These gains often are maintained long after the therapy has ended. If a patient is depressed or using tranquilizers, however, both of these conditions may decrease the effectiveness of or motivation for this therapeutic approach. Although medications may help a person achieve relief from the symptoms of OCD, there is a high risk of relapse when the medications are stopped.

DRUG TREATMENTS FOR OCD

Numerous nonspecific tranquilizers, antidepressants, and lithium are occasionally useful in the treatment of OCD, but controlled double-blind studies have shown that the most effective drugs are Anafranil (a tricyclic antidepressant with greater serotonin selectivity than the others in this class) and the selective serotonin reuptake inhibitors, which include Prozac, Zoloft, Paxil, and Luvox. These medications generally have to be used at fairly high doses, and the patient must typically take them for one or two months before they take effect. Although ongoing improvement is apparent at the three-month mark, the symptoms of OCD are only partially alleviated by drug therapy, unlike the symptoms of depression and panic, which respond more fully to medications. In fact, most drug studies have shown that the average patient achieves only a 40 percent reduction in the severity of OCD symptoms after two to two and a half months of treatment.

ANAFRANIL

The first drug shown to be effective for OCD was Anafranil (clomipramine), which is used outside the United States for the treatment of depression, panic, and premature ejaculation. Anafranil is a tricyclic antidepressant, which means that it has a three-ring chemical structure similar to the older-generation antidepressants, and shares many of the side effects of these drugs, including dry mouth, blurred vision, weight gain, constipation, and sexual dysfunction. There is also a small risk of seizures—about 0.5 percent at daily doses of up to 250 mg/day, and 2 percent at higher doses. Anafranil was the first drug to clearly distinguish itself from all other tricyclic antidepressants by being uniquely effective for OCD. Other tricyclic antidepressants, such as nortriptyline and desipramine, were often used as control drugs and found to be no better than placebo. The response to placebo (sugar pills) in OCD studies has been very consistently minimal. The presence of panic attacks along with OCD is a predictor of a good response to Anafranil; the presence or absence of depression does not affect the likelihood of a good response to this drug.

Anafranil is safe enough to be used long-term, and in one study patients who had a positive initial response to an average dose of 270 mg/day were able to reduce their dosage to 165 mg/day without reducing the drug's effectiveness. If the dosage can be reduced while maintaining symptom control, this should be done to minimize the burden of the side effects.

Prozac

Several early studies of Prozac (fluoxetine) showed that this drug was as effective as Anafranil in treating OCD when administered at average doses of around 80 mg/day. Although lower doses of this drug were not generally tried in studies performed in the 1980s, very recent research shows a modest difference in results, favoring the higher dose of Prozac over the lower one. The current approach to using Prozac for treatment of OCD is to begin with a modest dose of 10 or 20 mg, and then gradually work up to 60 or 80 mg/day. This practice is based on the assumptions that (1) higher doses are generally more effective, and (2) that building up to these higher doses over a period of several weeks is far more tolerable than trying to take very high doses in the first week or two of treatment. This is because the body has an opportunity to gradually adjust to side effects so they are not as intense as they would be with rapid dose escalation. As with Anafranil, the presence or absence of depression does not predict a successful response of OCD to Prozac.

A meta-analysis (literature review looking at many different studies) found that Anafranil was more effective in the treatment of OCD than Prozac, Zoloft, and Luvox, even though Anafranil has more side effects. This finding is controversial, since other studies show equal effectiveness in direct "head-to-head" randomized comparisons of Anafranil with each of the SSRI antidepressants.

Luvox

Luvox (fluvoxamine) has also been FDA approved for the treatment of obsessive-compulsive disorder. One of the main differences between this drug and Prozac is that Luvox has a shorter "half-life." What this means is that a dose of Luvox reaches steady-state blood levels fairly quickly, but that it also can be flushed out of the body somewhat rapidly if the side effects become intolerable. The disadvantage is that the drug must be taken twice daily at doses over 150 mg/day and that missed doses may cause a sudden drop in the level of Luvox in the blood. Luvox is usually used in the range of 100 to 300 mg/day, while Zoloft (sertraline) is used in the range of 50 to 200 mg/day, and Paxil (paroxetine) is used in the range of 20 to 60 mg/day.

BuSpar

Although BuSpar (buspirone) seems to be effective in the treatment of obsessive-compulsive disorder, studies on its effectiveness have been mixed. It appears to have a role in augmenting effectiveness when added to other OCD drugs, and it might even be useful by itself in those patients who cannot tolerate the standard OCD drugs, such as Anafranil, Prozac, Zoloft, or Luvox. The typical dose of buspirone is about 30 to 60 mg daily, given in divided doses. Other strategies that sometimes augment the effectiveness of OCD drugs include the addition of lithium carbonate to an SSRI. The antipsychotic or neuroleptic drugs are sometimes used in patients with OCD who also have a tic disorder, full-blown Tourette's syndrome, or schizotypal personality (strange, bizarre thinking and behaviors, and unusual perceptions). The atypical antipsychotic Risperdal used at a dose of about 3 mg/day has recently been reported to be of benefit when added to standard OCD drugs. Each of these augmenting strategies work for some patients and not others, and finding the best drug combination involves a fair amount of systematic trial-and-error collaboration with a doctor who is very persistent in trying new approaches to get the best possible response.

MAO INHIBITORS

On rare occasions, MAO inhibitors, such as Nardil or Parnate, may be useful in treating OCD, but they can never be combined with Anafranil or the SSRI antidepressants because they may cause a rare and potentially lethal interaction called serotonin syndrome. The MAO inhibitors appear specifically useful in patients with OCD and panic disorder.

To give you an idea of what it is like to experience symptoms of OCD and what sort of treatments are prescribed, we have put together several case histories taken from our files. These are real patients, with the names changed, and real outcomes. Sometimes the outcomes aren't ideal.

Joe: Obsessive-compulsive disorder

During his first session, Joe tells me that he has been diagnosed with obsessive-compulsive disorder and is seeking a second opinion. A forty-year-old lineman, he is currently living alone after separating three weeks previously from his wife of four years and their two children. Their marriage ended following a severe and chronic bout of OCD that Joe experienced after losing his job of fourteen years as a foreman with a major utility company. Losing his job, taking other jobs that felt demeaning, and being unemployed for a year has been very stressful for him, but he says that his real problem is that he has felt extremely lonely and heartbroken since his wife told him to move out. Over the past year, Joe has been in psychotherapy with Dr. K., whom he describes as very directive and confrontive. He feels that he has made a lot of progress during their time of working together.

A Catholic, Joe describes his main compulsive behaviors as saying prayers all the time and doing rituals that involve washing his hands and praying, although he says he has cut down on the hand washing a great deal. He feels that he has to pray a certain number of times in order to get it right, and he often feels the need to bless himself. He tells me that his OCD symptoms became much worse after his wife, then forty years old, became pregnant with their first child. At that time, he became obsessively fearful that the child might be born with a deformity.

When asked if he has ever had any other serious symptoms, Joe tells me that he had two panic attacks. The first was five years ago when he broke up with his former girlfriend, and the second occurred about a year ago. Both attacks involved shortness of breath, sweating, feelings of nervousness and anxiety, and becoming red in the face. For the last two weeks before coming, he has felt depressed and has been eating and sleeping poorly and waking up in the middle of the night. He is scared that his wife might meet someone else and that he might lose everything. These thoughts make him feel devastated and heartbroken.

Joe says that there had been no sexual contact in his marriage for a long time, partly because the Klonopin he has been taking for anxiety makes him sleepy, partly because he is concerned with praying, and partly because his sex drive has been decreased by his medications. His wife has taken all of these things very personally. Joe also says that there is very poor communication between them, as well as issues of codependence.

When I ask him if he has ever had symptoms of depression before, he tells me that he had a serious bout when he broke up with his previous girlfriend five or six years ago. He "was in a lousy mood and couldn't sleep." At that time his doctor prescribed Xanax.

Joe claims that he used to be much more social and would go to the theater and to parties, but that all this stopped when he got married to his wife five years ago. He stopped drinking and socializing, and no longer goes to the gym because of "low energy." The only hobby he has maintained an interest in is reading about and collecting African art. Although he admits that he doesn't have many friends, he has been spending time with his children three times a week since the separation. He describes his wife as a very competent woman who works at a day-care center.

Treatment Recommendations: To help Joe with his depression and obsessive-compulsive disorder, I suggested that he try taking Paxil. When he has reached a dosage of 50 mg/day and has been able to maintain that for a month, I recommended that he consider augmenting the Paxil with lithium or BuSpar for another month. The reason I suggested the lithium augmentation is that Joe's brother has bipolar illness (manic depression), which usually responds to lithium. Drug response often runs true in blood relatives. I suggested he consider trying the BuSpar augmentation because there are some reports of this drug being an effective treatment for OCD.

Nearly a year later Joe is taking 80 mg/day of BuSpar (as a "helper" drug for the OCD), 40 mg/day of Paxil (the primary OCD drug), and Klonopin (a tranquilizer to help with sleep). Despite the fact that he still hasn't found a steady job, he is doing well. Although he has tried to reconcile with his wife, she says she is burnt out with trying to deal with his illness and that she does not love him anymore. She told Joe that he didn't meet her sexual and emotional needs. His OCD symptoms are far better, but he continues to deny the finality of his wife's desire to end the marriage.

Conclusion: Joe is now taking 80 mg/day of BuSpar, 50 mg of Paxil, and no Klonopin. His biggest issue is that his wife has told him she is filing for a divorce. Even though she has been saying that for more than six months, he is still feeling shocked and hurt and suffering from massive denial. He keeps saying that he has "only been sick for awhile," and can't understand why she wants to end things when he has been so devoted to her and has done so much for her. He keeps wondering if marital therapy earlier in the course of his illness might have helped, but that is something we will never know. In spite of the stress of impending divorce, Joe says that he feels much better and is having much more success dealing with his compulsive behaviors. I note that the addition of BuSpar to his medication regimen has had a positive effect on what was a case of obvious and severe OCD.

One important lesson to be learned here is that chronic illness often affects the spouse as dramatically as it does the patient. The buildup of silent resentments in the face of having to deal with a loved one's compulsive, ritualistic behavior can take over a family's life. If care is not sought in time, the effect on the marriage can be devastating.

Andy: Fear of touching and of bad thoughts— severe obsessive-compulsive disorder

Andy is a fifty-two-year-old unmarried man who works as a supervisor at an entertainment center. He was originally diagnosed with severe OCD when he visited a psychiatrist fifteen years ago. Tragically, he received no long-term psychotherapy and no medication, and has been living with his symptoms for over two decades. Up until now, he has been unaware that there is any effective treatment for his condition.

He suffers from numerous symptoms, but he is especially afraid to touch things. In fact, when he came into my office, he was afraid to touch the pen so that he could complete the new patient information form, which he was also afraid to touch. He is fearful of sitting down because other people who had "bad thoughts" might have sat in the same place. Although he is a religious Catholic, he is afraid to go inside a church. He explains that he can't touch anything in the church, and that if anything in the sermon should upset him, when he got back home he would have to throw away the clothes he wore to avoid being reminded of what the priest had said. He has disturbing thoughts that he can't get rid of, and he compulsively washes his hands. Andy has so many ritualized washing and cleaning routines that it takes him over an hour to get ready for work in the morning, and about one and a half hours to get undressed in the evening. If a coworker has touched him during the day, he has to wash that part of his body first. He lives in a very small trailer, which is very dirty. Since he is afraid to touch anything at home, he can't clean it up. When he urinates, he has to use tissues or he is unable to touch himself. He can't use a public phone or sit on a public bench.

Andy's family history sheds some interesting light on his case. His father suffered from severe manic depression and was admitted to the hospital multiple times. Andy's mother was addicted to barbiturates, and would often stay in the bedroom and hide. While Andy was away at college, however, his mother and his two brothers were killed by the father, who then committed suicide. Andy was very tearful when he discussed this with me, and blamed himself for the deaths, claiming that his being away at school and using the family money may have been the cause for the homicide-suicide. He was unwilling to go into detail about any of this, but did tell me that he has never talked to anyone about this tragedy and has never had psychotherapy. This event has obviously had a devastating effect on his entire life, however. Andy lives alone, has never been married, and has never even had a major relationship.

Treatment Recommendations: When I opened the door to ask Andy into my office at the beginning of our interview, I found him standing up in the waiting room, and he remained standing throughout our half-hour session. He has a very intense, dramatic quality to him, and was extremely guilt ridden. As I mentioned earlier, he was unwilling to touch a pen or paper and said that he didn't know how he could possibly fill my prescription for medication because he couldn't go into stores and touch things. When he gave me a check at the end of the session, he signed his name with great reluctance and asked me to fill in the rest. Despite his very agitated appearance and behavior, however, he displayed no clear hallucinations or delusions; he did, however, carry an extraordinary amount of guilt about the death of his entire family.

I diagnosed Andy with severe obsessive-compulsive disorder and chronic post-traumatic stress disorder and asked him to start taking 20 mg/day of Prozac the first week. If he found he could tolerate this dosage, I suggested that he increase this to 40 mg. I also recommended that he begin psychotherapy as soon as possible to help him begin dealing with his guilt and anxiety issues.

After three months, Andy has worked his way up to 60 to 80 mg of Prozac per day but hasn't yet begun the BuSpar augmentation I suggested. He also hasn't been able to read any of the books on OCD I recommended because he is afraid of going into a bookstore. He is still worried about having impure thoughts and having his clothes touched by others (even the dry cleaner). Although his psychologist has suggested "real-life exposure treatment" and has offered to accompany him and give him moral support, Andy feels overwhelmed at the thought. I feel that he is showing only minimal improvement.

Conclusions: Although the psychologist and I both tried to work with Andy on an outpatient basis, the overwhelming nature of his post-traumatic stress disorder and his fear of beginning a behavioral program of exposure and response prevention led to a recommendation for long-term hospitalization initially and day treatment later. Only in this way could he really begin the battle with his illness. Two months ago, Andy was admitted to the hospital and is now undergoing day treatment. With the help of Luvox and Navane, he is starting to deal with the longtime post-traumatic stress caused by the loss of his family. He is also doing desensitization work by going into stores and touching things.

Pamela: Fear of killing others—OCD with panic attacks

Pamela is a thirty-three-year-old woman who is a college graduate. She is currently unemployed and self-referred. She tells me that she suffers from OCD and panic disorder, and that she has had major difficulties adjusting to her marriage (her first), which necessitated a move from the East Coast to California.

Pamela displays a variety of symptoms. For the last four years she has had dreams, fantasies, or fears of harming others. These began while she was sharing a summer house with a woman friend and dreamt that she would kill the woman. The feeling that she might do so was so powerful that she actually warned her housemate, got far away from there, and continued even then to be fearful that she would act on the impulse. She also has a terror of having knives in her home and must have them covered up, a condition that began after an earlier engagement broke up.

When she developed feelings of impending doom, her doctor treated her with up to 1 mg/day of Xanax. He prescribed Prozac when she complained of "bad thoughts," but this didn't help her because she claimed it made her fantasize her own funeral. Pamela also said that she felt toxic while taking Prozac, gained weight, and became severely constipated.

Although she has never acted on her impulses to harm other people, this fantasy has been a recurrent theme for her. Pamela says she also checks things a lot, and washes her hands when she is anxious because it makes her feel better. At times like these, she gets the feeling that if she doesn't do something such as touch an object, something bad will happen. Often she has to do so many ritualistic things that involve checking, washing, and touching that it takes her ten or fifteen minutes just to leave the house.

Pamela's OCD symptoms become worse on the days when she feels more anxious, but when she takes Xanax at doses large enough to control her anxiety, she feels stoned and sedated. Pamela says that she sometimes has thoughts of doing bad things to children and, because of this, has to have any knives in the house covered up and the tool drawer closed. She also has a fear that she might stab her husband.

At her worst, Pamela says, she used to suffer from frequent panic attacks, but she very rarely has them now. When she experiences an attack, she feels as if she is out of her body and has problems with her breathing. Her hands become cold, her hands and feet are numb, her heart races, and she sometimes sweats and feels the urgency to void. She also feels as if she is dying or going crazy and has an overwhelming sense of doom. These attacks last for several minutes at a time and because of them she avoided public transportation, crowds, and bridges for a long time. She also eliminated caffeine from her diet because she said it made her more anxious. Exercise helped her quite a bit, as did taking Xanax.

Pamela has not worked since she moved to California. She told me that the move was very traumatic for her because she was the marketing manager for a major magazine and had to give up her excellent job to relocate here with her husband when he was transferred. Being a housewife is not enough to make her happy but, until now, she hasn't been very serious about a job search because she didn't think that she could make nearly as much money here as she did in New York. She also didn't really believe that she and her husband would be staying in California long-term. Recently, however, she has gotten serious about job hunting and is actively seeking a well-paying position. Her husband is less concerned about the money and just wants her to find something that she will really enjoy.

Although she has made some friends since she came here, she has felt very bored. Her husband, who is an internist with an excellent job, is always working and seldom around. Pamela feels that many things about her life are good. She lives in a wonderful house and has a wonderful husband whom she loves very much. She would like to have a child, but she has agreed to wait because her husband is not ready and she wants to maintain a happy marriage. In her spare time, she enjoys exercising at the beach and going to horse races, antique auctions, and Japanese restaurants. She is impetuous, moody, and analytical, yet she is also a very good friend and extremely fun loving. Although her husband knows she is a hypochondriac and a constant worrier, he believes she is a basically good person, fun to be with, and caring.

Pamela admits that she was terrified of getting married but did so anyway in 1993. Since then she has had occasional thoughts of pouring Drano on her husband, and also has sometimes felt scared of other people. She says that she feels fearful about taking medications because "they might be contaminated," but also because, when she was younger, she witnessed her mother being very heavily drugged for her problems. Although Pamela is reluctant to take drugs, she says that her husband believes in them. He had to deal with an ex-girlfriend who committed suicide, and he feels that drug therapy might have saved her life. Pamela has recently noted a great increase in her anxiety level and feels this is directly connected with having to go on a fourteen-hour airplane trip with her husband.

Diagnosis and Recommended Treatment: Pamela clearly suffers from obsessive-compulsive disorder and panic disorder with avoidance, although the latter is currently in remission. I suggested that she continue taking her low dose of Xanax as needed, as well as the low dose of Inderal she takes to prevent headaches. I asked her to consider taking BuSpar and/or Anafranil, and told her that the latter would probably be the better drug for both OCD and panic. Pamela asked to return in one week for further discussion of these options after I had spoken with her former psychiatrist.

Six months later, Pamela is taking 10 mg of Inderal twice daily and 15 mg of BuSpar per day. Although she is hoping for a pregnancy very soon, her husband is still somewhat reluctant to start a family at this point, since he is currently very career focused. Pamela is still worrying a lot, but she may do biofeedback or cognitive-behavioral therapy in order to see if she can get off her medications. Two months later in mid-May, Pamela called me to say that she was three months pregnant, working, and felt strong enough to stop taking the drugs.

Conclusion: The fear, fantasy, or impulse to harm others, including children or sleeping adults, is very common to those suffering from OCD. Psychotherapists can spend years trying to analyze the roots of the conscious or unconscious hostility that comprise a part of these clients' ambivalent attachments to loved ones. What is fascinating about these compulsions, however, is their very lack of foundation in genuine malice. A classic characteristic of these impulses to harm is that they are so alien and repulsive to the person experiencing them. Although Pamela did have some conflicts with her husband, she was certainly never abused or murderously angry. It was always clear to her, myself, and him that she truly loved him. As she became more satisfied with her life by finding a job and getting pregnant, her OCD improved and she was able to get off the medications.

Amy: Severe obsessive-compulsive disorder

Amy is a twenty-nine-year-old housewife who has been married seven years and has one child almost two years old. Her obsessive-compulsive disorder began in high school when she began taking extremely long showers twice a day, spending forty minutes to shave her legs repeatedly. At the age of sixteen, she became obsessed with hair, plucking the hairs from her nose and eyebrows and shaving her hands and feet.

Beginning at age twenty, she worked as a paralegal, but her need to repeat all her actions many times made her the slowest worker in her office. Her next job was managing a food court at a mall. She stopped working when she got pregnant.

Although she had grown up with pets and, in fact, had two dogs in her home prior to her illness, she later developed severe phobias about dog hair. These fears became so bad that she had to give the dogs away. For an entire year, she felt compelled to shake the hair out of all her clothes before putting them into the washing machine, which took an extra half hour on the average. She frequently felt "dirty," and every time she came home, she would become obsessed with the idea that "there were cats around the house." The only way she could make herself feel comfortable again was to take off all her clothes and shower. Her obsession with cleanliness was apparent in her statement to me that "Nobody is as clean as I am."

All of these fears, of course, have severely restricted her lifestyle. For example, she and her husband bought a new house one and a half years ago, but she has never had a guest over because of her fear of dirt and animal hair. She cannot go to her parents' house because they have cats and dogs. Although she feels very guilty because she has to meet her parents and her in-laws at places away from their homes because of her terror of contamination, she believes that if she had a guest over she would "have to resterilize my house."

It is very difficult for Amy to go clothes shopping because when she sees dark-colored clothing, she thinks she can spot animal hair on it. When she goes out of the house, she has to check any car seat, bench, or chair on which she will be sitting to make sure there are no animal hairs on it. When she brings home groceries, she has to wipe them off before she will put them into the kitchen cabinet.

Beginning shortly after the birth of her son, her condition worsened and she began living in only one room of the house because she felt that the whole house was contaminated. She began taking ten showers a day, every time she left her bedroom. During this period, she became depressed and essentially housebound and would only leave her room to go out with her husband on weekends. At this juncture, she finally sought help and began working with Dr. P., who started her on 30 mg/day of BuSpar and 75 mg of Pamelor at bedtime. While taking this combination of drugs, Amy was able to lead a somewhat normal life. (Note that Pamelor is a tricyclic antidepressant and fine for depression but not generally effective for OCD.)

Amy's obsession with cleanliness and emotional instability has its roots in her family history. Her maternal grandmother had a breakdown after the birth of her second child. Although she is healthy at the age of seventy-seven, she spends three hours a day vacuuming, doing laundry, and scrubbing the floor. Amy's mother was also obsessively clean and mistreated her daughter when Amy failed to live up to her high standards. Everything in her mother's house had to be perfect and clean, and the rooms had to be dusted and vacuumed every day. Amy's mother, now fifty-five, has improved since menopause. Both the maternal grandmother and the mother have received medical help and are taking a thyroid replacement hormone. Amy's mother also took a tricyclic antidepressant after Amy's little brother was born.

Unfortunately, Amy's sister, now nineteen, has inherited the family obsession. All her closets have to be in perfect order, and once she has cleaned her room, no one can come in, not even her boyfriend. She is currently living with her parents. Amy's husband is an accountant whom she describes as a very normal person who is extremely patient with her; nevertheless, he has told her that he is getting tired of dealing with her illness. Since her disorder makes it necessary for both of them to have to shower before they can make love, sex can never occur spontaneously.

Amy's goal for her treatment is to be able to have people over to her home because she loves to cook and bake. She would also like to feel comfortable about allowing her son to play outside without having to worry that he's getting filthy. She very much wants him to lead a normal life.

Diagnosis and Recommended Treatment: Although Amy has severe obsessive-compulsive disorder, she is improving. She told me during our meeting that she had a breakthrough when she took her son to the park. Even though there was a dog present, she didn't bathe her son immediately on returning to the house, and she felt that this indicated significant progress. Eventually, she was also able to visit her parents' home and invite them to visit hers. She has begun to do things she hasn't been able to do in a long time, such as visiting others, and feels more in control of herself and more willing to try new things. She has experienced consistent improvement since she began taking Prozac. Although she is still "weird" about animal hair and has to wash her clothes twice to feel that they are really clean, she says she feels fine.

Currently, Amy has reached a dosage of 80 mg/day of Prozac, 50 mg of Desyrel at bedtime to help her sleep, and 10 mg of BuSpar twice daily to augment the Prozac. She has shown significant improvement in her obsessive behavior. When her parents gave her a refrigerator, she spent only two hours cleaning it to remove the "hairs." She was able to pet a dog briefly, and has reluctantly agreed to work on desensitization to dog hair prior to her visits to her folks, who have one. When she had guests come over on two different weekends, she cleaned up the day after they left, but didn't say anything if she saw some dirt or hair in the house or on someone's clothes during the visit itself.

Conclusions: A year later, Amy decided to take herself off Prozac for a few months. When she did, her headaches recurred, she gained 8 pounds, and she felt depressed, "bitchy," and complained of low energy. Regressing back to her old obsessions about cleanliness, she began throwing away any of her son's clothes that had animal hair on them, and was observed by her parents to be having problems with her "attitude." At this point, Amy began to confront her husband about the unfairness of her doing all the work around the house, and told him that she had decided that having one child was enough. She didn't feel that she could handle a second one.

Amy's impulsive decision to stop her medicine, and the worsening of her illness, has taken its toll on her marriage. She is separated from her husband and living with a girlfriend and planning to obtain a divorce. Her husband is angry and says that he should have left her five years ago when she had her breakdown. She's facing the reality of her impending divorce by moving out of the house and has seen her husband with his new girlfriend.

With a renewal of medicine, within a year, Amy has gone back to school and finished a nursing program, and is seeking a job in this field. Except for the few months that she stopped taking her medication, she has continued taking the drugs with favorable results. Soon after, she met a new man who has two dogs and began a relationship. She's doing desensitization work with them, but hasn't told him about her OCD problems and how much animal hair is a concern for her.

Once again, we can see the toll that obsessive-compulsive disorder takes on a marriage. Even a case of OCD this severe, however, can be overcome by medications and, now that the patient is dating a man with dogs, she is very highly motivated to aggressively do the exposure and response prevention work that she began early in treatment.

Ellen: Body dysmorphic disorder—the "distress of imagined ugliness"

Ellen is a twenty-four-year-old single woman who is currently living with her parents after having completed her master's degree in English. She is about to go to graduate school to begin work on her Ph.D. At our first meeting, she tells me that all her life she has experienced mood swings that seem abnormally extreme to her and that they have gotten worse in the last few years. She is not sure if these mood swings are driven by upsetting life events or a chemical imbalance.

Ellen has been on the East Coast for a year getting her master's degree and has just returned to California. While in school, she was in therapy for about three months to deal with anxiety issues. She recently had a therapeutic abortion after an affair with a man whom she really didn't love. Being in relationships with people whom she didn't love, but dated because she felt the need to be with someone, is a pattern for her. Currently, Ellen is having self-doubts about whether she is smart enough to be in a Ph.D. program.

When Ellen is in a depression, she feels slowed down, although this is not apparent to others. She feels apathetic, despondent, and hopeless. Her sex drive and concentration are lessened, and she avoids making decisions. Although she feels lonelier than usual, she also loses her desire to socialize with others, and experiences a decreased appetite accompanied by constipation. These symptoms last for weeks at a time. Although she can still get her typical six or seven hours of sleep per night, she has more frequent bouts of insomnia, a problem that has been with her for a long time. When she is depressed, she does feel some guilt around current issues, such as her abortion and her superficial dating relationships. She has no auditory, visual, taste, touch, or smell hallucinations.

Once Ellen falls into a depression, it seems that nothing cheers her up again because she feels no pleasure in anything during those times. Often she will make an effort to go through the motions of doing something she normally enjoys, but she will derive no real enjoyment from the activity. She does have diurnal mood variation, feeling better in the morning and worse at night. When she feels really down, she thinks about suicide but has never made a plan or attempt.

Ellen's emotional highs normally follow the appearance of a new man in her life, even if it is only for one date. Her high periods are less frequent than the depressions, however, and last from one to seven days. During those times, she feels as if her system is speeded up. She can't eat anything, and she feels six hours of sleep is plenty, although she can even get by on four. She is more social, calls her friends, has limitless energy, exercises more, and feels more spontaneous and relaxed. She also develops mild diarrhea and feels thirsty all the time. She has more mental and physical energy, less worry, and more confidence that she can handle things. Her sex drive is also a lot higher. She is more creative, and writes more in her journal.

While Ellen denies feeling symptoms of grandiosity and a racing mind during these periods of emotional high, she does admit that they give her more confidence. When she feels this good, she can easily imagine herself being successful as a professor and writer, and feels more certain that she has something to give in a relationship. She does find herself getting more irritable than usual, but there is no change in her spending patterns, nor does she talk faster or louder.

She does not engage in impulsive wild activities such as shoplifting, gambling, or any other behavior that could get her in trouble—except for driving 80 mph on the freeway. Typically she will drive 75. Her general mood is "exuberant, in love with life," and her behavior is more bubbly and self-confident.

Ellen's depressions and high periods have become more obvious since about the age of twenty. The depressions are becoming more common and more frequent, however. Over the last four years, she estimates she has been high about 5 percent of the time, has been in a bad depression about 10 percent of the time, and has been normal or very mildly depressed for 85 percent of the time.

Aside from her bouts of depression, Ellen also has obsessions about certain parts of her body. After she broke up with her fiancé when she was twenty-one, her hair started bothering her. Even when she pulled it back and it was firmly fastened, she was overly concerned that it might get loose and touch her face. On another occasion, she became obsessively worried that her breasts were sagging, even when she wore a bra. Her feelings of distress were so great that she couldn't even allow herself to look in a mirror. At one point, she consulted a plastic surgeon because she discovered that her breasts were asymmetric. He agreed that they were slightly different from each other, but told her that the difference was too little to justify a surgical procedure. More recently she has been concerned about her abdominal oblique muscles and has been exercising a lot to try and make them more even and less asymmetric. She has no history of compulsive hair pulling.

Ellen realizes that her concerns about her mild body defects are very excessive and she calls them "crazy." On the other hand, she admits that she is concerned that if she doesn't stay on top of her appearance, worrying about it and focusing a lot of attention on her hair and her clothes, she will look terrible. She denies engaging in any prolonged washing or grooming rituals, and claims that she is able to get up, take a shower, get dressed, and be ready to go in about an hour and ten minutes every morning.

Ellen admits that she is very concerned about her eating behaviors and has a difficult time having dinner with a new person because she is quite concerned about whether she can control her food intake. She doesn't want to eat too much or too little, or risk gaining weight or worsening her hiatal hernia.

She also freely admits that her concern about her bodily defects has gotten in the way of school. Her mind has been wandering to these issues so often lately that she has started worrying that she might be called on in the classroom while her thoughts are elsewhere, preoccupied with her physical appearance.

Although Ellen grew up locally and had a good childhood, there is a history of depression and bodily obsession in the family. A seventeen-year-old cousin named Mary used to spend hours in the bathroom taking showers or applying makeup. Even though Mary shaved off all her body hair, she claimed that she could feel it growing in and had to shave it again during the night. She also clawed at her face on occasion as a ritual to remove blemishes. Mary reportedly saw several psychiatrists who diagnosed her as having OCD. Ellen's paternal grandfather, a physician, also had problems with depression and had made a suicide attempt as a teenager. Although he went into a long-term remission from his depression, he developed manic depressive illness at age sixty and required lithium treatment.

At the end of my interview with Ellen, her mother spoke with me privately. Although she described her daughter as very smart, funny, and perceptive of subtle nuances, she told me that she thought Ellen had problems with emotional immaturity, and that she experienced considerable ups and downs in response to her life stresses, jobs, and relationships. Her mother said that Ellen exhibited a black, negative view of things at times, and said that she wasn't sure whether her daughter had a chemical imbalance or was simply a little spoiled. She told me that she is aware of Ellen's bodily concerns and wondered whether she has OCD.

When I asked Ellen to describe herself, she said she was intense, sensitive, and caring. She said that others saw her as cold, collected, even-keeled, giving, unselfish, very smart, and very together.

I perceived Ellen as a very attractive blonde woman who came across as articulate, warm and friendly, and appropriately concerned with and distressed by the issues that she described in the interview. She was also alert, well oriented, polite, and cooperative, and appeared mature enough to match her stated age. I saw no evidence of hallucinations, delusions, or thought disorder.

Diagnosis and Treatment Plan: Ellen has bipolar II disorder and body dysmorphic disorder. I suggested that she take one-half of a 20 mg tablet of Paxil daily, and at two weeks, she is tolerating this very well except for some dry mouth for which she carries a bottle of water. At this point, Ellen says that she has not yet had any significant response to the drug, but understands that it will take eight to ten weeks of treatment before she does. She told me that she is having difficulty with sustained thinking and concentration, and feels that if she tries to concentrate for too long she ends up looking haggard. This concentration problem is interfering with her ability to learn new material, especially in class. She also told me she harbors a fear that her mind will go blank if she is called on in class and doesn't have a well-prepared script.

I told her that she needs to learn how to deal with her fears of classroom catastrophe—that her mind will go blank or that she will answer a question incorrectly. She needs to desensitize herself to the feeling that if she makes a mistake or gives the wrong answer, something terrible will happen. Ellen also needs to practice speaking spontaneously in a group of people. To help her with this, I suggested attending Toastmasters' meetings or even an acting class. Either of these activities would be especially helpful in light of her tendency to socially isolate herself when she is in new places or situations. I also suggested that she use the techniques she is reading about in Foa's book *Stop Obsessing*.

Ellen also shared several other worries with me, many of them dealing with her need to follow fairly strict routines. One concern is that she might not be able to study enough or to be focused enough to do her homework during regular hours. She also expressed distress that her current logic class, which meets in the early evening, interferes with the ritual routine of her usual dinnertime. If she has to work past the usual hour at her current restaurant job, she is very worried that she might be too late to go for her scheduled workout after the job.

Although Ellen told me that she has spoken to previous therapists about her rituals around food and her ideal weight, she has been reluctant to share very much about her obsessions with body image. When she did work up the courage to discuss body image issues with her most recent therapist, the therapist told Ellen that she must be feeling a great deal of shame. She was very disappointed by the therapist's lack of empathy and understanding. No one actually ever diagnosed Ellen with body dysmorphic disorder or OCD, and no one has treated these illnesses directly.

Ellen said that I was the first person to ask her to read about OCD and body dysmorphic disorder, and that the Medline and articles I had provided her with made her feel very good. She said that giving her these things clearly indicated to her that I wanted to ally with her intelligence in fighting the illness, externalizing it, and making it something she could overcome. I told her that a big part of fighting her illness was arming herself with all the information she could possibly learn.

Conclusion: Sometimes having a clear diagnostic label attached to a problem is, in itself, helpful. In Ellen's case, this labeling provided clarification, and reading about the problem empowered Ellen by allowing her to learn from the experiences of others who share her illness. This educational process provides a way of externalizing the problem, making it something that can be dealt with rather than part of one's personal identity.

Ellen was obviously a very intelligent young woman, yet she was not at all informed about her illness. One of my therapeutic goals was to help her build confidence in her ability to conquer the symptoms and use her mind effectively in classroom situations. Ellen's immediate crisis of self-confidence was whether she could handle being in graduate school. Clearly, her body dysmorphic disorder was also a major problem. Like many people with the "distress of imagined ugliness," she looked like a fashion model. Her mood disorder was relatively mild, and she felt this was a much lower priority, though we discussed the fact that SSRI antidepressant drugs are effective for both OCD and depression. Months after leaving the state to attend graduate school, she wrote me a note telling me how well she was doing in adjusting to her new home and educational program.

John: Obsessive compulsive personality disorder—how it differs from OCD

John is a sixty-nine-year-old married Caucasian male who is currently leading a group whose major purpose is lobbying for social services for the elderly. His commitment to this cause is significant, since he has been caring for his elderly parents for the last ten years.

John told me that his childhood was very chaotic, since his parents had made and lost a great deal of money. He became involved in social welfare reforms in his youth. An Irishman, he was a heavy drinker, which led to a car accident as a young man.

John has never been on psychiatric medications, and he says that he has never had any major illnesses, operations, or hospitalizations, claiming that he has always been in excellent health. He has been married for forty-plus years, and he and his wife appear to get along well. She is very supportive of him and admits that they are both nervous workaholics.

John has always enjoyed being a wine collector, doing gourmet cooking, and giving dinner parties. Although he used to be very social, in his later years he has become a social recluse. He has lost touch with people in his own age group, most of whom are retired, because he finds them boring. John adamantly claims that the leisure pursuits of retirement don't interest him because they are not productive. Instead, he is completely committed to his cause and works seven days a week, sometimes twelve hours a day, in support of it. This gives him a sense of purpose in life. John has been involved with top political leaders in the liberal movement, and he enjoys these people, finding them to be as purposeful and goal oriented as he is.

John says that his obsessive-compulsive traits involve worry about what he is doing—the goals, the strategies, and the details of his work. He never has the intrusive thoughts about themes, such as sex, dirt, germs, aggression, or blasphemy, that would be typical for someone suffering from OCD. John's compulsive behavior is focused around checking for perfection in everything that leaves his desk because his reports are going to be challenged by numerous lawyers. He smokes two packs of cigarettes per day and enjoys it, saying that he has no desire to stop. He does not exercise regularly.

The only family history of emotional illness I was able to uncover was that his daughter has bipolar affective disorder. Her mood swings have been well controlled with lithium, however.

When I ask John to tell me about his personality over the long term, he describes himself as a perfectionist workaholic who is extremely honest and has been very level in his mood and his energy over the long haul.

We reviewed the diagnostic criteria for obsessive-compulsive personality disorder and John agreed that he does seem to have many of the symptoms. He is preoccupied with details and organization, perfectionistic, very conscientious and inflexible about moral and ethical values, a bit stubborn, and somewhat miserly in his spending for himself. In spite of all these things, John says that he enjoys life and his lifestyle and does not wish to make any major changes. He appears very intelligent, quick-witted, and alert. His major complaints are that he would like to be younger and to be able to sleep better.

Diagnosis and Treatment Recommendations: John has no acute psychiatric disorder, but rather a long-term lifestyle diagnosable as obsessive-compulsive personality disorder. I told John that I didn't feel that psychotherapy or long-term medications were indicated for him, but that he might occasionally benefit from sleeping pills when things became stressful and he felt he needed help to sleep.

Conclusions: There is a big difference between John and those patients discussed previously in this chapter who clearly suffer from obsessive-compulsive disorder. Although John does worry a good deal and display rigid, perfectionistic, moralistic, workaholic tendencies, these characteristics are very much a part of how he defines himself and his life's work. They are not symptoms that bother him or his wife, but rather part of who he is as a person. John came for consultation, not because he is bothered by "problems" or wishes to change his lifestyle, but because his daughter asked him to do so. He is functioning well, achieving his goals, and enjoying life, and really needs no medical treatment. This is the key difference between obsessive-compulsive personality disorder, as seen in John, and obsessive-compulsive disorder.

FAMILY ISSUES WITH OCD

How Obsessive-Compulsive Disorder Affects Families

When an individual is suffering from OCD, her behavior and the need for everyone to accommodate themselves to it can create great stress, as well as symptoms in family members that resemble other psychiatric disorders. An example of this dynamic can be seen in families who become very critical of the member who is exhibiting OCD symptoms. For instance, a spouse, sibling, or child may become filled with rage as she observes her loved one's need to engage in "meaningless" rituals before the family can sit down to eat a meal together, leave the house to go to an event, or even go to sleep at night. Soon this rage is turned against the person who engages in these compulsive rituals, and he becomes the butt of family jokes, anger, and torment. When this happens, a vicious circle is set up where this ridicule and criticism lowers the OCD sufferer's self-esteem, which in turn increases his need to ritualize.

Another common occurrence in such situations is that the family begins to assist the person in completing his rituals. Oftentimes, family members will do this simply to "get the rituals over with" so they can get the affected person to eat, leave the house, go to bed, or be more emotionally available. This really does not help the OCD sufferer and, in fact, actually perpetuates the unwanted behavior. By "helping" in this way, family members may be unintentionally encouraging the symptoms.

Whether the symptoms of OCD are spoken about freely or ignored and denied, it is not surprising that either way they remain the focal point of the family. It has been my experience that in some families this behavior is treated as a "white elephant sitting in the living room" that no one talks about. This kind of response is similar to that of families who are in denial that one of their members is alcoholic, and therefore refuse to deal with this fact.

Andrew, Becky, and Jessie: an OCD family

I work with one family in which the mother, Becky, and the father, Jessie, both have OCD, and the thirteen-year-old son, Andrew, is now exhibiting symptoms. Until entering therapy, Andrew had no understanding of his parent's bizarre behavior and, in fact, saw it as normal, although he is often annoyed, embarrassed, and sometimes frightened by it. His parents rarely talk about it even though Becky is receiving treatment specifically for OCD. Jessie remains in such denial about his own problem that he claims to know very little about it, despite the fact that his symptoms are the most severe in the family. In all fairness, Jessie apparently grew up in a family with a parent with untreated OCD. In families where such behaviors are accommodated or never discussed, obsessive-compulsive behavior is perceived as normal. When OCD is passed from one generation to the next, it becomes more difficult to identify these symptoms as a "problem."

As one might guess, it was easy for Jessie to be very critical and angry at his wife for her behavior because she mirrored the very traits that he felt uncomfortable with inside himself. Interestingly enough, Jessie was also often angered by the compulsive behavior displayed by his son, Andrew. As with his own behavior, however, when asked, he would deny that there was anything odd about Andrew's compulsions other than the fact that they annoyed Jessie.

This family situation presented me with a diagnostic dilemma with regard to Andrew. Does he actually have OCD, or is he just accustomed to living in a household with "don't-talk rules"? Do his excessive fears indicate some kind of disorder, or is he fearful because his parents have taught him to be this way? Talking openly about Jessie and Becky's behaviors, challenging the family communication style, working with Becky to recognize that Andrew, too, has a problem that is greatly affecting the family, are all ways of assisting each of the family members to shift their behavior. It is also important to identify how Andrew is receiving secondary benefits from OCD by identifying his family's issues of enmeshment. He needs to work with himself and his parents to help them realize that they have all received their own "secondary gain" by colluding with each other's rituals.

WHEN A FAMILY MEMBER REFUSES TO ADMIT THERE IS A PROBLEM

The question that often arises in family members is what to do when the person with OCD is in denial and refuses to get help, perhaps out of fear of giving up rituals or of medication side effects. The old saying, "You can take a horse to water, but you can't make him drink," truly describes someone who will not admit that he or she suffers from OCD. However, if the horse is exposed to the water often enough, perhaps he will eventually take a drink. He may even find that it tastes mighty good! Sometimes individuals must hit rock bottom before they are willing to finally accept help from family members and mental health professionals. When they do, however, they often find a sense of relief from their fears and compulsions that is very welcome.

Accepting that one has OCD is a process that takes time. An excellent place to start is with family therapy, even if the focus of this therapy is not initially on the person with OCD, but on the family members who are affected by these behaviors. This time can be well used to help the family become educated about this condition. Family members can begin to see how they participate in perpetuating the loved one's illness by understanding what kind of secondary gain is derived from this participation; for example, helping a family member hurry through mealtime rituals so that the whole family can sit down to eat as a unit. Once they understand the dynamics of the situation, family members can begin to *gradually* modify their own behavior so that it is less and less supportive of the loved one's rituals. In this way, they can slowly begin to place subtle pressure to change on the individual with OCD. This alone may be enough to get the "horse to drink the water you have placed before him"; in other words, to get the OCD sufferer to take an active part in his or her therapy.

In some cases, it may even become necessary to refuse to be involved in any way with the loved one's obsessions and compulsions. This means not assisting by checking or avoiding things, not giving reassurance about feared events, and not allowing time for extra checking or hand washing. Following the initial circumstance in which a family member refuses to get involved in the behavior, it is helpful to gently explain that she can no longer live by OCD rules, that it is time to obtain professional help for the entire family. She should also tell the loved one that following OCD rules doesn't help the problems to cease but, in fact, only makes them spiral.

The key here to helping the OCD sufferer is setting limits with empathy. Empathy means understanding how painful it is to be confronted with the information that you have a problem that is hurting others. It also means understanding how it feels to be asked to change a behavior that feels impossible to change. Empathy can be strengthened by observing the pain of the one who is ritualizing, as well as remembering the times in your own life when you were struggling to quit a habit such as drinking coffee, smoking cigarettes, or overeating. Then add to that memory of your own distress the feeling that you will suffer death or impending doom if you actually quit the bad habit. The fear of catastrophe if OCD rituals are abandoned creates such a double bind in the sufferer that he feels as if he will explode if he stops, that the whole world around him will crumble. Anyone who experiences fear and distress on this level is certainly deserving of our compassion.

A final word on getting the person to obtain treatment: It is most helpful if the entire family is included in this process, so that everyone is working as a team to help the affected person in the best way possible. It is also important to view getting the person into therapy as a process and not something that has to happen overnight. The family's goal should be to prime the person for treatment rather than to leave him feeling as if he has suddenly been thrown into the lion's den. Not participating in ritualizing means *gradually* decreasing involvement over time so as not to shock the loved one who has become accustomed to your participation. Remember, the objective is not to abandon the person with OCD, but to support him in changing instead of supporting him in ritualizing.

WHEN THE FAMILY MEMBER AGREES TO ACCEPT HELP

Once the person is ready to accept help for his OCD, it is beneficial for all the family members to become involved with exposure/response prevention training to help them understand the most effective ways to discourage ritualizing. The family can support the sufferer's own behavior therapy by acting as a therapist's assistant. The goal of family therapy should be reducing unwanted behavior over time. Everyone should be taught to recognize the targeted behavior, as well as their own behaviors that precede and follow the ritual. This gives family members more options about how to intervene in the compulsive cycle that they and their loved one have created. It also helps them to identify the signals that tell them when the OCD sufferer is having more difficulty than usual with his or her ritualistic behavior. These signals include the presence of large blocks of unexplained time, repetitive behavior, the need for reassurance, perpetual tardiness, increased concern for details, extreme emotional response to small things, insomnia, a change in eating habits, struggles to just get through the day, or the beginning of avoidance patterns. I then work with the family as a team to identify small areas where each member can make changes to gradually create healthier patterns.

Robert: Modifying rituals surrounding mealtime

Robert is a twenty-five-year old male who was still living at home with his parents. His OCD manifests as his having a great deal of difficulty around mealtime, and he expects his mother to have his meal prepared at exactly 5:30 each evening. She must prepare the exact same food on any given day of the week, and there must be an exact calorie count. She also has to have the food arranged in the exact same manner on the plate each time. In essence, Robert's mother has joined him in his OCD by developing her own ritualized behavior as she painstakingly tries to meet her son's demands.

If this mealtime ritual is not performed properly, Robert becomes obsessed with thoughts that he might die. Now, for his mother to suddenly stop preparing meals in this way would have devastating results. If, however, she learns to identify her behavior and to gradually begin to modify it over a period of time, with Robert's agreement that he would also gradually modify his behavior, this strategy would allow for the most success. It would also be necessary to identify what Robert's father contributes to the situation, whether compliance, criticism, disapproval, or added stress.

Perhaps the family can begin by agreeing that one food a day will be modified during the first week. This change will continue all throughout the second week with the addition of the agreement that the time of the meal will be varied by five or ten minutes each day. These sorts of small variations in the ritual can be adopted until gradually, over time, Robert and his mother are reassured that doom does not occur when one is flexible around dinnertime. Robert's father's role may be working to decrease his negative comments to Robert for causing so much stress in the family, and becoming gradually more supportive of the positive changes that occur as the family members work on their "behavior contract."

It is also likely that the OCD sufferer will be undergoing his own individual treatment involving medication and support for working toward changing his lifestyle patterns. It is important for family members to modify their expectations during time of stress, especially when they are working to make changes in their own behavior. Although everyone needs to be encouraged to work at their own pace, they should understand that they must continue working if they expect to go forward.

The family members need the therapist to supply them with and help create a supportive environment, and family communication needs to be clear and to the point. It is important for a therapist to be sensitive to the feelings of both the family members who are trying to change and the person with OCD. A normal family routine in which the needs of all family members are seen as just as vital as those of the patient is a reasonable goal. Humor is very important to help reduce tension and to remove some of the negativity from the situation. It is critical that the therapist and the entire family support the person with OCD in taking his medication as prescribed, and working on any issues of individuation and enmeshment that may be present.

CHAPTER 4

POST-TRAUMATIC STRESS DISORDER

Post-traumatic stress disorder (PTSD) begins following exposure to a traumatic event with the threat of injury or death, and experiencing a sense of intense fear, helplessness, or horror. It involves persistently reexperiencing the event in recollections or dreams, reliving the event in flashbacks, and a feeling of distress and physiological reaction to cues that are reminders of the event. There is a pattern of persistent avoidance of any reminders of the event and a kind of psychological numbing. The person avoids thoughts, feelings, activities, and memories that make him think of the event and becomes detached, with restricted range of affect and a shortened sense of what the future may bring. There is persistent increased arousal with insomnia, anger, problems with concentration, hypervigilance, and rapid startle response. Post-traumatic stress disorder may be acute with a duration of from one to three months, chronic with a duration of over three months, or delayed onset if it occurs more than six months after the stressful event. Acute stress disorder is the same difficulty; however, the duration of the problem is less than one month. The trauma that causes these disorders may be physical or emotional, may be an isolated event or repeated events, and may be experienced directly or witnessed by the patient.

Epidemiological studies suggest that 1 percent of the United States population has diagnosable PTSD, and 30 to 40 percent of Vietnam veterans suffer from it. The most common comorbidity is drug and alcohol abuse, which makes sense as the person attempts to decrease emotional responsiveness. Other frequent comorbid conditions are dysthymia or chronic depression, major affective disorders including major depression and bipolar affective disorder, obsessive-compulsive disorder, panic, phobia, organicity (difficulty with cognitive functioning in cases where head trauma has occurred), and antisocial personality or criminal behavior.

It is important to remember that there is a wide range of emotional responses to trauma that include rage, grief, a sense of helplessness, a suppression of feelings or detachment from feelings, selective attention, shock, disbelief, minimizing the importance of what happened, deadening feelings, and exhaustion. Later in the course of processing intrusive memories of the trauma arise intense emotions, overarousal, and use of defenses to cope with this overarousal. These defenses include emotional numbing with detachment, isolation, and avoidance of reminders. A fear of dissociation or flashbacks may also be present. Other psychological reactions that sometimes occur include a diminished sense of self-worth, damaged sense of identity, rage, fear, loss of control, blame, guilt, shame, despair, alienation, disconnection, and questioning the meaning of life.

The role of drugs in treating PTSD is controversial and most therapists agree that the primary treatment is through psychotherapy that allows abreaction and catharsis (retelling, reexperiencing, and reprocessing the story and associated feelings), and a sense of cognitive reappraisal of who one is and what life means. Often by doing the psychotherapy in a group of individuals who have shared similar experiences, it becomes possible to break down isolation, denial, self-blame, shame, and inability to forgive oneself. Individual therapy may focus on low self-esteem, negative identity, and fear of loss of control.

Studies of drugs that have been used in treating PTSD have shown that the antidepressants often help depression, intrusive recall symptoms, overarousal symptoms, and, sometimes, the emotional numbing. The antidepressants do not particularly help avoidance behavior. Numerous drugs including tricyclic antidepressants, selective serotonin reuptake inhibitors, and MAO inhibitors have been used and found helpful. It is not uncommon for a person with PTSD to self-medicate with alcohol or street drugs before obtaining treatment. Clearly, substance abuse must be stopped for the antidepressant to have a reasonable chance of having any benefit.

Tommy: Post-traumatic stress disorder with chronic major depression

Tommy is a forty-eight-year-old, twice-married Caucasian male Vietnam veteran referred by Dr. W. for medication evaluation. He is self-employed as a contractor.

Tommy came in with complaints of feeling very depressed and awful, and has repeated memories and flashbacks of his combat experience as a frontline hand-to-hand combat soldier in Vietnam. He was involved in killing people and several of his friends were killed during a major attack.

Tommy recalled that prior to going to Vietnam he was an attractive, smiling, friendly, charming, good-looking person. He indicates that on his return from Vietnam he was a heroin addict and was arrested twice, once for armed robbery and once for grand larceny. He has spent time in prison as well as in a drug rehab program. After his military discharge, he was working as a forklift operator and drinking a great deal. He had a daughter just before ending his relationship with his first wife. Subsequently, he remarried and his second wife, Jeanne, encouraged him to reestablish a relationship with his daughter. He feels guilt for having abandoned his daughter and for his mistrust of his current wife even though she is supportive. He hasn't had sexual relations with her in a very long time and doesn't feel close to her. He indicates that he devotes a great deal of time and attention to their four-year-old son.

His mother's birthday correlates with the date he was almost killed in Vietnam, when a tank fell from rotting trestles, and the anniversary of his admission into a drug and alcohol rehabilitation hospital to begin his five years of clean and sober living. This anniversary date continues to cause distress.

He states that despite being clean and sober, he has depressions, feeling constantly down, has a hard time getting to sleep, startles easily, has mood swings, is isolative, and has a lot of distressing memories of Vietnam.

He returned from Vietnam in 1967 and was honorably discharged with a Purple Heart. He was arrested that year and spent eleven months in jail, went to drug rehab, and then was rearrested and subsequently put on probation. He indicates long-standing problems of not trusting people and being very defensive and always on guard.

Tommy would like to get the horrible memories out of his head, have fewer flashbacks and less depression, and get a good night's sleep. At times of desperation, he plans ways to kill himself.

The Hamilton Depression Rating Scale was useful to assess the severity of Tommy's depression. The patient was given the Seventeen-item Ham-D on which he indicated that he was depressed 100 percent of the time over the last month. He has heard voices telling him to hang himself. He has had suicidal ideas, although he would not do this because of his son. In 1970, however, he did take an overdose of pills and alcohol. He has initial insomnia, taking thirty to forty-five minutes to fall asleep. He wakes up during the night and goes to sit in his office. He wakes up about half an hour before the alarm clock goes off in the morning. He has decreased his actual working time and indicates that a year ago he was working sixty hours a week but now is only working about three hours a day. He is turning down major jobs and only doing small ones. There is no psychomotor agitation or retardation. He is worried about minor things. He indicates he has physical symptoms of irregular heartbeat, shaking, feeling drained, hyperventilating, and headache. He indicates that he has had decreased appetite and has lost 5 or 10 pounds over the last month without trying. He describes his energy as about 25 percent of normal and his sex drive as 0 percent. He made the comment that he is not homosexual. There was no hypochondriasis. Tommy does have insight about his depression. He denied diurnal mood variation. He has very mild depersonalization and suspiciousness and no obsessive-compulsive symptoms.

Diagnostic Impressions: Tommy has major depression, which is chronic, and post-traumatic stress disorder, which is also chronic. He clearly requires multiple treatment approaches. His depression requires aggressive medication trials with a series of antidepressants until something helpful can be found. His profound sense of trauma could only be relieved by psychotherapy, and he was unable to tolerate the confrontive and sometimes uncaring approaches available from the Veterans Administration hospitals, so individual work with us was the treatment of choice. We would have to face his feelings of meaninglessness and thoughts of suicide head-on and teach him to find meaning in life again. Maybe church could help. Certainly his love for his son would be important. His desire to help other veterans in fighting for their entitlements would give additional meaning to his life, as would his search for some of his old friends from combat days. His relationship with his wife seemed supportive, but might not endure. His need for acknowledgment by the government might be aided by being awarded a service-connected disability pension; he surely deserved it, and we would support his getting it.

Conclusions: PTSD is often accompanied by substance abuse in an attempt to self-medicate and numb painful feelings. PTSD is also often accompanied by severe depression. This individual is stuck in the past, repeatedly reliving and unable to let go of the traumas of combat. Multiple antidepressant trials on tricyclics (Elavil, Pamelor, Surmontil), Desyrel, lithium, and high-dose Prozac as well as the MAO inhibitor Nardil have failed to be helpful, although Zoloft and Klonopin offered some slight relief. Reconnecting with old military friends, church, ultimately facing a divorce from his wife and a move cross-country, and surviving a potentially lethal overdose suicide attempt have left him a scarred man, yet one with a sense of hope and purpose for being alive.

He dreams and fantasizes about opening a healing retreat for others like himself who would benefit from a warm, caring, spiritually oriented alternative to the Veterans Administration hospital system. I have encouraged him in following through on the goals and values that give his life purpose and meaning, as he faces depression, flashbacks, and suicidal impulses that are part of his everyday life.

HOW PTSD AFFECTS FAMILIES

I have worked with many families where trauma has played a primary role in altering the family system forever. In some cases, the family was formed around a person who had already experienced the trauma prior to establishing the immediate family; in other cases, the trauma intruded on a family system that was once the picture of health. Traumatic events that affect families include child sexual abuse, physical battery, traffic accidents, miscarriage, war, murder or attempted murder of a family member, rape, life-threatening or deforming illness, observation of a traumatic event, suicide or attempted suicide, growing up in an alcoholic home, and many others. These events are all very real and I have seen them change a family permanently, but family participation in the treatment of the person bearing the symptomatology of PTSD is a strong motivation to heal and leaves these families eventually altered in a positive way. Most such family members I have worked with, about two-thirds of the way through treatment, say, "I would not change what has happened to us; I never would have believed when we began working on this that I could ever say that we are better than we were before the trauma, but here we are communicating and working together better than ever in our lives." Basically, the trauma pushes the family to work on issues that might have otherwise remained submerged, but once addressed allow the family to reach a new level of closeness.

EDUCATION ABOUT PTSD AND ITS EFFECTS

One of the most important aspects in the treatment of post-traumatic stress disorder is educating the person with PTSD as well as the family about the effects created by the trauma. This means learning what PTSD is all about, narrowing down the learning to the particular type of trauma that has occurred, and then further narrowing to understand how both the identified victim and the family are responding. It is important to note that the person who has been identified with PTSD is not usually the only one in the family who has at least some of the symptoms of post-traumatic stress. Heather was an adolescent who had been severely gang-raped and battered by a group of adult men. Her mother, Anna, had an inclination that something was wrong and had been driving around looking for Heather, and in fact, had unknowingly passed the car in which these men had Heather and were deciding whether or not they should kill her. Eventually, they dropped her off at the door of her friend. The next morning, Anna yelled at Heather for being out so late the night before; later in the day she found out Heather was severely injured and was out late because she was held captive by rapists. Anna then rushed Heather to the emergency room where they were further traumatized by being made to wait for hours and then treated like a "number" instead of compassionately. The saga of traumatic events continued. After Anna took Heather home, in her fury, she rushed over to view the scene of the crime which became fixed in her mind; she saw the doorway from which the eyewitness watched yet did not intervene until it was too late, the bed with sheets twisted and torn, and of course, the blood. She also saw the now-empty alcohol bottle they had used to get Heather drunk in order to lure her. This scene of hell never left Anna's mind; neither did the guilt of yelling and blaming the child. As if all this wasn't enough, a trial ensued that resulted in the perpetrators being released with only a "slap on the wrist" by the judge and petty misdemeanor convictions. One trauma led to another trauma and yet to another trauma. This particular saga is a tragic one, but not all are this bleak. I use it to illustrate that any members of the family where PTSD is lurking are at risk because they too have their own trauma. I spend a great deal of time in family therapy teaching people about their own post-traumatic stress as well as that of others in the family so they can begin to make sense of their feelings.

ANGER PLAYS A KEY ROLE IN FAMILY DISRUPTION

Families where trauma has disrupted the usual flow often have a great deal of anger. Anger may be displayed at the victim, who may be perceived as having placed himself in a dangerous situation or as having deserved what happened to him. Rage may also be self-directed, such as when the victim attempts suicide or when a family member feels guilty about not protecting her loved one. Anger also erupts when the victim is perceived as faking or exaggerating his grief, or using it to control other family members or to avoid returning to usual activities such as work, school, or family duties. Rage may also be directed toward the perpetrator of the trauma and, though reasonable and appropriate, may at times get out of hand to the point of assaulting the perpetrator. This, of course, creates a whole new level of trauma to both the family and the victim. It is important that family members talk about their rage and anger on an ongoing basis in a monitored and safe setting, so that it can be used in a productive manner to empower them to take charge over their lives again, rather than becoming a dangerous wedge that destroys the family unit. Trauma can either make a unit stronger or it can erode it very quickly. Unresolved anger and rage are usually the culprits. It is not uncommon to hear of people getting a divorce who do not obtain help or who cannot utilize help in a productive way soon after a major trauma. This is tragic. It is not the trauma that resulted in the divorce; rather, it is the poor communication, lack of understanding about post-traumatic stress, blaming instead of supporting one another, and pure rage that are often the causes.

TRIGGERS

Another very important element of treatment is learning what triggers set off the person with PTSD. By triggers I mean outside events, things that are said by others, smells that remind the victim of the perpetrator, or other stimuli. These may range from the classic example of a car that backfires and startles the person who feels as if she is being shot at again, to seeing a violent movie that leads to a series of nightmares, to a mother who makes a simple statement about her day that sets off a screaming fit in her adolescent child. Heather, mentioned above, went to the county fair and imagined she saw the faces of the perpetrators in every man she passed who was of the correct age group and ethnicity. She was terrified the whole day, but was unable to explain her terror to Anna or even understand it herself. Instead, Heather pestered her mother, poked at her, and made angry outbursts for no apparent reason. Later, in family therapy, it became important for both Anna and Heather to gain clarity about what was happening in the child's mind. This clarity shifted anger on the part of the mother into empathy for the child's suffering. To continue with this example, Heather was fifteen minutes late returning from a date with her friend. She walked in the front door as usual, and Anna went into a fit of rage at Heather for being late. Prior to the trauma, Heather was often fifteen to twenty minutes late and was never questioned. Heather's tardiness triggered the intense feelings Anna had after finding out her daughter had been raped. Anna's rage in turn triggered a sense of low self-esteem and guilt in the child that was symbolic of how the child felt after being raped.

Triggers can appear in other forms as well. A courageous woman, Terri, had been severely stabbed and was easily triggered by stabbings or other assaults that appeared in the news. Hearing of these events in society in the earlier stages of her treatment often led to depression, nightmares, physical complaints, and overeating. Being unable to identify the trigger led to petty arguments with her husband. Once she and her husband were aware of the trigger, other choices existed; they could talk about how she felt after watching the news and work through any feelings that arose, or she could avoid watching the news when she was feeling particularly vulnerable. Ongoing identification of triggers with the entire family creates new options. There are times and cases where avoidance is very key if the person is at particular risk of decompensation or she has not reached a point at which she can tolerate the situation. If family members are not clued in on what to avoid, they will not understand the needs of the affected person. They might even be angry that their family member won't attend certain activities with them if they don't understand what is happening to the individual. Please note: Avoidance is not ideal over the long run, but through therapy, a person can be desensitized to particular triggers, thereby gradually learning to tolerate these events or reminders.

Some triggers cannot be avoided. One woman I worked with had been molested as a child. Her own child was now the age she was at the onset of the molestation. Every time she looked into the eyes of her child, she reexperienced in her mind the entire molestation scene. Obviously, the woman could not avoid her child nor did she want to use avoidance. Identification of this trigger, however, allowed her to talk about her feelings openly with her therapist as well as with trusted friends, which eventually helped to alleviate the child as a trigger. Again, communication is the best bet to identify, reduce, and eventually eliminate triggers.

FAMILY HISTORY IS IMPORTANT

When looking at the family history of someone who has been traumatized, it is not unusual to find that a similar or equally catastrophic trauma has already occurred somewhere in the family tree; it is most always a trauma that has not been resolved by either the initial victim or by other family members. Children (including adult children) often engage in an unconscious repetition compulsion. This means they unconsciously attempt to recreate and then master traumas their parents or significant others have experienced. This is best illustrated in sexual abuse. Martha was molested at age eight by her father. She later married Stan and they had a daughter and a son. When the daughter turned seven and a half, Martha began to recall her own history of sexual abuse. This led to Martha not wanting to engage in sexual activity with her husband as well as Martha becoming terrified that her daughter might be molested. Her fear increased over the next six months; eventually Stan began molesting their daughter. In essence, the mother's worst fear came true. Both these people came into marriage with unresolved trauma. When their separate traumas became intertwined through marriage, they created a setup for the child to have to "work out" the parents' trauma. This may sound far-fetched, but I can't even count the number of times that the trauma reoccurs in the child at the same age it occurred in a parent. It can even skip around generations, and the child is traumatized at the same age as the grandparent. Also, the links between traumas may not be obvious, but they are nevertheless present.

SUBSTANCE ABUSE AND THE ALCOHOLIC FAMILY

We have already mentioned that substance abuse is a common problem with people who have PTSD as they seek to create psychic numbing in order to escape from their pain. The effect on the family is tremendous. The draw for people with PTSD to use substances is an attempt to control their overwhelming flood of emotions. Substances are also used to induce sleep and to reduce nightmares. In actuality, substances are ineffective to decrease arousal. If a person passes out from drinking, she will eventually become conscious and, hence, wake up in the middle of her sleep cycle; nightmares are very likely to occur.

Another example where family history plays a role that may be more recognizable is that of the alcoholic family. Cindy grew up with an alcoholic father and left home at age eighteen due to his abusive behavior. Instead of moving on to a better situation, she married an abusive alcoholic and spent the next five years of marriage trying to get him to stop drinking. This is unconscious repetition compulsion—she recreated the initial trauma so she could try old patterns in hope they would finally prove successful. If she has a child with her drinking spouse, she will be setting up the child to go through the same trauma she did. The key here is to work through a trauma when it occurs whenever possible rather than years later because it will have an effect on your life; it is up to you to make it a positive effect rather than a negative effect.

Sometimes it is not possible to work through trauma immediately. It may have occurred to a child who is not able to obtain outside help until adulthood, help may have been unavailable, or the trauma was felt to have had no lasting effect until one day it resurfaced. But addressing this once the problem is discovered will prevent repetition compulsion in both your life and that of your children. It is important to note that repetition compulsion is largely an unconscious process. I have included it in this section because by identifying these historical traumas of a similar vein, the family is then able to finally heal. The person who had the initial trauma may also be retraumatized when another family member is traumatized, and may have an onset of residual PTSD and require special attention as well. Again, when one member of the family is traumatized, the entire family is traumatized. The entire family can be part of the solution to bring resolution.

CODEPENDENCY

Another common dynamic that was alluded to above, but warrants further discussion, is when one person with post-traumatic stress disorder is attracted to and eventually develops a partnership with another person who has post-traumatic stress. Repetition compulsion is once again activated. One part of this attraction is clearly illustrated above in the description of Cindy. Other aspects of this attraction may be, "If I can't cure myself, I can cure someone else," and the dynamics of codependency. I found these aspects and others when working with partners of Vietnam vets who presented with PTSD; many of these wives had at least symptoms of post-traumatic stress from childhood or a previous marriage. Common histories for these wives included child sexual abuse, children of alcoholic parents, women battered in previous marriages, and women who were raped as adults. It was up to these women to work on their own issues in order to be most effective in helping their husbands. Many of these wives exemplified codependency as they were the sole breadwinners, walking on eggshells to avoid setting off any triggers in their husbands, and catering to the husband's every need with little regard for their own needs. Codependency can be a way of avoiding dealing with one's own issues. In fact, it can make one feel like she has no problems at all except for supporting her husband and coping with his issues. This enhances the spouse's symptomatology. In other words, if your wife doesn't expect you to get better, you won't be motivated to do so. I have discussed this concept of secondary gain in detail in the chapter on panic disorder. Family therapy as well as group therapy can be very effective in helping a partner gradually remove herself from the role of caretaker to that of an equal partner. When someone is considered an equal, he is inclined to work to operate in that manner.

PTSD is a family issue and needs to be treated as such in order to bring about full healing. Including the family in treatment decreases the person's isolation, allows greater understanding of the trauma and triggers that enhance the trauma, allows the opportunity for all family members to work through their own traumas, and helps to identify repetition compulsion. This path can turn victims into survivors, and survivors into people who are healed and able to conduct life without negative constraints.

CHAPTER 5

GENERALIZED ANXIETY DISORDER

■ **DRUGS DISCUSSED:**
BuSpar, Librium, Valium, Xanax, Ativan, Klonopin

This disorder is characterized by excessive anxiety and worry which are present most days for at least six months, with a key feature of uncontrolled worry. In addition, the person will typically feel restless, keyed up, and fatigued; have difficulty concentrating; and demonstrate irritability, muscle tension, and insomnia. These symptoms cause distress or impairment and typically these symptoms may be differentiated from panic disorder, social phobia, and OCD by their very gradual, insidious onset, the focus on very chronic worry about things that could happen in everyday life, and the lack of acute episodes coming "out of the blue."

Some psychiatrists consider generalized anxiety disorder rare or hard to find for clinical studies and look at it as a kind of "wastebasket diagnosis" for anxious patients who don't have OCD or panic attacks. Often, very chronic worriers present with multiple somatic complaints to the family primary care physician.

BENZODIAZEPINE

The most traditional standard treatment for generalized anxiety disorder is use of benzodiazepine antianxiety drugs such as Librium, Valium, Ativan, or Xanax. These drugs share a wide spectrum of activity including cutting anxiety, helping a person to relax and fall asleep, and having some anticonvulsant activity when used in the context of drug withdrawal; they have muscle-relaxant properties and also share cross tolerance with alcohol, so they are frequently used as part of the detoxification process for alcoholics. The side effects of these antianxiety drugs include sedation, so some people will report that their anxiety is lessened while others will feel sleepy or tired all day while taking them. The drugs can induce incoordination and, in elderly people, this may involve a risk of falling. The drugs also slow reflexes. Some of the high-potency benzodiazepines such as Xanax, Ativan, and Halcion can cause learning or memory impairment (called anterograde amnesia). This means that things learned shortly after taking a dose of the drug do not get put into long-term memory. This can be a great advantage for the anesthesiologist who gives this drug preoperatively and finds that the patient does not remember going to the operating room. Amnesia can be a great disadvantage for the individual who receives important phone calls during the night that require decision-making skills; the person cannot remember these calls the next morning. Rarely, people will become confused while taking minor tranquilizers, and tests show that reaction time, vigilance, and performance on speed-sensitive tests are the most significantly affected by these drugs. These functions are critically important to driving an automobile. There is substantially greater impairment when benzodiazepines are combined with alcohol, so this is a potentially deadly combination for the automobile driver. A person taking a benzodiazepine minor tranquilizer should never drink and drive. An occasional drink taken when the person won't be driving is acceptable.

There are some difficult patients that psychiatrists see who have borderline personality disorder and among these are individuals who have repeated self-injurious behavior, such as superficially cutting on their arms or burning themselves. These patients often receive prescriptions from their physicians for tranquilizers such as Xanax because they seem so anxious and overwhelmed, but this is usually not a good idea. Although they have a mixture of chronic anxiety and depression, they are far more at risk for impulsive self-injury than an individual with generalized anxiety disorder. One study has shown that Xanax (alprazolam) caused disinhibition, so these patients performed more self-injurious behavior while taking the antianxiety drug. This behavioral disinhibition is akin to the disinhibition from getting drunk.

Benzodiazepine minor tranquilizers are best classified by their half-life and their potency. Half-life is the time it takes, during the drug elimination phase, for the blood level to fall by half. It is a measure of how long it takes the body to "get rid of" half of the drug present after a single dose is taken. Potency is the strength of the drug, as measured by how many milligrams are typically given per day to an average patient. A drug with an average dose of about 2 to 5 mg/day (such as Xanax) is more potent than a drug with an average dose of 20 to 40 mg/day (such as Valium).

Half-life is a function of whether there are active metabolites of the drug and how long the body takes to excrete them. Long–half-life drugs are characterized by dosing once a day, gradual buildup of steady-state blood levels, and a gradual tapering out of the blood when the drug is discontinued. Long–half-life drugs typically have active metabolites, and the low-potency ones require a relatively large milligram dose on a daily basis. Long–half-life drugs with active metabolites include Valium, Librium, and Tranxene. The long-acting high-potency drug on the market is Klonopin (clonazepam), which is officially FDA approved as an anticonvulsant but widely used in treatment of panic disorder and mania.

The short-acting benzodiazepines have no active metabolites and typically have a half-life of five to fifteen hours, and so require multiple daily dosing. The low-potency, short-acting drug is Serax and the high-potency, short-acting drugs include Ativan, Xanax, and the sleeping pill Halcion.

BUSPAR

The alternative drug for treating generalized anxiety disorder is BuSpar (buspirone). When BuSpar came on the market, some doctors said that it caused no sedation, no psychomotor effects on coordination, no dependence or withdrawal problems, no muscle-relaxant effects, no anticonvulsant effects, no risk of abuse, no rebound anxiety, no behavioral disinhibition, no alcohol interaction, and, many psychiatrists would jokingly add, no effectiveness. Formal studies actually demonstrated the drug was as effective as the benzodiazepine minor tranquilizers such as Valium for patients who had generalized anxiety disorder. What was not recognized initially was that the complete lack of cross-reactivity between this drug and the benzodiazepine minor tranquilizers meant that a patient who was taking a minor tranquilizer such as Xanax and was switched to BuSpar would have very significant withdrawal anxiety from going off the minor tranquilizer that BuSpar would not prevent or relieve. As a result, BuSpar was incorrectly considered ineffective for anxiety because it did not prevent withdrawal from the minor tranquilizer and because an individual dose of BuSpar had very little subjective effect.

As we learned more about using this drug, it appeared that it is very effective for the cognitive, psychological, and ruminative symptoms of chronic anxiety (perhaps more so than the physical symptoms), but the drug takes two to four weeks to be effective and has to be used two or three times daily. It is an excellent drug to use in patients who have a history of substance abuse and a high risk of abusing (or addiction to) minor tranquilizers. The side effects of BuSpar include nausea, dizziness, and headache, and the average dose in treating generalized anxiety disorder is about 30 to 60 mg daily, divided into two or three doses per day.

Two very important considerations with BuSpar are that it does not work to eliminate panic attacks and that it does not work on a single dose as-needed basis. These factors make it very different from the benzodiazepine antianxiety drugs. It clearly takes a few weeks to become effective and its onset of effect is gradual and subtle.

Lea: Generalized anxiety disorder with occasional panic attacks

Lea is a bright, forty-five-year-old, divorced woman who completed law school thirteen years ago. Just prior to attempting the state bar exam to be allowed to practice law, she was informed that her husband planned to divorce her. During the lengthy divorce, she failed the exam several times because her extreme anxiety made it impossible to concentrate and do the analysis and writing required to demonstrate her knowledge.

During this time, she moved up to become the first female executive and the only woman involved as a director at her company. She felt distressed about working for a tobacco company because she is much more interested in liberal causes, such as health care for poor people.

Lea has chronic worries. She tries to get places exactly on time and she is worried about whether people will like her. She worries that the bumps on her skin might be cancer or that cardiac symptoms might mean that she is having a heart attack.

Lea describes herself as a warm, caring, honest, bleeding-heart liberal; says "my word is my bond" and "you can count on me—I always come through." She describes herself as introspective. She loves to read, bake, make presents for people, and cook for friends.

Lea indicated she wanted medicine that would cut anxiety when she faced exams but didn't want something that would change who she is. She wanted to stop the chronic worrying.

Her panic attacks are classic but quite infrequent. She feels she can't get enough air and will suffocate, feels claustrophobic, and feels the walls and ceilings closing in on her. She has a feeling that she is going to die. Her whole body is in crisis and on "red alert." She has overwhelming fear, feels faint, and feels she'll disintegrate. These attacks have occurred in an airplane twice, in a conference room at work, and at the library.

Diagnostic and Treatment Plan: Lea has generalized anxiety disorder with occasional panic attacks. I believe she suffers from fairly chronic anxiety with exacerbation under stress of taking the bar exam or traveling in an airplane, or in a work situation that involves conflict. She doesn't meet the full frequency criteria for panic disorder because her attacks are quite rare. She is reluctant to take medication every day. I suggested to her that a trial on BuSpar or imipramine might be very helpful for the chronic anxiety, however. I gave her a prescription for BuSpar.

A year later, Lea has been on BuSpar 20 mg/day long term. She had one more failed attempt, then finally called to share the good news that she'd passed the state bar.

In just six months, I was happy to receive a call from Lea's therapist telling me that Lea is now engaged and working as a law clerk for a federal judge.

Conclusion: Lea's panic attacks were very rare and her chronic anxiety was drastically increased by the stress of taking a major examination. While using the BuSpar she was able to confront her fiancé assertively on issues of emotional growth, commitment, and intimacy, and was able to study hard and finally pass the examination that would allow her to practice law. I have had other patients who have used BuSpar to cut chronic anxiety prior to taking a major test, and they have appreciated the lack of sedation or memory problems while on it.

Linda: Generalized anxiety disorder

Linda is a forty-seven-year-old female attorney in her first marriage. She is living with her three-year-old child and her husband.

Linda states she was normal until age forty-four, at which time she had a baby after the fifth *in vitro* fertilization attempt.

She subsequently had severe anxiety and medication intolerance.

Prior to age forty-four, Linda had never had any psychiatric treatment, taken any psychiatric medications, or experienced any persistent anxiety or depression. The pregnancy went very well. The labor also went well until she was given droperidol for nausea; then she felt very dizzy and as if she were going to crawl out of her skin. The baby was healthy and is an easy child. She took six weeks off work after having the child. This was a stressful time because she was preparing to go in and argue her first case in front of the California Supreme Court, her house-remodeling project was still in progress, and she had the new baby. She slept poorly, felt tired and overwhelmed, and she also found that her work schedule was no longer loose and free because of the need to take care of her baby.

She consulted a psychologist who encouraged her to work out day-care arrangements. She was able to find an excellent part-time nanny who gets along well with her three-year-old son.

During this stressful time, her internist prescribed Ativan, which she used off and on for about a year. She found that about one to two days after taking a dose she would overreact emotionally. She was taking about ½ mg at bedtime to get to sleep. She went off Ativan gradually with no problem, and for six months felt recovered and happy with no medication.

Later, when symptoms returned, a psychiatrist prescribed Anafranil based on the fact that her brother had OCD; Linda was sure she didn't have OCD and was drowsy and perhaps had a panic attack on it. She next tried Prozac and had agitation on 20 mg/day. With lower doses, she was getting a positive response, feeling happy, and sleeping longer, but had some agitation and then stopped taking it. It was unclear during the time of taking Prozac at reduced dose, about 10 mg every four days, whether her anxiety was due to the Prozac or due to the underlying illness. Nonetheless, at that time she was sleeping longer and feeling happier.

She tried Klonopin, which worked to curtail anxiety but did not completely eliminate it. She took BuSpar at a dose of 20 mg/day and this seemed to work fairly well to decrease anxiety. She felt fine at 20 mg/day but at 35 mg/day she felt very "crazy." She had an episode after ten weeks on BuSpar when she was also taking penicillin and developed hives, and three days later developed what she thought was a BuSpar reaction with her head, chest, and neck all feeling tight. In retrospect, she doesn't really know if this was due to the BuSpar or to a penicillin allergic reaction.

She tried the beta-blockers (to stop the physical symptoms of anxiety) Inderal and Corgard and they did nothing to help her anxiety and caused trouble breathing if she exercised. She then switched to working with another psychiatrist and tried Zoloft 50 mg for two or three days only and took this along with 0.75 mg Klonopin; she slept a full night but felt extremely nervous in the morning. She tried Paxil 20 mg/day for only two days along with 0.75 mg Klonopin and slept through the night but woke experiencing extreme agitation. She took Sinequan 25 mg at night and felt very drowsy the next morning. She took Tofranil recently, 10 mg/day for one week and then 20 mg for three days and then 30 mg, and was unsure if this caused some nervousness. Thus, many of her medication trials had been too brief to get a therapeutic response and often limited due to side effects.

Linda came to me giving the above history and was clearly frustrated with past treatment attempts, stating clearly that she is not depressed but is enthusiastic for life and projects, yet her concentration is impaired by anxiety. Her feelings vary throughout the day. In the morning she feels nervous with her stomach turning, is shaky, and unable to relax. She states that she used to be able to relax, read the newspaper, enjoy her yard, feel a sense of fulfillment and calmness, and feel glad to be alive, but these things are missing now. She states these good times do come back momentarily; for example, when she is on a trip with her husband. She appreciates having a good marriage and financial security.

Generalized anxiety disorder criteria were reviewed with her and it is clear she has long-standing anxiety. She has a feeling of being "keyed up," a problem concentrating, muscle tension, and sleep disturbance.

Linda described herself as independent, having friends but being somewhat of a loner, and enjoying doing things by herself, yet being outgoing, assertive, and determined. Her husband is more sociable and she enjoys more time alone.

At the time I met her, she was taking Klonopin averaging about 2.5 mg/day.

Diagnostic and Treatment Plan: Linda has generalized anxiety disorder.

I suggested that she use the Klonopin as a relatively short-term medication while waiting for the BuSpar to become effective, and that she resume BuSpar and work her way up to 20 mg daily in divided doses (half in the morning and half at night) over the next week or so. I suggested that she take steady, level doses of Klonopin at the lowest effective dose for her and that she plan on tapering off of this medication over the next few months.

Conclusion: A half-year went by and we could see that Linda's stormy period of medication trials was not finished. Often a patient who is very sensitive to medication side effects requires several medication trials to find just the right combination to be effective without intolerable side effects. She had been unable to taper off of Klonopin, felt oversedated on Serzone, had started Effexor and gradually worked her way up to 168 mg/day, with Klonopin now at 2.75 mg/day. She is doing well, is looking forward to a vacation in Northern California and going to a family reunion this summer, and is working hard. She's feeling Effexor is a miracle drug for her anxiety and depression and has come to accept that she'll be on Klonopin for quite awhile longer. She attributes her improvement to finding the right medication combination and settling in to acceptance of taking medications rather than trying to taper off of them.

OTHER ANXIETY DISORDERS

The *DSM-IV* includes other diagnoses such as anxiety due to a general medical disorder or substance-induced anxiety disorder. These are best treated by dealing with the underlying medical or substance use problem.

DRUGS TO AVOID WHEN TREATING ANXIETY DISORDERS

There are some drugs that will lower anxiety, but their use is simply not justifiable because of their side effects. The typical antipsychotic drugs such as Haldol and Stelazine fall into this category because of the risks of tardive dyskinesia (abnormal involuntary movements) and neuroleptic malignant syndrome (very high fever), and the subjective response of feeling like a "zombie" while taking them. The barbiturates and meprobamate (Miltown) are obsolete in the treatment of anxiety because of the risks of severe withdrawal reactions and of death from overdose. The antihistamines may have some role as sleeping pills (especially in those who have abused alcohol or other substances and want to stay away from habit-forming drugs), but again the side effects tend to outweigh therapeutic effects for most people.

CHAPTER **6**

INSOMNIA AND MINOR TRANQUILIZERS

■ *Drugs discussed:*
Halcion, Restoril, Dalmane, Sonata, Ambien, Doral, Xanax, Ativan, Valium, Librium, Desyrel (trazodone)

Insomnia is divided diagnostically into three general categories. The first category is acute stress-related insomnia. This usually occurs in the context of traveling across time zones or in the face of a major situational upset such as a move or loss of a relationship. In acute situational insomnia, it is quite reasonable to expect that use of a sleeping pill for a week or two will be beneficial and very effective.

The second category is insomnia due to another psychiatric disorder, such as a mood disorder (mania or depression), anxiety disorder, or psychotic disorder (such as schizophrenia). This type of insomnia is best treated by treating the underlying psychiatric disorder. Sometimes a sleeping pill will be helpful short term while waiting for the antidepressant, anxiolytic, mood stabilizer, or antipsychotic drug to start working.

The third category is more debilitating. Chronic insomnia may be related to a true sleep disorder or sleep phase disturbance. Major sleep disorders include sleep apnea, in which there is often heavy snoring, obesity, older age, hypertension, and, most important, periods in which breathing stops during sleep and the person awakens with a gasp several times during the night. Other important sleep disorders include periodic leg movements in which the sleeper is described as running or kicking in his sleep. The rapid eye movement (REM) sleep disorders can include sudden motor activity of a violent nature, and this has been described in patients with post-traumatic stress disorder. Other individuals with chronic insomnia have a circadian rhythm disturbance in which they can sleep and awaken rested but are not on the same sleep-wake schedules as others in the household. People who are retired or on vacation often stay up later than usual, sleep late into the morning, take a nap, and don't usually consider this a problem until they need to conform to the schedule of others who work "regular" job hours of 9 A.M. to 5 P.M.

Because of the wide variety of potential causes of chronic insomnia, it is well worth considering behavioral approaches and a sleep laboratory evaluation in anyone who reports months or years of sleep problems. The behavioral approaches to chronic insomnia involve a program of good sleep hygiene. This means control of distractions and annoyances at night that might interfere with relaxing. Furthermore, it is necessary to eliminate naps, caffeine in the afternoon or evening, and alcoholic beverages. Alcohol can help a person get to sleep but then cause waking up as the alcohol effect goes away over an hour or two. Often, circadian (twenty-four-hour clock) rhythm disturbances are treated by changing the sleep-wake times. Bright artificial light or exposure to sunshine may be used in the early mornings as a way of cueing the body to the appropriate wake-up time. Relaxation training may help in getting to sleep. Exercise that is done in the morning or afternoon may help to produce a normal sense of tiredness in the evening. Going to bed and getting up at the same time each day, including weekends, can lead to more normalized sleep-wake rhythm. Using the bedroom for sleep and sexual activities and not for work, study, and arguments can help to avoid an association of the bedroom with stressful activities.

There are many different classes of sleeping pills. The over-the-counter ones are mostly anticholinergic (causing dry mouth and blurred vision and sometimes memory impairment) or antihistamines. The prescription sleeping pills are in the benzodiazepine minor tranquilizer family. They differ from the minor tranquilizers discussed earlier more in how they are marketed than by what they do to the brain. Phillip Janicak, a renowned psychopharmacologist, has commented on benzodiazepine hypnotics, saying that "careful, time-limited, intermittent prescribing is the only reasonable management strategy." It is indeed far too common to see patients who have been taking sleeping pills for months or even years who present saying that they cannot sleep without them, yet they don't really work very well. All this really means is that they have rebound insomnia as part of their withdrawal syndrome and dependency if they don't take the drug. Most of these drugs are recommended for use for only two to four weeks. There have been no real studies of sleeping pills that have gone past three months and even that is considered an extremely long time to take these drugs.

Drug half-life is an important concept. After a drug is first taken and distributed to the body tissues, its blood level falls from a near-maximal level toward none over a period of time. The time required for the level to drop by half is called the half-life. Drugs with a half-life of a few hours have a short duration of action, while those with a half-life of a few days have a long duration of action and the risk of accumulation if the drug is taken every day.

The long half-life sleeping pills include Dalmane (flurazepam) and Doral. These drugs have a half-life for elimination from the body of approximately two to four days. This has several implications. The first is that the drug is present in very substantial quantities the day after it is taken; this may lead to daytime sedation or interactions with alcohol if the person drinks. The second is accumulation of the drug in the body with repeated use, with subsequent risk of toxic side effects such as confusion or incoordination. Elderly persons are especially at risk for accumulation of the drug because they tend to metabolize drugs more slowly. Long half-life also means that if the drug is taken long term and abruptly stopped, it leaves the body very gradually and so there is less risk of rebound insomnia and severe withdrawal symptoms.

Restoril (temazepam) has a half-life of approximately seven to eight hours; this appears to be a very reasonable time for a sleep medication. Halcion (triazolam) has a half-life of two or three hours. This makes this drug particularly useful in initiating sleep in those who have a hard time falling asleep, such as travelers who have crossed several time zones. Unfortunately, when the drug wears off, chronic users sometimes find themselves waking up in the middle of the night and needing to take a second or even a third dose in order to sleep until morning. Halcion has been associated with behavioral problems including confusion, psychoticlike behavior, disinhibition, amnesia, and drug-induced hostility. For these reasons, it is especially important to limit the dose to the FDA-recommended maximum of 0.25 mg per night in adults and only half of this in geriatric patients. Rare side effects of Halcion include blistering, sore throat and tongue, vasculitis, asthma, and facial edema.

Ambien (zoldipam) has a half-life of two and a half hours and a total duration of action of about six hours, while Sonata has a one-hour half-life and a duration of action of about three hours. Sonata is the only sleeping pill approved for use in the middle of the night or early morning.

The need for repeated large doses of Halcion or other sleeping pills to sleep through the night is a clear warning that the drug has caused tolerance and should be discontinued. The usual remedy for this tolerance is using a longer half-life drug for a taper in addition to behavioral relaxation techniques. The question often arises as to how to treat the chronic insomniac who refuses to get a sleep lab evaluation or who lacks adequate insurance coverage to provide this. Many psychiatrists now favor the use of a low dose of very sedating antidepressants as chronic sleeping pills because of their lack of addiction risk. Commonly used drugs are Desyrel (trazodone) 50 to 100 mg, Sinequan (doxepin) 25 to 50 mg, or Elavil (amitriptyline) 25 to 50 mg at night. Some individuals find these medications very helpful. Substantially higher doses are safe and quite commonly used in the treatment of depression. Some people will try these medications and feel particularly drugged or report a tremendous hangover the following morning. For them, these antidepressants are intolerable as sleeping pills. Fortunately, most people tolerate low doses quite well.

Keith: Insomnia and depression (not otherwise specified)

Keith is a thirty-seven-year-old, single male who works as an academic advisor at a local school. He has a master's degree in educational counseling and is currently a Ph.D. student. He has been in therapy for personal growth and relationship issues. He sought treatment complaining that he has periods of a couple of weeks of severe insomnia in the context of a family history of depression.

Family History: Keith's mother has had depression but has never been manic. She was treated with ECT when Keith was a child and has also been on unknown antidepressants in the past. His brother, who had severe depression but was never manic, did not do well on psychiatric drugs and committed suicide five or six years ago after several psychiatric hospitalizations and failed trials on medications.

Keith told me that when he experiences severe depression he has initial insomnia with difficulty getting to sleep before 4:00 or 5:00 A.M. He sleeps for only two or three hours and then wakes up to go to work. He starts work at a variable hour between 8:00 and 11:00 A.M. He does not take daytime naps. His energy, sex drive, concentration, and decision-making abilities all remain the same and he is still able to enjoy things. His mood is about the same. His interest in doing things decreases. He feels less motivated. He is irritable, anxious, and has some palpitations, and very recently has had some panic symptoms. He denies feeling suicidal.

Keith denies any history of spontaneous depressions lasting more than two weeks or any depressions that were incapacitating relative to school or work. He emphasized that these episodes of insomnia are commonly stress related. They typically last a couple of weeks and had their onset about two years ago, although there is one episode that he can recall having had as an undergraduate in college.

He has benefited from aspirin, antihistamines, L-tryptophan (which is no longer available), Sinequan, and Doral.

Diagnosis and Treatment Plan: Keith has a significant family history of depression, but does not meet the criteria for major depression. He appears to have insomnia and depression not otherwise specified with no personality disorder, medical cause, or significant stressor. ("Not otherwise specified" is a *DSM-IV* term for a disorder that does not meet full classical criteria.) I prescribed trazodone, a nonaddicting sleep medication.

When I saw him two years later, Keith told me that he had done well on trazodone prescribed by his family doctor. A lot had happened. He had gotten married recently, had sold his home and moved to Chino, and had cut back to part-time on his job hours. He was about to begin writing his Ph.D. dissertation. He has had occasional mild irritability, some tiredness, and decreased sexual interest. He states that his appetite and energy are good and he is able to enjoy activities. He has no side effects on the trazodone. He indicates he continues to feel that insomnia is his main problem and still questions why this is ongoing. In light of his family history of mood disorder and his chronic insomnia, I believe the long-term use of trazodone at low dose has demonstrated that it is both beneficial and very well tolerated; therefore, we decided to continue this medication.

A couple of years later he had an evaluation in a local sleep disorder clinic which noted that he had sleep-onset insomnia beginning five years earlier after the stress of receiving a poor grade, with three hours of initial insomnia. Suspicion was psychological dependence on medication with low level of tolerance for insomnia. He was given stimulus control instructions; asked to limit caffeine, increase exercise, and allow wind-down time in the evening; and given a relaxation tape. Over the next few months he continued to do well after tapering off the medication, and was pleased to have completed his Ph.D.

Conclusion: In this case, there were hints of depression coupled with the strong family history. There also was a fairly chronic insomnia that returned whenever the trazodone was discontinued. Because of this, the use of the low-dose antidepressant was far more beneficial than any sleeping pill would have been. There was no addiction, no tolerance or loss of effectiveness with chronic use, and no concerns that he might overuse the medication. When he finally completed his Ph.D., he was ready to taper off the medication using a behavioral strategy.

FAMILY ISSUES WITH INSOMNIA

Impairment in Relationships

Insomnia often accompanies other psychiatric disorders, yet has some distinct characteristics of its own that it brings to families. Insomnia can lead to impairment in families and relationships. First, the person may be less accessible to family members and less available for family activities if he is irritable due to lack of sleep. He may be rendered unable to function at work in a productive manner, thereby unable to maintain a family income. His energy, concentration, and decision-making abilities may be impaired, leaving a great deal of responsibility for the family on the spouse or even the children in some circumstances. The insomniac may not be safe to drive at times, making her often unable to help out with errands and transportation, which of course can lead to anger and resentment. The person with insomnia may also detach from parental responsibilities, causing a variety of ramifications on both the spouse and children.

In addition, marital discord may erupt when insomnia continues over a prolonged period of time. The person may have a lower sex drive or may use sleep disturbance as an excuse to withdraw from sexual contact. Also, sleep patterns in which people have different sleep cycles tend to cause couples to miss opportunities for sexual contact, affection, and visiting time. Indeed, this can be caused by outside forces, such as when individuals in the couple work opposing shifts or when a child who has nightmares or has insomnia herself is allowed to sleep with the parents, thus creating insomnia in one or both parents. A child I know requires a great deal of attention from her parents at bedtime. They are often awakened in the middle of the night, with the child requesting interaction since she can't sleep. An expectation of the child to awaken them leads to disrupted sleep for the parents as well. This can play havoc on the intimate aspects of a marital relationship. It can also be a matter of each partner having a different internal sleep clock; this leads to the question as to whether this is a real difference or if this is imagined as a way of avoiding intimacy. Furthermore, insomnia can lead to the affected person feeling inadequate, insecure, and dependent. A declining self-image can gradually erode any relationship.

FAMILY DYNAMICS

It is important to address some of the dynamics that can be created in a family where insomnia plays a key role in creating family problems. Secondary gain arises when someone in the family derives benefit from another family member being sick. Hence, both family members and the person with insomnia are unconsciously gratified by the problem. Secondary gain may also arise when the ill family member is relieved of certain undesirable tasks due to the insomnia. This can be difficult to pinpoint when you are a participant and may require an outside observer. A clue that secondary gain may be a culprit is when you find yourself beginning to feel particularly angry at the person who seemingly cannot help his illness, when the family is most often focused on the illness instead of sharing concern around equally to all family members, and when the family accepts the ill person's excuses and rationalizations for avoiding responsibilities. Other clues are when family members may not expect the patient to get well or may not genuinely desire improvement, since they may unconsciously prefer the patient to be uninvolved in family activities or to have less power in family decision making.

A double bind is created when family members want the patient to get well, but at the same time expect the patient to remain ill. Double binds are difficult to break and lead to confusion that results in the patient becoming even more ill. These dynamics that get set in motion in families are noteworthy because identification of them can lead to a healthier-functioning family as well as to added relief for the person with insomnia. Secondary gain issues for all members of the family can be resolved if they are identified and worked through.

Good sleep hygiene is very important to a satisfying and restful sleep life. It is best if the bedroom becomes a place of peace and relaxation and not the scene of family fights, resentment about missed sex, or a place of work. It is best to avoid alcohol or caffeine in the evening. Regular bedtime and time of awakening should be employed even on weekends and vacations. Naps should be avoided. For children, a system of rewards can be utilized to encourage sleeping through the night.

In short, when one person in the family is ill, it affects all members of the family. The entire family must be willing to look at its own participation in keeping the family member ill, habits, and underlying issues that keep the patient locked into his symptoms. Just as all members may unknowingly participate in the problem, they can learn to be a part of the solution.

BENZODIAZEPINE TREATMENT ISSUES

Because benzodiazepine tranquilizers and sleeping pills are often prescribed by physicians of many different specialties, it is important to include a special note about them. These drugs generate a great deal of controversy concerning their appropriate use versus abuse.

The benzodiazepine antianxiety drugs all work quite nicely for generalized anxiety disorder, although now we have BuSpar as a very good alternative. Benzodiazepine tranquilizers are not effective for the anxiety experienced in obsessive-compulsive disorder, and they may not be particularly helpful in post-traumatic stress disorder other than as short-term sleeping pills. The high-potency benzodiazepines, including Xanax and Klonopin, are clearly effective in panic disorder and probably also quite effective in social phobia. Ativan (oral or injectable) and Klonopin are sometimes used to help calm down people in the manic phase of bipolar affective disorder and get them to sleep early in treatment, before the mood stabilizers have had a chance to work effectively.

Risk Factors

The benzodiazepines clearly have associated problems that must be balanced against their benefits.

The principal problem of these drugs is rebound or withdrawal symptoms. For example, a person taking Xanax may report feeling hints of anxiety increasing and a strange, uneasy feeling six or eight hours after the last dose of medication. This kind of mini-withdrawal is similar to what cigarette smokers and alcoholics experience as drug craving when the drug gets out of the system. Individuals who take benzodiazepines long term and then stop them may have numerous withdrawal symptoms, including return of the original anxiety or even intensification beyond the original level of symptoms. Often, withdrawal involves insomnia, irritability, headaches, muscle aches, flulike symptoms, sensitivity to noise, loss of appetite or weight loss, poor concentration, strange feelings, oversensitivity to light and wanting to be in a dark room, oversensitivity to smell, ringing or buzzing in the ears, upset stomach, sweating, restlessness, and depersonalization. Sometimes these symptoms progress to a full-blown delirium with extreme confusion, hallucinations, and seizures. Along the way, involuntary muscle movements and feelings of panic and depression are common. Seizures may occur as part of benzodiazepine withdrawal and the highest incidence of seizures, according to FDA reports, has been with the use of the short-acting drugs Xanax and Ativan.

Other risk factors for seizures are history of seizures and using other drugs that can lower the seizure threshold such as alcohol and theophylline (for asthma) or antipsychotics. The abuse of cocaine can also cause seizures. High doses of the tranquilizers taken regularly for more than four months and abruptly discontinued lead to the highest risk of seizures, however.

The incidence of minor tranquilizer withdrawal symptoms is fairly low with use for only a month or two, but at four to twelve months of the standard dose of a tranquilizer, about 5 to 10 percent of patients will have some withdrawal symptoms. When the drugs are used for more than a year on a regular basis, 43 to 57 percent of patients will experience withdrawal symptoms. The two approaches to dealing with this are prevention (by using the drugs on a time-limited basis for only a month or two during extreme stresses), or if the drugs have been used long term, to taper them off very gradually over a period of one to four months. It is frequently reported that there is a plateau when the original dose has been cut down by about 50 percent after a few weeks, and it can be very difficult to lower the dose beyond this plateau. Patience is required in maintaining this level for a few weeks or a month before reattempting the gradual tapering off.

Approximately 1.6 percent of the adult population in this country uses benzodiazepine tranquilizers regularly for more than one year. Often these individuals have multiple medical problems including cardiovascular, musculoskeletal, and psychiatric difficulties.

Sometimes the medical benefit of these drugs more than outweighs the side-effect and withdrawal risks and there may not be any urgent reason for discontinuing these drugs. If they are to be discontinued, these drugs should always be tapered gently and slowly over a few weeks to months to minimize the risks of withdrawal symptoms. The American Psychiatric Association (APA) task force on benzodiazepines recommends individualizing the decision about their long-term use based on the disability caused by the anxiety, severity of illness, quality of the treatment response, and the drug's ability to normalize the person's life. The APA does acknowledge that panic disorder is a justification for long-term treatment with benzodiazepine tranquilizers.

Martin: Benzodiazepine abuse leads to severe consequences

Martin is a thirty-nine-year-old man who repairs dry cleaning plants. He has had two stormy marriages and complains that he "lives life in the fast lane" with symptoms of insomnia, headaches, and drinking alcohol to get to sleep along with taking Xanax 4 mg/day. Martin has a history of excessive drinking, past drug abuse, lying, and being a con artist. He was recently arrested for drunk driving. I suspected depression due to his alcohol use. I recommended trials on Mellaril 25 mg (a very low dose of a major tranquilizer) or Desyrel 50 mg (an antidepressant) for sleep, and I suggested relaxation tapes and that he continue the low dose of Xanax until life was more stable. His priority should be to eliminate alcohol and work in supportive psychotherapy to decrease his chronic stress levels.

A year later Martin reported using various herbs to try to cleanse his body, lower cholesterol, and treat a sinus infection. He said he had been using the herbs also in an attempt to cut down his alcohol use but is still taking Xanax to 3 to 4 mg/day.

He wants to taper off his Xanax, and I strongly supported this effort.

Twenty months after his initial evaluation Martin told me about his drunk driving arrest, his recent diagnosis of hepatitis B, and that he was still using Xanax up to 4 mg/day. I also learned that he was in prison in the past for seven years for being an IV drug abuser and related crimes. A few months later he told me that he had increased his Xanax on his own up to 6 mg/day and had a new diagnosis of pancreatitis (which could have resulted from cleaning fluid chemical exposure or drinking heavily).

Three years after the initial evaluation, I got a call telling me that Martin apparently drank on top of medications the prior evening and had a seizure and was taken to a hospital emergency room where Dilantin was prescribed. I told him to taper off Xanax and phase in Valium while using Dilantin as prescribed by the E.R. doctor. I recommended inpatient drug and alcohol rehabilitation, which he declined.

A few months after an unsuccessful outpatient detoxification attempt by another doctor, I got a call to tell me he had been in an inpatient rehabilitation program in a local hospital for detoxification under the care of still another doctor.

Conclusion: Martin didn't tell all at the start of treatment. He had long-standing problems with a history of IV drug abuse, a drunk driving charge, using codeine and minor tranquilizers, and drinking on top of them while escalating the doses of the minor tranquilizers. He repeatedly called for phone prescriptions, and he did battle with me about my insistence on his coming for appointments and about his requests for extra prescriptions for minor tranquilizers. He had hepatitis and pancreatitis problems as a result of his drug and alcohol abuse (perhaps complicated by his work-related chemical exposure), and ultimately paid the price in having had a couple of seizures before finally getting into a detoxification program. If I had it to do over, would I have given him minor tranquilizers? Probably not, unless we had a treatment contract that they were for very time-limited use, that he would not drink alcohol with them, and that they were given as part of a detoxification program and AA participation.

CHAPTER 7

DEPRESSION

■ **DRUGS DISCUSSED:**
Prozac, Zoloft, Celexa, Paxil, Serzone, Effexor, Wellbutrin, Tofranil, Elavil, Desyrel, Nardil, Parnate, Lithium

HOW A PSYCHIATRIST DIAGNOSES DEPRESSION

The diagnosis of depression always follows two clear, simple pathways. First, a psychiatrist will decide whether an individual's depression stems from *primary* or *secondary* causes; second, whether or not the particular type of depression is *unipolar* or *bipolar*. Primary depression is an illness more severe than normal grief, disappointment, or adjustment to life stresses. It cannot be explained as due to medical illness or substance abuse. Primary means that it is not caused by, or developing in close relationship to, a major medical illness, substance abuse, or another psychiatric disorder. Often there is a genetic predisposition.

Secondary depressions are those that have a physiological cause at their roots and can only be diagnosed by taking a patient's medical history and giving him a physical examination and a laboratory evaluation. This type of depression usually involves either mood disorders caused by substance abuse or disorders caused by general medical conditions. Sometimes prescription drugs can also cause depression. Usually, these individuals have never experienced serious depression prior to their abuse of alcohol and/or drugs, or their current physical illness. For example, a person with no previous history of depression might begin to experience this state after periods of heavy drinking. Another might begin taking a blood pressure medicine that acts on the brain in such a way that she becomes despondent after a few months. In both of these situations, it is reasonable to assume that the depression was due to the addition of an outside toxin to the person's body chemistry.

DRUGS THAT CAUSE DEPRESSION

Some of the drugs commonly known to cause depression as a side effect include those blood pressure medications that act on the brain, such as Catapres (clonidine), reserpine, Inderal (propranolol), and Aldomet (methyldopa). Steroids, often used to control severe arthritis, autoimmune disease, or asthma, may also contribute to problematic changes in one's mood by causing feelings of depression, euphoria, or irritability. All of the "recreational drugs" people commonly abuse, such as alcohol, cocaine, methamphetamine, and opiates, are capable of causing depression. Fortunately, one can usually treat a mood disorder caused by substance abuse by removing the substance that caused it. In such cases, an individual's depression will often clear up on its own within a month.

Sometimes, however, the medical causes of depression are not so easy to detect. These conditions include chronic infections; endocrine problems, including over- or underactive thyroid, parathyroid, or adrenal glands; various forms of cancer, especially cancer of the pancreas; and various forms of neurological degenerative diseases, such as multiple sclerosis.

Also under consideration in the differential diagnosis of depression is normal human sadness that is a part of adjustment disorders and bereavement. Adjustment disorders are reactions to stressful life events that go beyond the normal, average, expectable reaction. Bereavement is the culturally expected normal sadness in response to the death of a loved one or another major loss. Sometimes the "grief work" of letting go of a loved one is done during a prolonged terminal illness and there is a sense of relief rather than profound sadness at the time of the actual death. Nevertheless, there is usually a great sense of loss.

The types of depression that are secondary to medical problems, substance abuse, or life adjustment and grief often do not require medication. The use of antidepressants, however, might be considered in cases where such depression is unusually persistent; keeps recurring in a form similar to previous bouts of depression; runs in the family, such as when a blood relative has the same problem; or worsens rather than improves after a period of a month or two of "watchful waiting" and emotional support.

UNIPOLAR AND BIPOLAR MOOD DISORDERS

If people experience depression in the absence of drug or alcohol abuse, prescription drugs known to cause depression, or any other obvious medical or biological causes, it may be an indication that they are suffering from a *primary mood disorder*. This may develop anytime from childhood through middle or late adulthood. The primary mood disorders are divided into two basic groups: unipolar (single episode or recurrent major depression) and bipolar. Both terms describe types of major depression that often recur throughout the person's lifetime, but bipolar affective disorder, the modern name for manic depressive illness, describes those individuals who also have episodes of hypomania or mania that are separate from their bouts of depression. Hypomania and mania are periods of unusually high mood and energy. (For more details, see chapter 8, which discusses bipolar disorders.)

A psychiatrist will diagnose someone with major depression when the patient exhibits, for a period of at least two weeks, at least five symptoms or "indicators" for this condition. A despondent mood, and a loss of interest or pleasure in most activities, are always key diagnostic elements. Additional symptoms include changes in appetite, weight, sleep patterns, or psychomotor activity (either an agitation or an extreme slowing of thinking and movements); fatigue or loss of energy; feelings of worthlessness or guilt; problems with thinking, concentration, and making decisions; and suicidal thoughts or attempts. Interestingly, some people may develop insomnia and loss of appetite and weight, while others have the opposite symptoms during a major depressive episode.

Before a psychiatrist will make a diagnosis of major depression, he or she must be convinced that these symptoms are causing significant impairment in an individual's normal functioning.

SUBTYPES OF DEPRESSION

When planning a patient's treatment, it is important for a psychiatrist to establish which *subtypes* of major depression a person is experiencing.

1. *The melancholic subtype* is diagnosed when a client exhibits a marked loss of interest or pleasure in life, an inability to enjoy pleasant events or to be cheered up by a compliment or positive attention, and at least three of the following symptoms: feeling worse in the morning, waking up too early in the morning, showing signs of either physical agitation or slowed physical movements, and significant anorexia or weight loss. When a person in this subtype has symptoms that include severe slowing of physical movements and responses, an inability to respond emotionally to life events in an appropriate way, and consistent inability to experience pleasure, he or she will usually respond well to antidepressants or electroconvulsive therapy.
2. Another subtype of depression associated with a specific treatment response are those with *atypical depression,* which is currently defined as persistence of mood reactivity so that the individual is capable of responding to pleasant life events and being cheered up, plus two or more of the following symptoms: weight gain or appetite increase, oversleeping, feeling of

leaden paralysis taking away the energy to do things, and long-standing rejection sensitivity—depression that is often triggered by criticism or romantic rejections. Atypical depression predicts that the patient's response to monoamine oxidase inhibitors, such as Nardil and Parnate, will be better than her response to tricyclic antidepressants, such as Pamelor and Elavil, and might also predict a positive response to the selective serotonin reuptake inhibitors, such as Prozac, Zoloft, and Paxil.

3. A third subtype of major depression includes those patients who exhibit *catatonic symptoms,* including immobility, or stupor; excessive physical movements or peculiar ones, such as unusual posturing; negativism or refusal to speak; and a tendency to repeat the words and movements of others. Catatonic depression often responds extremely well to injectable Ativan (lorazepam) or electroconvulsive therapy.

4. The category of major depression referred to as *psychotic* is associated with a great amount of guilt and more evidence of psychomotor changes. In this case, there will often be a family history of bipolar illness, and the patient usually suffers severe impairment at the time of illness and afterward. Psychotic depression also always involves the presence of hallucinations or delusions, although deciding whether or not the client is really suffering from delusions can be a difficult clinical judgment call for the psychiatrist. Typical depressive delusions involve thoughts of guilt, sin, evil, or punishment by God, as well as remorseful statements such as, "If only I hadn't done such and such, this would have never happened to me." The treatment of psychotic major depression is different from all other forms of depression because it frequently requires both an antidepressant and an antipsychotic drug, or the use of electroconvulsive therapy.

5. Sometimes a major depressive disorder recurs only at certain specific times of the year, typically worsening in the fall and winter. Most often, individuals suffering from *seasonal depression* are women who already have bipolar II disorder

(depressions and hypomanic episodes), and whose symptoms might also include overeating, oversleeping, social withdrawal, and craving carbohydrates and sugars, with chocolate as a favorite self-treatment. Recent research has shown that seasonal affective disorder, as this condition is called, frequently responds to bright artificial light. The typical treatment is usually 10,000 lux, the equivalent of sitting by the window on a bright summer day, administered for one hour each morning. Light boxes designed for this purpose, using full-spectrum fluorescent bulbs, are commercially available from several companies.

ILLNESS AND DEPRESSION

Certain neurologic illnesses are associated with episodes of major depression, including Alzheimer's disease, Parkinson's disease, and stroke. Although these depressions are secondary to medical problems, all of these may respond well to antidepressant medications. Sometimes, however, when one is suffering from a major illness, the symptoms of depression can be missed. For example, someone in a rehabilitation program following a stroke might seem unmotivated or uncooperative. In reality, he or she might be severely depressed, a very treatable component in the factors that are presently making him "disabled." Major depression following a heart attack should definitely be treated, as it raises the risk of death over the next several months.

Major depression should always be thought of as an illness that has a high potential of recurring. Because of this, an important part of evaluating any depressed individual involves looking at his or her lifelong history of depressive episodes, even if those episodes were never treated. This "big picture" may be an important factor in making a decision as to whether the patient should take medication short term (six to twelve months) or for his or her entire life. Individuals who have had particularly recurrent and severe episodes of depression, resulting in impairment of their ability to function, incapacitation (being unable to work, go to school, or take care of everyday family or self-care responsibilities), and/or loss of their jobs or families certainly deserve consideration for long-term preventive medication treatment.

The research data available on the recurrence of episodes of major depression, especially a collaborative study of depression done by the National Institute of Mental Health, emphasize this point strongly. Researchers at NIMH found that patients treated for an episode of major depression in a series of university clinics by a psychiatrist, and who were well for a period of at least eight weeks following their treatment, had frequent recurrences of this condition. When these individuals were followed up over the long term, they had an average relapse rate of 33 percent at the one-year point, 46 percent at two years, 54 percent at three years, and 60 percent at four years. Thus, the recurrent nature of major depression typically makes itself known within a few years of recovery from the initial episode.

DEPRESSIONS UNRESPONSIVE TO DRUGS

The coexistence of major depression and substance abuse is particularly difficult to treat. Recent studies have shown that even a moderate use of alcohol can interfere with an individual's responsiveness to antidepressants.

Major depression superimposed on long-standing dysthymia may also cause less than ideal treatment response. *Dysthymia* is defined as a condition where one has experienced a depressed mood or mild background depression for at least two years, and has never felt well for more than two months during that time. Dysthymia also includes at least two symptoms from the following list: poor appetite or overeating, insomnia or oversleeping, low energy or fatigue, low self-esteem, poor concentration or difficulty making decisions, and feelings of hopelessness. An individual suffering from dysthymia may have a slower and less complete response to medications than those suffering only from bouts of major depression. The onset of dysthymia may occur early, before twenty-one years of age, or it may develop later in life. Often the patient reports, "I've been depressed all my life," when asked how long he has had a problem.

A few years ago the treatment of dysthymia was controversial. Some psychotherapists maintained that very chronic mild depression did not justify medications and was frequently a result of early childhood developmental problems, and so could best be treated with psychotherapy. In an extensive research program, Hogop Akiskal, however, demonstrated that some of the biologic markers of more severe depression were also present in those suffering from chronic mild depression, such as changes in sleep patterns resulting in a shortened time between falling asleep and going into rapid eye movement (dreaming) sleep. Other patients suffering from dysthymia showed abnormal response to biologic tests for depression, such as the dexamethasone suppression test. More important, many individuals with dysthymia do respond to mood-normalizing drugs, including antidepressants and lithium, if these are given for a period of at least a few months. About 60 percent of patients with dysthymia will respond to Zoloft, Serzone, or imipramine if they continue taking the medication for a period of three months, so any patient with very chronic depression deserves an antidepressant trial rather than simply labeling the illness as chronic and unlikely to respond to anything short of several years of psychotherapy.

PSYCHOTHERAPY OR MEDICATIONS?

A very frequent question asked in clinical practice is how much of a role psychological factors versus biological factors play in the development of depression, and whether one should choose psychotherapy or medications to treat it. Many studies that have looked at various specific forms of psychotherapy, including cognitive behavioral therapy and interpersonal therapy, have shown that these very specific forms of psychotherapy are just as effective as the tricyclic antidepressant imipramine in treating mildly or moderately ill outpatients with major depression. In patients who suffer from more severe depressions, however, the tricyclic antidepressant drugs have a greater effectiveness in treating their conditions when compared to various forms of psychotherapy.

Although it is a matter of personal style as to whether, and to what extent, a clinician believes that either psychotherapy or medication should be tried first in the treatment of depression, most generally agree that if a treatment modality fails to yield a reasonably good response after a couple of months, then the other type of treatment should be tried. Most clinicians also agree that the combination of psychotherapy and medications is more effective than either alone. While the following suggestions clearly reflect my own personal opinion, I think that they are also reasonably valid summaries of the recommendations made by many experts in my field.

Many health care professionals agree with me that individuals who have experienced major psychosocial issues in their past and present may need psychotherapy. These types of issues might include childhood emotional, sexual, or physical abuse; growing up with a parent who abuses alcohol or drugs; or the death of a parent during childhood. Such experiences certainly cause long-term emotional scars, and psychotherapy can substantially help people to overcome the damage done by them. People who are suffering from severe job-related stress or stress within important relationships in their lives may also greatly benefit from having someone with whom to talk over these problems and explore new coping and problem-solving strategies. Another category of people who might benefit from psychotherapy are those who feel a tremendous social isolation. Such individuals suffer from a lack of family and friends, which translates into a lack of the natural stress-buffering effect of having people to turn to and talk with in difficult times. Psychotherapy may play a role for these individuals, both in helping them with their current problem and in changing their long-term lack of social interaction. When issues of social isolation accompany depression, they might be the cause of the depression, the result of it, or even the reason the depression has been so prolonged.

On the other hand, some of the patients that I see do not really want or need psychotherapy, feeling that medication is enough for them. Typically, these people tell me that life is good, that they generally enjoy their work, that their relationships with their friends and family are satisfactory, and that they have enough money to feel comfortable. In spite of all these things to be happy about, however, they feel that they are not really enjoying their successes in life.

For these relatively happy and successful individuals, depression seems to come out of the blue. They might currently be undergoing life stressors or changes, but these situations are not overwhelming and certainly within the range of problems that the person has handled without undue distress in the past. As a rule, these people also have strong coping abilities and good support systems. They see any changes or circumstances that occurred prior to their current depression as issues that they could readily deal with under normal circumstances, if only they were feeling as well as they usually do.

Many of these types of individuals also have a history of previous episodes of depression and a family history of mood disorders or other related conditions, including alcoholism or suicide. In spite of this, in my experience, all they often need or want is a little bit of support for a few weeks while waiting for an antidepressant drug to work. For them, psychotherapy seems unnecessary. They may even have attempted psychotherapy in the past and found that it was interesting and taught them a lot but did not really help them to get over their depression. It is hard to justify the expenditure of time and money for such individuals.

SUICIDE

The greatest risk one encounters when undergoing a severe mood disorder is suicide. Over the long term, individuals with untreated mood disorders run about a 1 percent per year risk of dying by suicide and about a 10 to 15 percent lifetime risk. These suicides always occur when a person is in a state of tremendous emotional distress, but are needless because such feelings almost always pass within a few days.

The risk factors for suicide are very well established. Those most likely to become so depressed that they end their own lives are the elderly, those who live alone, substance abusers, and those with debilitating medical illnesses. More men than women commit suicide. Those with a personal or family history of suicide attempts, or those who have a sense of hopelessness that things will never get better, are at especially high risk for suicide. Individuals whose past attempts to end their lives involved a true intent to die and a setting in which there was little chance of being rescued are especially at risk.

If you are reading this now and thinking about suicide, please remember that depression is an extremely treatable illness, that the harm done to your surviving relatives and friends is incredibly traumatic, and that there is every chance in the world that in a few weeks you will no longer want to be dead if you can just hang in there and continue on medications. If you are not in treatment, see a psychiatrist as soon as possible, even if it means going to a psychiatric hospital emergency room. If you feel like you just can't go on living, the best thing to do is to ask your doctor for hospitalization; a hospital can both protect you from self-harm and provide an intensive interaction with staff who can teach you new coping mechanisms to help you to genuinely overcome your desire to end your life.

LABORATORY EVALUATION OF DEPRESSION

While there are no precise guidelines as to how much of a medical evaluation is appropriate to diagnose an individual with depression, there are some very simple basic tests that anyone can request of the doctor to screen for common physical causes of depression.

These include:
- a complete blood count
- a chemistry panel
- thyroid functions
- a urinalysis

For older patients or individuals who are at risk from having multiple sexual partners, smoking, or using intravenous drugs, a chest x-ray, electrocardiogram, and possibly an HIV test may be appropriate.

There are many tests to discover biologic markers of depression that have been popular at times. These, however, are best reserved for research studies because they are fairly expensive and often miss cases of depression. The biologic markers these tests are looking for include the dexamethasone suppression test, the thyrotropin TRH-TSH test, the rapid eye movement latency (REM latency) sleep test, the amphetamine challenge, brain electrical activity mapping by computerized electroencephalogram, and spinal tap to assay cerebral-spinal fluid 5-HIAA, which is the serotonin metabolite that might predict suicide risk.

Although there was once hope among researchers that these kinds of tests might accurately predict an individual's responsiveness to various antidepressant drugs, this information can easily be discovered anyway during the course of treatment. Another downside of these tests is that their results may not be reliably reproducible by the average laboratory.

The lab is best used to screen for underlying medical illness, while the clinical history and family history give the best guides to medication selection.

CHOOSING THE PROPER MEDICATION FOR TREATMENT OF DEPRESSION

Making the right selection from among the many available antidepressant drugs is a very great challenge for the psychiatrist and an extremely important issue for the patient. An interesting analogy for this process is that of a lock and key. Say that I walk up to a new building with the custodian's key ring and want to open the front door lock. I don't know which of the twenty keys will do the job, so I inspect each of them to decide which one looks as if it's about the right size, and then I proceed to try each of this subgroup in turn until I finally find the right one.

In the same manner, when I am working with a new patient suffering from depression, I don't know which of about twenty available antidepressants will work, but I can make some intelligent guesses and then begin a systematic series of trials until I find the right one. The right one is the medication that gets rid of the vast majority of symptoms with only minimal side effects.

One of the most helpful things you can do to make your own treatment successful is to bring the psychiatrist a list of every medication you have taken in the past, including its name, your dosage, the duration of use, your response to the drug, and any side effects you may have experienced. The same list should be made for any blood relative who has been on antidepressant medications, since their responses and yours might be very similar. Compiling these two lists is well worth the effort because they can make a world of difference in choosing the very best medication for you to start with.

SIDE EFFECTS: HELPFUL OR HARMFUL?

A major issue in medication selection is whether side effects might be helpful or harmful to the patient. One such example can be seen in medications that act as sedatives. Drugs such as Elavil (amitriptyline), Sinequan (doxepin), and Desyrel (trazodone) are highly sedating. New-generation drugs such as Serzone (nefazodone) and Remeron (mirtazapine) share some of these sedating properties. Some individuals who take these drugs say that they are finally getting a decent night's sleep for the first time in weeks or months. Others will take the same drug and report that they absolutely cannot tolerate the extreme side effects of drowsiness and drug hangover that they feel, leaving them tired all the next day. The response to sedating antidepressants tends to be highly individualistic and, unfortunately, is not always predictable. The sedating effect of these drugs may be used to advantage when a person takes them to get to sleep, but these same effects may also serve to limit the intake of the drug. The dose that helps with sleep yet lets one feel awake during the day might never be high enough to adequately treat the individual's depression. Sadly, it is a common experience for people taking one of the most sedating antidepressants, even at a low dosage of 50 or 100 mg/day, to complain to their doctors that their depression never really got any better even though they are sleeping a little better and have been gaining weight on the drug. The occurrence of such underdosing was very common a few years ago when tricyclic antidepressants were the only drugs available for the treatment of depression.

Weight loss is another potential side effect of antidepressants such as Prozac (fluoxetine) and Wellbutrin (bupropion). The mild weight loss effects of these drugs do not justify using them as diet pills but can be of some benefit, especially in treating an individual whose obesity makes control of diabetes or high blood pressure very difficult. On the other hand, weight gain is a substantial side effect of Elavil (amitriptyline), Sinequan (doxepin), and Remeron (mirtazepine). This weight gain might be helpful in treating an individual with anorexia nervosa or one who has had major loss of appetite due to a chronic systemic illness such as cancer.

The anticholinergic side effects of drugs such as Elavil (amitriptyline), Sinequan (doxepin), and Vivactil (protriptyline) include dry mouth, blurred vision, constipation, and difficulty urinating. They can also include a worsening in someone suffering from glaucoma. The effects of such medications may be a major problem in an elderly man suffering from an enlargement of the prostate gland and chronic constipation, but they may be very helpful in the individual with irritable bowel syndrome or chronic diarrhea.

Another consideration in selecting the appropriate antidepressant drug is whether monitoring a person's blood levels during a drug trial will be helpful. Blood level monitoring might especially be appropriate for individuals who take anticonvulsants, smoke cigarettes, drink a lot of alcohol, or take other drugs that might have a significant interaction with the antidepressant that will cause them to metabolize the drug either much more slowly or more rapidly than usual. Blood monitoring can be especially important in the elderly or in individuals who have already tried several drugs that have proven to be ineffective.

Tests for antidepressant drug levels can serve as a guide to the psychiatrist for appropriate dosing and help the client to achieve optimal blood levels of a drug fairly quickly. These kinds of tests are available for all the antidepressants but really only give meaningful information about the tricyclic antidepressants—Elavil (amitriptyline), Tofranil (imipramine), Norpramin (desipramine), Pamelor (nortriptyline), Sinequan (doxepin), and Vivactil (protriptyline). Blood levels obtained for the selective serotonin reuptake inhibitors such as Prozac, Zoloft, Paxil, and Celexa, as well as for Wellbutrin, Serzone, and Effexor, represent measurements without valid standards for their interpretation. In other words, I might get a number from the lab, but I really would not know what to do with it. Only if the patient was taking a drug that was a tricyclic antidepressant would the blood level help to adjust the dosage.

Another area of concern in selecting antidepressants is whether the individual has any cardiovascular risk factors. Standard tricyclic antidepressants may cause what is known as postural hypotension. What this means is that the patient has a drop in blood pressure when going from lying or sitting to a standing position. Most young people experience this as a brief moment of dizziness from which they rapidly recover. This reaction can be much greater in elderly individuals, however, who may feel as if they are about to pass out, especially if they are taking blood pressure medicines with the antidepressant. If this reaction occurs, one runs a substantial risk of having a brief loss of consciousness accompanied by a fall and possibly a broken hip. Fortunately, the risk of developing postural hypotension is very low with the selective serotonin reuptake inhibitors, Wellbutrin (bupropion), and the two tricyclic antidepressants Pamelor (nortriptyline) and Norpramin (desipramine).

For some individuals, the risk of having a seizure is another important issue to consider when deciding what medication they should take. In one to four cases out of every thousand, the standard antidepressants pose the risk of causing a seizure in a person who has never had one before. This danger is even higher in individuals who are taking other drugs that can lower the seizure threshold. High-risk medications include theophylline (aminophylline), taken for asthma or chronic obstructive pulmonary disease; antipsychotic or neuroleptic drugs taken to treat psychotic symptoms; short-acting minor tranquilizers, which might be causing withdrawal symptoms; excessive alcohol; and stimulants, such as amphetamines or cocaine. People who have any of these risk factors or who have a history of significant head trauma or previous seizures should generally avoid any antidepressant that is labeled with a seizure risk of four or more people per thousand. These include Wellbutrin (bupropion) immediate-release form (the slow-release form is safer at a dose of 300 mg/day or less), Ludiomil (maprotiline), and Anafranil (clomipramine). For these individuals, their depression may be best treated with anticonvulsants such as Tegretol (carbamazepine) or Depakote (divalproex), or the SSRIs (Prozac, Zoloft, Paxil, Celexa), or MAOIs (Nardil or Parnate).

When finding an "ideal" antidepressant, the psychiatrist and patient must consider what sort of side effects it has on sexuality. Anafranil and selective serotonin reuptake inhibitors (Prozac, Zoloft, Paxil, Celexa) might cause delay in sexual response as a common side effect, with some people unable to achieve orgasm or reporting loss of sexual desire. This orgasmic delay can be a major problem if orgasm cannot be reached at all, but it might prove to be a major sexual enhancer if orgasm is delayed in a man who has premature ejaculation. Both men and women who have experienced drug-related loss of sexual drive, excitability, or orgasm while on antidepressants may find that their sexual response normalizes if they are switched to Wellbutrin (bupropion), Serzone (nefazodone), or Remeron (mirtazepine).

Additional factors that a psychiatrist and patient might consider in the selection of an antidepressant include other types of psychiatric conditions that might be present. Obsessive-compulsive disorder, bulimia, and panic disorder all respond well to the selective serotonin reuptake inhibitors used to treat depression. Attention deficit disorder in adults may be a persistent chronic condition from childhood that responds well to Wellbutrin, MAO inhibitors, and possibly to tricyclics such as Norpramin (desipramine) or to the stimulant drugs such as Dexedrine (dextroamphetamine) or Ritalin (methylphenidate). Individuals who have a history of mania or hypomania should consider taking lithium, an anticonvulsant such as Depakote or Tegretol, or certain antidepressants that will be discussed in the next chapter that are less likely to induce a switch from depression into mania.

THE NEW GENERATION OF ANTIDEPRESSANTS

Repeated comparison studies done as part of the premarketing evaluations of the new generation of antidepressants are remarkably consistent in showing that all of these new medications have a response rate comparable to the standard tricyclic antidepressants. Studies typically randomly assign patients in double-blind fashion so that neither doctor nor patient knows if the patient will be receiving the new drug, the comparison drug (tricyclic antidepressant), or placebo (sugar pill) during the experimental trial. At two weeks, patients on the active drug (new drug or old tricyclic antidepressant) are better than those who get randomly assigned to the placebo, and this difference between drug and placebo gets progressively greater at four and six weeks. Sixty to 70 percent of the patients who are taking the active drugs are rated by their doctors as either improved or very much improved at the end of four to six weeks of treatment. Only about 30 percent of the patients in these studies tested on the placebo got better. There are, however, major differences between the new drugs and the old tricyclic antidepressants in regard to side effects and dropout rates of the individuals taking them; all are in favor of the new drugs.

A recent comparison study has shown that when the new-generation drugs Prozac (fluoxetine) and Wellbutrin (bupropion) are randomly assigned to patients participating in the study, these drugs show about equal effectiveness and equal dropout rates. Studies of Desyrel (trazodone), a relatively new drug, versus Tofranil (imipramine), a classic tricyclic antidepressant, have shown these drugs to be equally effective.

SAFETY AND OVERDOSE RISK

The safety of the tricyclic antidepressants is an important consideration because they can be lethal when taken in overdose. Asendin (amoxapine), Ludiomil (maprotiline), tricyclic antidepressants (Tofranil, Elavil, Pamelor, Norpramin, Sinequan, Vivactil), and lithium carbonate can all be dangerous or even fatal if a patient takes a two-week supply all at once. The new generation of drugs, however, which includes Desyrel (trazodone), Wellbutrin (bupropion), and the selective serotonin reuptake inhibitors (Prozac, Zoloft, Paxil, Celexa, and Luvox), as well as Effexor (venlafaxine), Serzone (nefazodone), and Remeron (mirtazapine) are all relatively safer when taken in an overdose.

HOW TO BEST UTILIZE MEDICATION TRIALS

Unfortunately, even when a doctor and a patient have the very best selection of antidepressant drugs to choose from, and even based on all that we know about them, a medication trial is still just that, an educated trial-and-error process to determine if a drug will be helpful. There are a few things, however, that a patient can do to make this process a much more effective and collaborative effort. The first is a regular charting of mood and depression ratings throughout a drug trial. One tool that will help with this is the Seventeen-item Hamilton Depression Rating Scale, which a psychiatrist can perform in about five minutes during a routine office visit. Yet another is for a patient to do a Beck Depression Inventory self-rating, which takes just a few minutes and can be done either in the waiting room or at home. By doing such tests and plotting the results of a medication trial over a period of four to six weeks, both psychiatrist and patient should be able to see, obviously and clearly, whether or not a drug is working and if a patient's moods are changing for the better. We typically define an adequate antidepressant trial as four to six weeks at the maximum tolerated dose, or at the therapeutic blood level for tricyclic antidepressants, or at the usually effective dose for the new-generation drugs. For example, if a selective serotonin reuptake inhibitor (SSRI) antidepressant is being used, then a standard dose of 20 to 80 mg/day of Prozac, 50 to 200 mg/day of Zoloft, or 20 to 50 mg/day of Paxil would constitute a typical trial. Wellbutrin is typically used in doses of 150 to 450 mg/day.

Flexibility in drug trials is very important. Both psychiatrist and patient should have a clear sense that the goal is to treat the patient with a drug that is both effective and very tolerable, rather than a drug that is the doctor's personal favorite. If a drug causes intolerable side effects, such as agitation, insomnia, sedation, hallucinations, sexual dysfunction, or suicidal tendencies, it is the patient's responsibility to tell the doctor immediately. Simply stopping the drug and waiting a week or two until the next appointment is not taking responsibility for the doctor/patient collaboration. If a medication trial of four to six weeks does not lead to a good clinical response, it is time to change treatment by trying another drug.

WHAT HAPPENS WHEN THE MEDICINE DOES NOT WORK?

Sometimes a patient might take a maximum tolerated dose of a medication for four to six weeks with little or no response. At this point, the psychiatrist and patient will face a difficult decision. At this juncture, the patient's charting of his or her moods and depression ratings is especially valuable because it can help the doctor to sort out the difference between no response and a partial response to a drug. If a patient has had a partial response to a drug, noticeable enough to lower his or her depression ratings, yet has not experienced a complete remission of symptoms, then the psychiatrist should consider the option of *augmenting,* adding a secondary mood-normalizing drug to one that is already being taken. This avoids starting over with a drug that works by a different mechanism and might not be effective at all.

Another factor that will help the patient and clinician to decide on the next step is that, by the four-to-six-week point, they should now have some additional data that may not have been available at the beginning of treatment. Hopefully, by this time there will be a complete set of lab results on the patient and a very detailed family history of any other individuals who may have had similar problems. This information can serve as an important guideline in choosing the next step in treatment. For example, if the clinician discovers that a relative of the patient has a history of bipolar (manic depressive) illness that has responded well to treatment with lithium, then he or she will know that an intelligent strategy would be to try the patient on lithium augmentation therapy. The typical dose in such a case would be about 900 to 1,200 mg/day with the most important factor being the blood level achieved; typically, serum levels of around 0.5 to 1.0 milliequivalents per liter of serum. When lithium is added to a drug to which a patient has already shown a partial response, some individuals will respond favorably within a couple of days while others might take two to four weeks. Augmenting a medication that has already shown an initial partial response to gain added benefit is the preferred strategy of most psychiatrists.

Another example of how drug augmentation works can be seen in the treatment of individuals whose lab tests reveal that they have even the slightest elevation of the hormone that stimulates the thyroid gland (TSH), or who have a family history of thyroid disease. A helpful strategy in this case would be the addition of a low dose of the thyroid hormone triiodothyronine, also known as T3 or Cytomel. Again, if an individual is going to respond favorably to this augmentation, the results should be apparent within one to two weeks.

A third augmentation strategy, useful in individuals who were taking a selective serotonin reuptake inhibitor in the first medication trial, is to add a selective norepinephrine reuptake inhibitor such as Norpramin (desipramine) in a low dose. This is usually very energizing. This augmentation must be done cautiously because it is possible that Prozac and Paxil, more than Zoloft or Celexa, may increase the level of the tricyclic antidepressant to the point of causing risky side effects. Typically, augmentation with desipramine is at a dose of only 25 to 75 mg/day. When this drug is used by itself in the treatment of depression, doses are frequently in the 100 to 300 mg/day range. The blood pressure medicine Pindolol has been used with SSRI antidepressants to augment the response or make it faster; reports of results have been variable. Pindolol would be a good choice in a patient with high blood pressure. Occasionally BuSpar (buspirone) is used with an SSRI for augmentation; this would be a good choice in a chronically anxious patient.

If a patient really has not shown any response to the initial drug trial, then switching him or her to a different drug at the four-to-six-week point makes sense. Some clinicians advocate switching from one selective serotonin reuptake inhibitor to another. Although some recent studies have shown this strategy to be occasionally effective, it is not clear if this is because of subtle differences between the drugs themselves or simply the result of taking this type of drug for a longer period of time.

When an initial drug trial is ineffective, most clinicians simply change the kind of antidepressant being administered. Broad classes of antidepressants include the tricyclic antidepressants (Tofranil, Elavil, Pamelor, Norpramin, Sinequan, or Vivactil), the selective serotonin reuptake inhibitors (Prozac, Zoloft, Paxil, and Celexa), the atypical antidepressants (Wellbutrin, Desyrel, Serzone, and Effexor), and the monoamine oxidase inhibitors (Nardil and Parnate). The choice in moving from one antidepressant to another is often governed by an attempt to choose a drug from a different family and with a different mechanism of action. While this is debatable, I would never waste time with a third or fourth SSRI in a patient who had not responded to a four-week or longer trial on one or two others in the past.

RESPONSE LAG

The most common question I hear from a patient with depression is, "How soon will this treatment work?" The best answer I can give is this: In randomized studies in which half the individuals get a drug and half get a sugar pill, it takes about two weeks for a drug to show its superiority to a sugar pill. This is statistical and not clinical superiority, so that on average the people who got the drug were a little bit better off than those who got the placebo, but most were not yet well. The maximum effect of most drugs, however, usually occurs somewhere around the four-to-six-week period. An occasional, lucky individual will respond to a drug in less than one week, and others may take more than six weeks. This is why we say that a fair drug trial is four to six weeks long. During that time, the patient and clinician should also be monitoring the drug to make sure that it is well tolerated—that the side effects are a minor nuisance rather than severe symptoms.

Unfortunately, all that most people experience from a psychiatric medication for depression in the first two weeks is a few side effects. I urge the reader taking a new drug for the first time to stick with it, however, because this is one case where patience and perseverance pay off, and where there is little evidence that there is any way to get a drug to work faster.

Antidepressants are never used as needed like aspirin. Using a few pills when emotionally upset is a major mistake and a strategy that won't be effective beyond the placebo effect. Such misuse is usually based on lack of doctor-patient discussion. These drugs are used on an everyday basis to treat depressions that have gone on for weeks. The only rare exception that I will make to this strategy is the occasional use of a few days of antidepressants during the worst depressions of rapid-cycling bipolar affective disorder patients, in whom this may be adequate to push them out of a brief depression and not be enough to make them manic.

DURATION OF TREATMENT

The second question I am frequently asked is, "How long do I have to take this medicine?" The most honest answer I can give is that the advice of experts has changed over the last decade. Ten years ago, depression was viewed as an illness that might occasionally recur and should be treated each time it did for six to twelve months. In general, the strategy was for the patient to wait until his or her depression was in good control with no residual symptoms, take the medication for another six months, and then taper off gradually sometime over the following three to six months, preferably at a time when life stresses were relatively low. During the tapering-off period, the patient would be monitored to determine whether the medication was still needed, based on the presence or absence of any depression symptoms.

As we have seen, however, more recent studies show that depression tends to recur in a high percentage of cases. For this reason, some individuals do best with a lifetime regimen of maintenance medication. The strongest argument for long-term maintenance comes from the work of Kupfer. He discovered that patients who had been successfully treated for recurrent depression with the drug Tofranil (imipramine) fared far better with continuing drug treatment than with a placebo. This was not only true in the first one to three years of treatment, but even beyond this to five years. This study was accomplished with the help of a few brave individuals who were willing to be randomized to a drug or to placebo after three years of treatment on imipramine. The next two years showed that those who remained on the actual drug had a far greater chance of staying well than those who took the sugar pill. Other studies done on the new generation of antidepressants have also been extremely consistent in showing that individuals who have gotten well for about two months and then were randomized to a year of treatment on either the drug or placebo also do much better if they continue taking the drug. The difference in recurrence rate between those who take the medicine and those who are given placebo shows up as about 30 percent fewer recurrences of depression in the drug continuation group. Kupfer's imipramine data made a strong point that "the dose that got you well is the dose that will keep you well," and that cutting the dose in half for long-term maintenance actually decreases a drug's effectiveness in preventing a recurrence of depression, though the effectiveness is still better than that of placebo.

DRUG DOSING

What constitutes an appropriate dose of an antidepressant varies from one drug to another, and from one condition to another. For example, when Prozac is used to treat a panic disorder patient, a psychiatrist will typically begin with a very low dose using the liquid form of the drug. The average patient might start at 2 or 4 mg/day, and then work up the dose by 2 mg per week until his or her panic attacks are controlled or until side effects become noticeable. Often 10 or 20 mg of Prozac a day is plenty.

In contrast, individuals suffering from depression typically require about 20 to 60 mg of Prozac per day. Although studies where the dose is randomized within this range tend to show that people have equal response rates to any level of dosage, clinical experience shows that some individuals do notice a major difference in the way they feel on Prozac when they are in the 20 mg range, as compared to the 40 to 60 mg range. In still another context, when Prozac is used for the treatment of obsessive-compulsive disorder or bulimia, high doses appear to be substantially better, and doses of 60 or 80 mg daily are quite typical.

A similar situation applies to the dosage of other selective serotonin reuptake inhibitors. Zoloft is typically prescribed in the range of 50 to 200 mg daily, and Paxil in a dose of 20 to 50 mg daily. Celexa dose is 10 to 60 mg/day, with most people taking 20 to 40 mg/day. Prozac, Zoloft, Celexa, and Paxil may all be taken once a day, and the timing of this dose is very much a matter of individual preference. The manufacturer typically recommends taking the drugs in the morning because there is some risk of insomnia early on in treatment, but I have certainly heard many individuals say that they prefer to take it after their largest meal or at bedtime. Because these drugs are reasonably long acting, there is no point in dividing the dosage up throughout the day, except to minimize side effects such as upset stomach.

Wellbutrin (bupropion) is typically prescribed in the range of 150 to 450 mg/day, since 150 mg/day is the lowest dose that has been proven to be better than a placebo. The upper limit of 450 mg/day was chosen by the manufacturer because the seizure risk at this dose or lower is 0.4 percent, while the seizure risk at doses above this ranges from 2.3 to 2.8 percent using the immediate-release form. Because of these risks of seizure, and the desire to avoid very high peak blood levels, which may increase seizure risk, the manufacturer strongly recommends that Wellbutrin never be taken in an individual dose of more than 150 mg of the immediate-release form at a time. Therefore, a higher dosage of the drug may require that the patient take it two or three times per day. It is best if these doses are separated by at least six hours, with the last dose before 5:00 P.M. to minimize the risk of insomnia. A slow-release form of Wellbutrin (called Wellbutrin SR) is now available, and the seizure risk of this formulation appears to be only 0.1 percent when the dose is limited to 300 mg/day. For individuals requiring a higher dose, 200 mg may be given twice daily. This medication is not usually given after dinner or at bedtime because it is activating and may cause insomnia.

Because Wellbutrin has a slightly higher seizure risk than other drugs, the manufacturer recommends that it not be used in individuals who have a history of seizures, head trauma, bulimia, recent withdrawal from the benzodiazepines or alcohol, or who are taking other seizure-provoking drugs such as aminophylline. Zyban, which is used as a prescription medication to help people stop smoking, is Wellbutrin under another name, and so should never be used with Wellbutrin.

Wellbutrin has several good points in its favor, including the lack of sexual dysfunction as a side effect, its benefit in the treatment of childhood and adult attention deficit disorder, its usefulness in helping individuals who wish to stop smoking, and its effectiveness in the treatment of those who have bipolar II disorder. It may cause some weight loss, especially at a dose of 400 to 450 mg/day.

Effexor (venlafaxine) is an interesting drug that acts in some ways like a mixture of serotonin and norepinephrine reuptake inhibitors. Although it achieves its results without many of the standard side effects caused by tricyclic antidepressants, it can cause side effects such as feelings of weakness, sweating, nausea, constipation, loss of appetite, vomiting, sleepiness, dry mouth, dizziness, nervousness, anxiety, tremor, blurred vision, and abnormal sexual response. Often, however, these side effects can be avoided by starting at a very low dose for the first few days and very gradually working up to a higher dose. Because the immediate-release form of this drug has a short half-life of only five hours, and a metabolite half-life of eleven hours, it has to be given two or three times a day. Its side effects may also be lessened by taking it after a meal. A typical daily dose is 75 to 225 mg/day for outpatients, and a maximum of 375 mg daily for nonresponsive or severely ill patients. A new extended release form of Effexor (Effexor XR) has a more gradual release into the bloodstream, fewer side effects, and better tolerability, and may be given once daily.

The percentage of people who respond favorably to Effexor increases as the dose increases; yet, as we have seen above, the dose is typically limited early in treatment because of the side effects. Thus, the strategy is to start at a very low dose such as 37.5 mg XR once a day and gradually increase the dose to the maximum that the individual is capable of comfortably tolerating. A very important experiment was done by researchers Nierenberg and Feighner in which they worked with patients who were extremely resistant to previously tried antidepressant medications. They demonstrated the effectiveness of Effexor by showing that one-third of those who took it in their study got well at eight to twelve weeks by taking an average dose of 245 mg/day. This study indicates that Effexor might very well be a rescue drug for people who have failed multiple other antidepressant trials.

Another important study on Effexor done in French hospitals demonstrated that individuals suffering from melancholic major depression showed some initial response to high doses of the drug within four days. These individuals actually showed a better response to Effexor than patients who were randomized to receive Prozac. During the four to six weeks these inpatients were studied, they received high doses of Effexor, in the 200 to 350 mg/day range.

Effexor might be effective for panic disorder, obsessive-compulsive disorder (OCD), attention deficit hyperactivity disorder (ADHD), and chronic pain or fibromyalgia. These uses are supported by case reports but not yet by double-blind controlled studies, and so they are considered "off label" relative to the FDA approval process. Also, like the selective serotonin reuptake inhibitors, Effexor should not be combined with an MAO inhibitor (Nardil or Parnate) because of the potential for a serious negative interaction. Just as with the short-acting selective serotonin reuptake inhibitors, when the patient has taken Effexor for more than a couple of months, it is highly recommended that he or she taper off of this medication to minimize any withdrawal symptoms.

MAO INHIBITORS

In the United States, there are currently only three MAO inhibitors on the market that have been approved for the treatment of depression. Nardil (phenelzine) is the most widely used, and typically a dose of 1 mg per kg of body weight per day is recommended. The side effects of this drug are substantial sexual dysfunction, weight gain, and sometimes sleep disruption, with the patient typically not feeling sleepy at bedtime, getting only a few hours of sleep at night, and being tired during the day. The alternative drug Parnate (tranylcypromine) has less severe side effects, but has a stimulating effect, somewhat like an amphetamine. Typically, Parnate is taken in a dose of 30 to 90 mg daily. Marplan, the third drug, is rarely used. Both Nardil and Parnate require strict adherence to a diet that eliminates aged or fermented foods, which have a high tyramine content. Such foods include beer, wine, cheese, sour cream, fava beans, pickled herring, and others. Combined with the drugs, the tyramine in these foods might lead to hypertensive (high blood pressure) reactions, including severe heart palpitations, headache, flushing, and the potential risk of catastrophic consequences such as stroke. Often, psychiatrists who prescribe Nardil or Parnate will also prescribe a few 20 mg capsules of the blood pressure medication nifedipine for the patient to keep handy in case this high blood pressure reaction occurs. The nifedipine tablet can be punctured and placed under the tongue where it rapidly decreases blood pressure, potentially eliminating the need for an emergency room visit.

In much of the rest of the world, two selective reversible inhibitors of monoamine oxidase-A, moclobemide (Aurorix, Manerix) and brofaromine, are used because of their effectiveness in treating depression and their lack of any specific dietary requirements. Although their safety is far superior to that of the nonspecific MAO inhibitors Nardil and Parnate, they are not marketed in the United States and probably will not be in the foreseeable future for economic reasons.

BUSPAR

BuSpar (buspirone) is a useful alternative drug for treatment of individuals with mixed depression and anxiety. Typically, the dose is 30 to 60 mg/day (sometimes even 80 mg/day), which is often very well tolerated and is very effective in treating outpatients with depression, especially if uncontrollable worry is a major feature. Sometimes BuSpar is added to conventional antidepressants in an attempt to augment their effectiveness.

SEASONAL AFFECTIVE DISORDER

Seasonal affective disorder describes a condition in which an individual suffers from a noticeable onset and remission of major depression at very specific times of the year, with the onset usually occurring during the fall and winter seasons and lifting in spring and summer. This condition becomes a "disorder" when a person experiences at least three episodes of this type of major depression within a five-year period. Four times more women than men suffer from seasonal affective disorder, and it most frequently occurs in individuals with bipolar II illness, or with a family history of depression or alcoholism. The symptoms of this disorder include sadness, decreased activity, interpersonal difficulties, anxiety, work problems, irritability, weight gain, increased appetite, a craving for carbohydrates, drowsiness, decreased sex drive, and menstrual difficulties. One of the interesting characteristics of these individuals is that they will often find that they are "light seekers," especially during dark winter days. Usually, if they go on vacation to a very sunny area, they feel better quickly. Seasonal affective disorder appears to respond nicely to bright artificial light given for about an hour a day, typically in the early morning. Many companies sell light boxes capable of providing 10,000 lux at 3 feet for use for about one hour each morning during the dark seasons; this is often as effective as an antidepressant for these individuals.

REFRACTORY DEPRESSION

There is a lack of consensus agreement in much of the research literature in the psychiatric field about how to actually define refractory depression. The term *refractory* means that the depression is not responding to the usual treatments, and there are many possible reasons for this. Many experts say that refractory depression consists of a combination of biological depression and personality factors that inhibit the satisfactory enjoyment of life and relationships, often complicated by substance abuse and chronic stressful situations in one's life. When medication is prescribed for this condition, the most frequent causes of a lack of response are an inadequate dosage and duration of treatment, and the complicating effects of substance abuse.

When psychiatrists say that a person is not responding to an antidepressant, this might mean many things. There may be either no improvement of symptoms or only partial improvement; improvement, but with intolerable side effects; short-term improvement followed by recurrence of symptoms; or improvement of the symptoms in a person who still feels quite miserable about his or her life circumstances. Refractory depression always requires a careful rethinking of the diagnosis; a very careful look at all the treatment options that have been tried and those that have not been tried, including dose, duration, and response of each medication trial, and whether these were done at a time when the person was clean and sober; and reconsideration of medical and substance abuse issues.

The psychosocial issues of refractory depression are best addressed by meeting with an individual's family or significant others. It is always helpful to spend some time with these individuals and to obtain their perspective on any history of substance abuse, mania, or suicidal statements that the patient might have made. Those who are close to the patient and have seen him at his best and his worst will also be able to give a valuable description of the patient's level of functioning or impairment when he is both well and ill, in addition to the client's illness behaviors and family expectations. For example, the family may describe a normally energetic, hard-working individual who just lies in bed when depressed, and expect that person to return to full functioning. On the other hand, a person who is barely coping with minimal stressors and is chronically unemployed might not be expected to do much more when her depression clears.

When a patient is extremely depressed, nonfunctioning, and not responding well to outpatient treatment, a psychiatrist might consider carefully discussing the patient's option of being declared legally disabled. Obtaining temporary permission to be in a sick role and be freed from one's overwhelming responsibilities and life stresses might be justified in cases where the "time out" for disability is limited in duration, and the patient agrees to use the time to make some meaningful life changes. Assuming a sick role is not appropriate for everyone, however. Labeling oneself as disabled, albeit only on a temporary basis, may take away a major source of self-esteem in very achievement-oriented individuals and cause more problems and sense of failure than it is worth.

A psychotherapist might sometimes encourage a patient to request medical disability during times of very intense regressive work with traumatic early childhood memories. Assuming this role might lead an individual to move from functioning at his or her home and work responsibilities to being frequently hospitalized in the service of doing intensive psychotherapy. This kind of regression work is very controversial, yet psychotherapy is sometimes practiced in this way by individuals whose ambition is to resolve early life traumas at the expense of everyday functioning. I favor a slower working through of painful memories at a rate that the patient can tolerate without falling apart in terms of facing "here and now" responsibilities.

Situations that might potentially encourage a condition of refractory depression might include a family that rewards regression and dependence, a lawsuit arising out of an injury or worker's compensation case, or any other situation where there is a societal message that getting well will involve potential loss of the benefits of being sick. Some examples of the latter are an individual who is stressed and harassed at work, gets depressed, and then is advised by her attorney not to resume working until a lawsuit against her employer is resolved. The lawyer must advise her that a large judgment against the employer is more likely if the person is disabled for a long time and requires very extensive therapy, thus discouraging her from getting well.

ELECTROCONVULSIVE THERAPY (ECT)

Electroconvulsive therapy (shock treatment) is still very much a part of the psychiatrist's armament in the treatment of severe depression. Usually it is reserved for patients who are psychotic (hallucinating or delusional), suicidal, nonresponsive to medications, or who have done well with it in the past after failing medication trials. ECT is done under general anesthesia and typically a course of treatments involves six to twelve sessions over a period of two to four weeks. The most common complaint is poor memory for the time period of getting the treatments and a few weeks before and after. Unilateral electrode placement over the half of the brain that is not dominant for speech minimizes the memory complaints.

George: A man suffering from a serious single episode of major depression

George was a forty-seven-year-old attorney who came to me for treatment of depression. He had been married (for the first time) for four years and was concerned because he was experiencing attacks of rage that he either internalized or acted out in front of his wife. George had only experienced minimal, mild problems with depression up until two years ago when his mother had died after a chronic illness involving repeated minor strokes, congestive heart failure, blood clots, almost debilitating arthritis, diabetes, and high blood pressure. Being around her during her final months had taken a terrible emotional toll on George and, in the two years following her death, he had been constantly depressed, although he did remember one happy, relaxed period when he and his wife took a vacation in Russia.

Although George felt that he had a good relationship with his mother, he felt guilty that he hadn't spent more time with her and hadn't given her more attention or appreciation. Because his mother had never believed in funerals, she insisted that she not have one. George felt very strongly that this had prevented him from reaching some kind of closure about her death. George's living relatives include a father, a brother with whom he shares his home, a full sister, and a half-sister. Although his blood family pulled together around the time of his mother's death to give one another support, afterward George was only able to talk about his feelings a little bit with his wife. Since then, he told me, he had experienced feelings of rage over minor, inappropriate things, and suffered from crying jags, uncontrollable fatigue, and listlessness. He felt no enthusiasm for anything and took little pleasure out of life.

When I gave George a standard Seventeen-item Hamilton Depression Rating test, it showed that he was depressed about 75 percent of the time, had some guilt, repetitively replayed past events in his mind, and had feelings that he had let people down. Although he wished that he were dead, he had never attempted suicide, never made a suicide plan, and admitted that any ideas he might have about killing himself were very vague and not really serious. George typically fell asleep five to ten minutes after he got into bed, but woke up around two or three in the morning in a cold sweat, sometimes getting up to watch TV when he couldn't get back to sleep. He also occasionally woke up earlier than his alarm clock. Since this sleeplessness left him feeling lethargic, he was generally slow to get up and get dressed in the morning, and he usually didn't get as much done during the day as before. Even though he had decreased the time that he spent working, he still felt a sense of exhaustion when he got home. George typically brought work home from his office, but then left it in his car and felt guilty about not doing it. During the interview it was apparent to me that George's speech and motor skills were slightly slower than normal.

George said that he felt irritable and worried much of the time, and also had a lot of physical symptoms along with his depression, including upset stomach, diarrhea, dry mouth, sweating when under stress, headaches, and muscle aches. He said, however, that the headaches were neither new nor were they more painful than they had always been. George's appetite hadn't suffered too much. He was still able to feel hungry and sometimes enjoyed food, but he said that he also ate more fatty foods when he was depressed, and had gained 30 or 40 pounds over the last couple of years. George had some concerns about his obesity and his general health because of a family history of heart problems and diabetes.

When I asked him if he ever had panic attacks, he said no. He did feel that his energy level was only 70 percent of normal, and that his sex drive felt less than half as strong as it used to be. In fact, his sexual desire had gone down steadily over the last two years, and had become even worse recently in response to attempts at *in vitro* fertilization in which he had to provide sperm samples on demand at his wife's most fertile time each month. Although George said that he wanted a child, he also feared the possibility he would not be a good parent. He also felt that providing sperm samples for injection was a very unnatural sexual activity, one that made him feel extremely uncomfortable.

He freely admitted that he was depressed, but he experienced no morning to evening pattern of variation, or psychotic symptoms. Although he felt stressed and overwhelmed at times, he had no paranoid symptoms nor any compulsive behaviors. His only obsessional thought was that at some point he might scream at a judge or his opposing counsel in court.

When I asked George if there was any seasonal pattern to his depression, he admitted that he felt worse around Christmas for a few weeks and said that this had been going on for a very long time. George felt good about the fact that he was still able to enjoy a few of the things he did in his spare time, such as going out for dinner with friends and going to a gem and mineral show recently. When asked why he was seeking help, however, he said his depression was worsening and he felt that he had to do something because it was affecting his marriage. When I asked George to describe himself, he said introverted, introspective, and insecure. When I asked his wife how he was before his depression, she said that he was wonderful, happy, loving, and supportive.

Diagnosis and Treatment Recommendations: I diagnosed George with a single episode of moderately severe major depression, most likely set off by the issues generated by his mother's death. I felt that medication would help him. One of the factors that led me to the conclusion that drug therapy was called for in his case was George's Seventeen-item Hamilton Depression Rating Scale. This score was 23, five points above the cutoff of 18 that usually signifies that antidepressant medication should be administered. I suggested that George take an antidepressant; when I asked him what the qualities of his ideal medication would be, he said that he would like a medicine that would give him more energy and enthusiasm and bring an end to the periods when he was in a low mood. I told him that Prozac or Wellbutrin were my first choices because they had the potential side effect of weight loss rather than weight gain.

In addition, I strongly recommended that George consider some psychotherapy and possibly a support group to help him deal with his unresolved grief issues around his mother's death. I also suggested that he seriously consider beginning a regular exercise program to get some stress relief and to help him begin controlling weight.

When I mentioned stress relief, George was quick to confess that he experienced a great deal of stress as an attorney because no matter how well he prepared a case and how good or bad the case might be in terms of facts, he didn't ultimately have control over the outcome. For this reason, he had become very demanding of himself and had developed a tendency to beat himself up. After realizing during the course of our discussion that he had no outlet for his stress, George came up with the idea that he might try learning a craft or a hobby. I strongly encouraged him in this.

I also provided George with some moral support in confronting his assumptions that mental illness is a weakness or that he could choose to not be depressed. He will obviously continue to need some support in this area.

Five months later, I took stock of George's progress. Over the course of twice-monthly therapy, he had shown a prompt response to Prozac, and we had been able to adjust his dosage to a point that was optimal for him, 40 mg/day. George had also been able to talk about some of the stress he experienced in his office. In spite of the fact that he had many employees, he did not feel that he was getting the organizational help, quality paperwork, or team effort that he needed from them. To alleviate the situation, he eventually decided to fire one office worker and spend more time learning how to talk to and train the others, describing what he needed from them. In addition, he found ways to become less angry when tense situations arose.

He and his wife also discussed a restructuring of their financial priorities—whether they were happy with him working more hours and making more money versus working less and being at home more. By this time, his wife had become pregnant and they were confident that she would be able to carry the child to term because she had passed the three-month period, so issues of how much he was going to be at home and help her with the baby had also arisen. From this need to rebalance his home time with his work time, George began to learn that it was okay to say no to clients, and filed motions to get out of representing clients who abused his time, made great demands, and did not pay their bills. He also started to realize that it was all right to refer clients to other attorneys if he did not really want to work with them. When he made these changes, he began to experience a sense of control and challenge in his work and personal life and no longer felt like dying.

Conclusion: As George's depression began to clear, he was finally able to process the issues in therapy that were major stresses for him. Increased assertiveness and less fear of displeasing others are common personality changes that people on SSRIs or other antidepressants often notice. This newfound courage can be life transforming, as the need to please others and avoid rejection becomes less central, and the person can begin to take care of herself emotionally.

Jane: Double depression—when major depression is superimposed on a dysthymic disorder

Jane is a thirty-seven-year-old psychotherapist who came to me complaining of serious depression. She told me she began getting depressed at the age of thirty. When I asked her if she had experienced any significant substance abuse or major medical illnesses at that time, she said that the only two precipitating events she could think of might have been the breakup of another of a series of dysfunctional love relationships and the stress of failing part of her licensing exam. Jane confessed that her inability to find a good relationship and get married in the last three years had made her fear that she was socially deficient.

When I asked her about her current feelings, she said that she felt as if she were a "black hole" filled with negative thoughts. Even though her life was going well and her therapy was helping her, she was concerned about being so depressed most of the time. In spite of the fact that she was very busy with leisure activities that included shopping, taking care of her home, cooking, theater, and movies, and was excited that she had begun dating a new person she met through a singles group, she still felt unhappy at times. She said she felt somewhat isolated socially and that she didn't really experience a sense of community in the California area.

When I asked Jane if she had taken any kind of medication in the past, she told me she had tried several over the last three years. Although Desyrel made her feel slightly better after she had taken it for three weeks, she developed inner ear problems. When she took Desipramine, she could only tolerate it for a week because it made her feel tired, fuzzy, and unable to function. She tried taking 20 mg of Prozac for a few days, but felt sedated and experienced decreased concentration and memory problems. When she took Xanax for a few days, she felt slightly worse than she did on the other drugs. Although she was able to take Nardil for a slightly longer period than the other drugs, at a dose of two or three pills per day, she felt no benefits from it. She also tried BuSpar for awhile but was unaware of whether it had helped her. I was not surprised at these results, since her medication trials were extremely sporadic. She had never had a regular long-term psychiatrist working with her. As we have seen, all of these medications take more than a week to give a person beneficial results.

When I asked Jane to tell me about her medical history, the only major condition she could remember was measles encephalitis at age three. She did say that her mother had been very preoccupied with her weight and had started putting her on diets at age seven. Jane's weight went up to 160 pounds in her teens, but she was able to get down to 120 pounds by the end of college, with no bingeing, purging, or anorexia.

Jane told me that her periods of depression had been with her a long time. During her worst bout, approximately three years ago, she had stayed in bed all day on weekends. If she went to work, she would often find herself falling asleep there. Her appetite increased and her weight went up about 10 pounds in six weeks. During this time, Jane remembered having no energy or sex drive, and decreased concentration. Her moods always seemed to get worse in the evenings, as well as her ability to respond emotionally to people and events around her. Although she felt worthless, she did not have any delusions of sin, evil, or guilt; nor did she have any auditory, visual, taste, touch, or smell hallucinations. She felt physically ill during much of this time and had recurrent ear infections.

Her current feelings of being a "black hole" intensify on the weekends when all her negative thoughts come to the surface. During such periods she feels tired, bored, and lonely; overeats; questions whether she should stay in this area or move; and spends a lot of time thinking of herself as "fat and ugly" and unlikable. When I asked her to describe herself, these negative images surfaced as she described her personality as having a "shitty, rigid, uncomfortable, forced quality."

An important life area that Jane is working on is learning to be single, not dependent, helpless, or reactive. Her current sadness is intensified the day before the start of her menstrual period, when she finds herself crying and generally feeling in a very bad mood.

Diagnosis and Initial Treatment Recommendations: It seemed clear to me that Jane was suffering from what is called "double depression," a major depressive episode superimposed on an already existing dysthymic disorder. Although at the time I chose to defer my diagnosis of her personality until I had more information, I could see that Jane had very chronic and significant self-esteem issues.

Because of the need for a medication that would neither sedate her nor cause her to gain weight, I suggested that Jane try Wellbutrin, beginning at a very low dose of 100 mg/day and gradually working up to 100 mg three times per day. If she could not tolerate this drug, my next choice was another try with a very low dose of Prozac, approximately one-third capsule daily with a gradual increase in dosage. I asked Jane to return in about two weeks.

By the second visit, she was doing well on 100 mg of Wellbutrin per day, with no discernible side effects. Her appetite was down and her mood was good, with no recurrence of black holes. She did have one migraine that necessitated an emergency room visit, a condition that recurs with her about every two months, but she experienced no PMS that month. She also told me that she was seeking a boyfriend with "mind and substance."

Unfortunately, even though Jane seemed to be making good progress on Wellbutrin, the following month she decided that she didn't feel good on the drug and that it was making her migraines worse. I lost track of her at that point because she decided not to come back for any follow-up visits.

Reevaluation—Two Years Later: A little over two years later, Jane returned to my office saying she had once again become depressed and felt she needed some kind of antidepressant medication. During the last two years she had continued to work at the hospital half-time, and had also developed a private practice with a group of psychologists and a psychiatrist that she found very enjoyable.

During this time, she had become involved in a serious relationship, which quickly led to her and her new partner living together with the expectation that this arrangement would result in marriage. After a time, however, she said they both came to realize that the relationship was neither suitable nor appropriate for them and wasn't working out well. Jane told me one day her boyfriend suddenly announced, out of the blue, that he had decided to move out of their home. She was distressed that he hadn't even bothered to talk this decision over with her, but admitted that this was a pattern with him. He often made decisions without consulting her. The excuse he gave her initially for wanting to end the relationship was an allergy to her cats, but he subsequently confessed that his feelings had changed about the relationship.

Although Jane had remained in psychotherapy and indicated that her therapy was going well, it was clear that something serious was amiss in her life. She was quite rational about the fact that her relationship hadn't worked out and that she wanted to get on with her life, but she was very depressed and had significant emotional problems. A certain emotional lethargy was creeping over her life. She told me she didn't want to get out of bed in the morning, didn't want to go to the gym, didn't care about her practice anymore, and felt as if she had no friends. The reason she gave for deciding to try antidepressant medication again was a conversation she had with one of her clients. He had told her that shortly after he started taking antidepressants, his mood had changed dramatically.

Jane described her present mood as "like crap." Her lowest times of depression were now coming in the mornings, the opposite pattern from the last time I had seen her. When I asked her to describe her current symptoms, she said that her sleeping patterns were "a mess," and that her rest was fitful and fretful, with frequent times of awakening. She had begun to use food to self-medicate and had gained 10 pounds. This weight gain might also have been worsened by her decision to quit smoking. She complained of fluctuating energy and was concerned that she had begun to decrease the times she went to her gym. She also said she has experienced some sudden mood shifts into sadness and anger, and premenstrual syndrome. Although she never thought about suicide, she did have a recurring fantasy in which she escaped to the Midwest to work and live near her brother. Her only current medical conditions were her usual migraine headaches and hypothyroidism, both of which were being treated by her family physician.

My overall impression of Jane was that she was an attractive, well-dressed, articulate, intelligent woman. She showed no evidence of hallucinations, delusions, or any psychomotor agitation or slowing. Aside from her depressed feelings, she said her life was really going extremely well, both in her private practice and in her hospital job. She also told me that she was starting to think about dating some other people.

Second Diagnosis and Treatment Recommendation: On this visit I diagnosed Jane with a recurrent major depression of moderate severity. When I asked her what her ideal medication would be, she said she would like a medicine that would lift her overlay of feeling so "junky." Because of her past intolerance of the standard doses of Prozac and the tricyclics, I suggested that she begin on Zoloft at 25 mg/day for about one week and then increase the dose to 50 mg/day, as tolerated.

In a follow-up visit two weeks after beginning the Zoloft, Jane told me that her "inner screaming" was gone, and that her overall mood was better. In her own words, she had gone "halfway from shitty to happy." The only side effect she was experiencing on the current dose of Zoloft was some increased tiredness. When she returned for a visit six weeks later, however, she told me that she had been off the Zoloft for a week, even though the drug had been working for her. Jane told me that she had recently ended a relationship, but continued to emphasize her desire to find someone emotionally available for marriage and to start a family. I could see that this goal was very important to her.

Conclusion: Jane represents a good example of a person who suffers from recurrent depression even though the general context of her life is good—although in Jane's case she felt bad about lacking someone with whom to share her life. Despite her ongoing personal psychotherapy and her excellent coping skills and specific talent for helping other people to deal with their depressions, her condition kept returning. Although Jane's responses to medications were positive and dramatic, her desire to get off the medications quickly put her at risk for more episodes. Jane would certainly have benefited from a long-term preventive medication, but she was unwilling to stick with one, so her depressions always recurred.

Sandra: The "night eater"—a moderately severe single episode of major depression

A thirty-one-year-old woman named Sandra came to me for a consultation. When I asked her to tell me a little bit about her life, she said that she had a career in marketing and public relations, and two children by her current marriage, which had lasted for nine years. Her main complaints were experiencing symptoms of depression and anxiety, and a tendency to eat snacks in the middle of the night. For the last six years she had gone to bed about 10:30 P.M., only to awaken about two hours later, very hungry. At this time she would go into the kitchen and eat a snack of potato chips, toast, or peanuts. I did not really categorize this behavior as an eating disorder, however, because her need to eat wasn't so bad that she went out to the store to buy special things, and she never binged to the point where she felt sick, nor did she feel the need to purge (throw up) afterward.

During her initial visit, Sandra was unable to identify any emotional issues that might have precipitated this eating behavior, such as how she was getting along with her husband at the time, whether they had experienced satisfying sexual relations, or how her workday had gone. Although the amount of food she ate each night was only equivalent to a normal snack, she spent a great deal of time thinking and worrying about how this habit was ridiculous and out of control, beyond her ability to stop it. She was also worried because her weight had increased about 10 pounds over the last year.

As mentioned above, when I asked Sandra questions that might shed some light on whether she had an eating disorder, she didn't seem to fall readily into that category. She didn't use laxatives, diuretics, or diet pills, nor had she ever had a period of severe weight loss. She was 60 pounds overweight at about age thirteen but went to Weight Watchers and was pleased about losing the weight in a healthy way. Each time she was pregnant she gained 50 or 60 pounds, but she was also able to lose that weight in a normal fashion. Her regular dinnertime is around 5:30 or 6:00 P.M. and is shared with her husband and two children, as well as the husband's grandmother who lives in the household and takes care of the children five days a week. All of Sandra's meals are very well balanced and she always ate a normal breakfast and lunch.

Sandra told me that her current depression had lasted about a year and a half. She felt that part of the reason for it was her husband's long-term unemployment on two separate occasions. When he did work, he had a position on-site doing construction management. Another factor that had contributed to her depression in the past year was her disappointment at being passed over for promotion by the insurance company she had worked at for fourteen years.

Over the past year, Sandra had been depressed about 70 percent of the time. Although she was able to fall asleep without difficulty, her sleep was interrupted and she felt tired in the mornings, which were also her most intense times of depression. Her other symptoms included an increase in appetite and a decrease in energy to the point where it was hard for her to go to the gym. Even when she felt unhappy, however, she told me that she tended to just tune out her feelings and keep going on. Her most important symptom, she said, was her inability to enjoy things (anhedonia) and a feeling that she was just going through the motions of living. She was able to concentrate most of the time, but sometimes she caught her mind drifting a little, although she was still able to make decisions. She experienced decreased reactivity, could not be cheered up, and was more sensitive and tearful two days before her menstruation, although she had never had any suicidal thoughts.

On the plus side, Sandra had no panic attacks or history of auditory, visual, taste, touch, or smell hallucinations. Her only obsession was her nighttime eating, and she confessed that she sometimes felt a compulsion to keep busy. Other times, she felt anxious, immobilized, stuck, and had a tendency to startle easily. Her chronic eczema had flared up again lately, and she had begun to feel a sense of impending doom, as if something bad was going to happen.

When I asked her if anyone else in her family had ever shown any psychiatric symptoms, Sandra said that her mother had received behavioral treatment for agoraphobia, but that she did not know if her mother's condition had ever been accompanied by panic attacks. To her knowledge, no one else in her family had ever had any psychiatric problems.

Aside from her job and her worry about her nighttime eating, another major area of stress in the past year involved Sandra's marriage. Last summer she had asked her husband to leave because she found out that he was maintaining contact with his former girlfriend. Sandra had discovered a résumé her husband had written for this woman on his computer, and noticed that the ex-girlfriend's phone number was on their phone bill. These incidents had made Sandra afraid that he was still emotionally connected to the girlfriend. After a one-week separation, however, Sandra and her husband reconciled, and their relationship had been getting better. Something that contributed to the improvement of their relationship was the fact that he was working steadily. A remaining tension in their marriage is the presence of her husband's grandmother who lives with them and helps take care of the children five days a week. Usually, Sandra appreciates this, but occasionally there are problems, such as differing parenting styles.

When I asked Sandra to describe herself, she said she was busy, witty, tough, and responsible, although she had a tendency to avoid things. She thought her husband would describe her as independent, strong, stubborn, and someone who could live without him even though she didn't want to do so.

Diagnosis and Recommended Treatment: I diagnosed Sandra with a single, moderately severe episode of major depression, along with a slight eating disorder. Her major life stressors clearly circle around her marriage and her job difficulties.

When I asked Sandra what she would like to have from psychotherapy, she said that she wanted to be able to feel more, and we agreed to weekly sessions together. She also wanted me to prescribe a medication for her that would help her to feel calmer and less anxious. I gave her a prescription for Prozac with instructions to take 10 mg daily for the first week and then to work her dosage up by about 10 mg each week until she started feeling better or her side effects became bothersome. I also suggested that she take 2 mg of diazepam, one or two daily as needed for anxiety.

A month later, Sandra was taking approximately 20 mg/day of Prozac and doing very well with it. She was so pleased with her improvement on the drug that at one point she shared a fear with me that I'd take it away from her. I reassured her, pointing out that staying on the drug was really her decision.

Sandra opened up about her life quite a bit over the next month, and during those visits voiced her concern about the absence of intimacy in her marriage and the lack of cooperation her husband gave her in dealing with their son's problems. She also felt her husband did not listen to her needs, using as an example the time when she had told him that she was unwilling to consider moving only to find out that he had gone ahead anyway and made an appointment for a realtor to take them house-hunting. She commented repeatedly on how negative her husband was about her psychotherapy sessions, and how he resisted her suggestion that they might benefit from psychotherapy as a couple.

During this session, after telling me this story, Sandra confessed that it was easy and familiar for her to give away her power because she hated conflict so much. She also admitted that she felt sorry for herself, never seeing herself as someone deserving of a break or help. She told me that she saw me as the wise doctor who might be able to assist her.

On the plus side, Sandra had begun actively dealing with the dissatisfactions she feels in her life, especially those that center around her job and her family. She confessed that raising her children was stressful at times, and that she might have to set some priorities. She felt that she was always putting others first, juggling others' demands with her own and trying to fix everything, not taking enough time to acknowledge her own feelings and needs.

For the first time, she admitted that she had recently envisioned life without her husband. Far from alarming her, this idea had given her a sense of peaceful relief, as if a burden had been lifted. In the past, she has always felt responsible for the fact that he is miserable, unhappy, and never has fun. When she tried to talk to him about her feelings, he would either give lip service to her needs or act as if he didn't understand them.

Two months later, Sandra told me that she had finally asked her husband to consider moving out and paying some child support. She had finally accepted the fact that he was never going to be responsive to her emotional needs, or ever be a partner either sexually or in caring for their children. Sandra has been taking 40 to 50 mg/day of Prozac, and handling her stress well with it.

Five weeks later, when her husband was demoted and subsequently quit his job, she came right out and told him that she couldn't support him through another period of prolonged unemployment and that she wanted a divorce. Two months later, in March, when her husband had finally moved out, Sandra felt no dramatic sense of relief, but was sure that she had made the right decision, even though she was disappointed to be getting only minimal child support.

When I saw her in August, Sandra said she and the children were doing remarkably well. She had begun seeing a man she was attracted to at work, but had pulled back from the relationship because she suspected that he drank too much. She also observed that he was not very interested in her children. Her kids were having no problems with the divorce, and were feeling alright about only seeing their father part-time.

Sandra had gone off Prozac abruptly a couple of months earlier and had felt fine for a brief time, but had become much more depressed again. Although she had been reluctant to call me back to resume therapy and medication because of financial considerations, she felt a rapid sense of relief when she did so and began taking Prozac again. When she asked me if we could do only low-intensity therapy, I told her that was acceptable.

By mid-January of the following year, Sandra was experiencing a feeling of loneliness and a lack of supportive nurturing since she had been single for a year, but also a new sense of strength and self-reliance in her career and child rearing.

Conclusion: Sandra's mysterious desire to get up and eat in the middle of the night served as a "ticket of admission" to therapy for her need to deal with the long-standing stressors she felt in her marriage. At the start of her treatment, she was depressed and not ready to admit that these things were bothering her so intensely. Her depression rapidly responded to Prozac, however, and once her emotions leveled off, her marital issues came into clear perspective. She was able to feel brave enough to confront her husband, tell him what she wanted and needed, and finally ask him to leave after she put a major effort into trying to improve their relationship.

Martha: A highly refractory case of major depression

I had a consultation with a forty-four-year-old, single, psychiatrically disabled woman named Martha. Martha was well known to me from numerous admissions to our nearby medical center over the last two years. She had a very long history of depression that dated back to her college years, but she had recently done extremely well with maintenance electroconvulsive therapy (ECT) on an outpatient basis. She had tried numerous antidepressant medications and lithium over the years without long-term benefit. Martha told me that her current medications included one 20 mg tablet of Prozac daily, two 50 mg tablets of doxepin at bedtime, and 1 mg of Klonopin three times a day, although she said she did not feel any different on Klonopin than she did when taking Valium, which was much less expensive for her. The medications were given in a long-term effort to decrease the frequency of recurrences, and were only partly successful. She had briefly used Ritalin in the past, one or two tablets a day for one or two days at a time. Although she felt rather sleepy and somewhat nauseous on it, it did help her to make it through some depressed days.

When I asked Martha about her medical history, she said that her menstrual periods had gotten irregular, falling at about one to one and a half month intervals. Sometimes she would stop menstruating for awhile, only to have her periods resume after she received an ECT treatment.

Martha has had three separate long-term lithium trials in combination with some tricyclic antidepressants. Although two of these lithium trials went on for at least a year, they were not helpful. For a couple of months, she responded positively to Wellbutrin, but then it stopped working. The same was true of Prozac. When Martha went off these medicines and then restarted them, however, she did feel better for awhile. She tried three different MAO inhibitors in the 1970s without a response.

Diagnosis and Treatment Recommendations: Martha had a case of major depression that is highly refractory; that is, resistant to treatment. I suggested that she continue to take 20 mg of Prozac once per day, but that she substitute 10 mg of diazepam, one to three times per day, for the Klonopin. I initiated a comprehensive hormonal evaluation to check for early menopause or pituitary tumor, but found no significant abnormalities.

Conclusion: Martha asked if she could see me on an outpatient basis in my private practice for medication maintenance, and I agreed. She will also work with another doctor for inpatient bilateral ECT at our medical center when this is necessary. Martha repeatedly told me that, in the past, other doctors had refused to listen to her when she said she only needed one or two ECT treatments when her depression became unbearably intense. Over her protests, other psychiatrists had insisted on a full course of six to eight treatments, which, she said, had never kept her well for a longer period of time than one or two treatments. She told me that when she could enter the hospital and have one, or occasionally two, treatments, she would feel much improved and could go home shortly thereafter. We worked out a good balance with her where we used medications for the long term and ECT treatments occasionally. In this way, Martha was able to improve greatly, and she and her family repeatedly thanked all of us involved for giving her a good several years and helping to keep her alive despite her sometimes unbearably intense depressions. Martha has often told me that if I ever needed anyone to talk with a potential patient who is reluctant to accept a recommendation for ECT, she would volunteer.

Carolyn: Recurrent major depression with psychotic features

Carolyn is a twenty-nine-year-old third-year medical student who has been married for four years and has no children. When I first saw her, her husband and parents came with her to the interview. Carolyn told me she would be meeting with her school's dean the following day and that she needed a psychiatric evaluation and medication in order to return to school. Although she had taken antidepressants on and off for a few weeks at a time, her family really doesn't believe that they were necessary. With their support, she resisted taking them because she really didn't want to be on them.

Although Carolyn had been born in the Mideast, the family moved to England when she was a year old and to Southern California when she was nine. She graduated college at age twenty-one, and had no psychiatric problems throughout high school and college. In 1991, she started medical school on the East Coast, but left after only one year so that she could marry her husband. During that year she felt very depressed, missed classes, and had difficulty studying. Other problems included frequent crying, oversleeping, decreased appetite, and a waning interest in activities. When she spoke with someone in the psychiatry department in Boston, they told her that she should receive psychotherapy and medications, but she refused to do so, fearing the stigma attached to someone who needed this kind of help.

She was delighted to be accepted for transfer to a local medical school, but realized once she got there that she needed to make up a course in neuroanatomy. She told me she "cracked a couple of years ago." She began feeling she was overdoing the studying for her classes, yet she couldn't stop herself; and although she took extremely meticulous notes, she became fearful about failing. Her husband tried to convince her to just get through the year, but she was having great difficulties functioning and found herself crying all the time.

That spring she began to see a psychologist and a psychiatrist. They both encouraged her to take medicines, but she clung to what she called "my stupid ideals of no medication" and never actually took the drugs they prescribed for her. She had another episode of depression a year later in the spring of the following year, at the end of her second year at medical school. Fortunately, she had managed to pass all her classes except one, and even achieved honors in one. Although she felt she wouldn't be able to pass her medical board exams, she came close on her first try, took a review course, and passed on her second try.

A family doctor gave her Xanax, which relieved some of her tension and helped her get to sleep, but she only took it for a few nights. She had no memory problems from it, yet she blamed it for making her fail a class exam.

Carolyn confessed that she had a great fear of things being much more difficult for her than they actually turned out to be, and that her faculty always had to give her a great deal of reassurance. Because of this fear, she spent a year in research, partly out of interest and partly as a break before she began her clinical training. During that year, she felt her coworkers were not cooperating with her and were giving her difficulty.

When she began her third-year hospital rotations, she again had a sense they would be much more difficult than they actually were, although she continued to receive great encouragement from the faculty to offset her fear of failing. In fact, by the time of our first meeting, she had passed two rotations and would probably pass her third, although she hadn't yet received her evaluation there.

Carolyn told me she felt as if her coworkers were not teaching her properly and were misguiding her, and that the faculty had labeled her as doing poorly. She was also having trouble in surgery, where she had difficulty understanding things because of her illness and her lack of confidence in herself. When she asked questions in front of patients, however, she was told that she should stop doing this because it was undermining the confidence patients had in the treating physicians. One of her mentors had told her there were concerns about her performance, and she had told him about her depression problems. After confessing this, she felt as if she had been forced to see a psychiatrist and psychologist.

At this time, Carolyn had begun taking medications again. About eight weeks ago she had started taking Zoloft, but stopped after only a few days because it gave her the shakes. When she started taking Paxil, her husband said that she slept better and seemed much brighter. Carolyn also said that Paxil made her feel calmer, less irritable, and more energetic. She stopped it after five days, however, because it made her forgetful and gave her diarrhea, nausea, headaches, insomnia, and some muscular tremors.

Carolyn did much better when she resumed Paxil. She began taking a dose of 20 mg for about three weeks. She then cut the dose to 10 mg and stayed on it another month. She felt good on the Paxil, got a lot of sleep, felt calmer and less irritable, and found that both her memory and her concentration were better. She experienced some tremors while taking 20 mg daily, but got rid of that side effect on a 10 mg daily dose. Nevertheless, when she had trouble trying to remember a phone number, she used this as an excuse to stop taking Paxil.

This was unfortunate because her husband said she was doing much better on the drug and seemed to go downhill after she stopped it.

When I asked Carolyn to describe herself, she said she was usually worried, that sometimes she was mellow, and that other times she panicked inappropriately. Her husband described her as someone who worried and cried for no reason. Her father was somewhat protective of her, stating that all his kids were good and that there was nothing wrong with any of them. He said that crying and worrying were normal; he had experienced those emotions many times during his own career, and thought they were part of immigrating and being a member of a minority group.

Diagnosis and Recommended Treatment: Carolyn is suffering from recurrent major depression. Because she had a response to serotonin antidepressant medications but was sensitive to side effects, I suggested that she use Prozac liquid at a strength of 20 mg per 5 ml. I asked her to start with just 1 milliliter (4 mg)/day for the first week or two, and then to see if she could work up to 2 milliliters the next week and then 3 milliliters the following week. I told her that this would allow her to work up to the dose that was best for her based on both her response and the side effects.

When I saw Carolyn one month later, her condition had worsened. She had become paranoid about water, refusing to drink it, and was concerned that people had been putting some kind of drug in the food she ate at her home and at her parents' home where she was now staying. The reason she gave for this belief was that someone had been trying to get her to drop out of medical school. Now, she said, they intended to kill her. She told me she thought the drug in her food was a slow neurotoxin that would impair her memory and coordination. She didn't know why she had been singled out for this but thought it might relate to her being a nonwhite woman who was not on a scholarship, claiming that white people with psychological problems would never have been treated like this.

I told Carolyn that her fear of being poisoned was an indication that she needed antipsychotic treatment, and I strongly suggested a low dose of Risperdal. Even though Carolyn refused to accept the prescription, her husband asked me to write it anyway. I felt I couldn't go against her wishes, but I told her if she decided she'd be willing to take the drug to call me, and that I would phone it in to the pharmacy for her.

Although Carolyn was organized and cohesive, her thinking had taken a definite paranoid turn. She told me that she could not resume her clinical rotations unless she had a letter saying that she was under my care and able to go back to school. I thought that she would have a difficult time doing so, but told her I would consider it. At this point, she clearly had paranoid delusions so I rediagnosed her with major depression with psychotic features.

When I saw Carolyn a week later, she was still feeling afraid that she was being experimented on, poisoned, or would be killed. In spite of her obvious need for help, her family told me that she was not taking her medications regularly. I had a serious talk with her and told her that we had reached the point where I had to make a medication decision for her. I said it was vitally important for her to take her medications, and that these must include the antipsychotic drug Risperdal.

When I saw Carolyn two months later, she told me she was eager to meet with the dean and return to school, but she was still reluctant to accept her ongoing need to take an antipsychotic to prevent getting paranoid again. This need became even more apparent when, a few weeks later, she saw me after a trip she and her husband had taken to Hawaii. While there, she had a couple of fights with him because she became convinced that he was communicating secretly with people by gestures; for example, by wiping his lip. She had also become concerned that he was having an affair. In addition to these stresses in her marriage, Carolyn had developed a fear of sex. Since she was married in a civil, not a religious, ceremony, she had begun to believe that it was wrong to have any sex with her husband until they could have a religious ceremony. In spite of this, she told me she still wanted a normal marriage.

About three and a half months later, Carolyn was doing well and was back in school, but still worried that her husband might be having an affair. She was still celibate in her marriage because she hadn't yet had a religious ceremony in addition to the legal one. Her plans for the future were to start applying for residencies and she hoped to have a child during residency. In spite of her resistance to any type of drug, I was able to convince her to keep taking Desyrel 150 mg/day, which had replaced the Prozac as her antidepressant, and Risperdal 1 mg at one-quarter tablet daily.

Conclusion: Unfortunately, despite her obviously high intelligence, Carolyn was never able to develop any insight into her own paranoia. Instead, she remained convinced that no one could see her side of things, that she was being persecuted, and that people were attempting to get her to leave school or to kill her. I felt that simply getting her to stay on an antidepressant rather than complain of side effects to everything she tried was a major accomplishment, and, with encouragement, she was reluctantly willing to take a tiny dose of the antipsychotic that she so desperately needed to allow her to remain in good contact with reality.

She did have a normal desire to be a wife and have children, yet she continued to feel a strong religious prohibition against having sexual relations in her marriage until she could have a religious ceremony. This was an ongoing source of tension between her and her husband, since the official services and celebration would be extremely expensive and elaborate, costing tens of thousands of dollars. At this juncture, I was not so willing to dismiss her concern that her husband might be having an affair simply as a symptom of her paranoia. Under these circumstances, who was to say that the idea of her husband being unfaithful was unthinkable?

Irene: A case of geriatric depression

Irene, an eighty-two-year-old Caucasian woman, came to see me on August 10, 1992, complaining of depression and requesting medication. She had two sons from a marriage that had ended in divorce after eighteen years, and she had never remarried. A creative and active woman, even at her age, she currently worked as an interior decorator and was developing a new business selling painted furniture. Irene was referred to me by a friend from her Alcoholics Anonymous group, which she had been attending for the past two years.

When I asked her to give me a little history that might help me to put her present illness into context, she said that she had taken pep pills, drank, and partied a lot in her forties.

At this time in her life, Irene developed a sense of terrible anxiety and foreboding. She began questioning what life was all about, and lost the desire to do anything. Around the age of forty-eight, she had what sounded like a severe depressive episode. The doctor Irene was seeing at that time treated her with lithium and also with Elavil. Irene said the lithium did not help, and that she was unsure whether the Elavil had made her feel any better. She went to live with a friend who had been involved in doing interior decorating in the desert. That friend took away her pep pills and alcohol, and within a few weeks she felt better than she had in several years, and the depression lifted. Unfortunately, she and her friend were involved in a car collision shortly thereafter. Although Irene was hospitalized for only a few days, her friend was killed.

Irene had no recurrence of any emotional illness from age forty-eight until very recently when she developed her current depression, which began approximately eight months prior. At that time, she had agreed to decorate a large Christmas tree, and had spent two entire months making elaborate ornaments for it. Even though the Christmas tree sold for $1,300, she said that instead of enjoying this work as she usually would, she felt as if it were a real chore and felt very lonely doing it. When she visited her sons in Montana six months later, she felt even more depressed.

At that time, she felt her depression was worsening, although she denied having any manic episodes. She felt frantic and unreal, and told me she could easily understand how people could take their own lives. Her friends told her she looked very pale and shaky.

When I asked Irene to tell me about her current medical history, she said she had leukemia. Fortunately, she did not require any chemotherapy for it and was under the care of Dr. V., who gave her a very good prognosis. This was a kind of leukemia that would allow her to live for a long while, feeling pretty good physically right up to the end. She had tonsillitis as a child, which led to rheumatic fever; bowel disease; and a damaged heart valve that she had to have replaced five years ago, although she does not have to take an anticoagulant drug for that. Over the last six weeks, her internist has had her taking Xanax, at a dose of about one-half tablet three times daily. She was also taking Premarin for sweats, Lanoxin to strengthen her heart's pumping ability, and Vicodin as needed for pain.

Irene has been an active member of AA in the past two years, and has not used any alcohol in the last fifteen years, nor any stimulants in the last several years.

When I asked her to tell me about her family history, Irene remembered that her mother, who was thirty-nine when she was born, would often lie around the house and cry a lot. Both parents were extremely long lived. Irene's father died at age ninety-five and her mother at age eighty-nine. Her parents were devoted to her and gave her a normal, pleasant, happy childhood. She has one sister, aged ninety-four, who is feeble and in a rest home but has no psychiatric problems. She also has a brother, aged eighty-five, who has had no psychiatric problems and is as physically healthy as any thirty-five-year-old.

When I administered a Hamilton Depression Rating Scale, Irene had a score of 17 on the Seventeen-item Ham-D Rating Scale. Usually a score of about 18 is used as a criterion for someone to enter outpatient antidepressant drug treatment. Over the last couple of weeks she had felt depressed 100 percent of the time. Although she was normally hard on herself, and that hadn't changed, she was experiencing other thoughts, feelings, and symptoms that she never had before. She described a sense of terror and confessed that she had thoughts about death, although she didn't have the "courage" to end her life. This death wish was so strong at times that only her religious convictions and her desire not to hurt her family prevented her from killing herself. On the plus side, however, she had no hallucinations, delusions, thought disorder, or cognitive impairment. Irene's sleeping habits were also disturbed. Although she got to sleep easily enough, she frequently woke up at 4:00 A.M. She said the Premarin she was taking had helped her with the sweats.

While she experienced no psychomotor agitation or slowing, she felt as if her energy level was very decreased. Her job had suffered, and she had cut her workweek down from eight hours a day to only ten or twelve hours a week. Her appetite had decreased and sometimes she had to push herself to eat, resulting in the loss of a couple of pounds. When I asked her if there was any change in her sex drive, she said it had been absent for at least ten years. She had no excess worry about physical problems, but she did acknowledge that she was depressed and was seeking treatment for that.

Beneath her depression, Irene seemed a very youthful and energetic person. She looked and sounded at least ten or twenty years younger than her age and was very talkative, bright, and articulate, although she seemed under a certain amount of pressure. She had some financial concerns, but no worries about her health. Most important, she had a strong motivation to get better.

Diagnosis and Treatment Recommendations: I diagnosed Irene with a recurrent major depression of moderate severity, with a history of alcohol and stimulant abuse in long-term remission. She asked if I could give her an antidepressant. Irene had already tried Zoloft, one-half of a 50 mg tablet daily for two or three days, but claimed it made her feel detached, and that she was not able to think clearly. Because of her intolerance for Zoloft, I recommended that she try 25 mg Desipramine once per day, and suggested that she gradually up the dose to six pills per day. If she was unable to tolerate this drug, I told her my second choice would be Wellbutrin. My selection of these medications was based on the fact that she apparently had enjoyed taking stimulants in the past and appeared to be an individual who liked to remain very alert and energetic. These drugs would have that effect on her.

I maintained her dose of 0.25 mg/day of Xanax, but encouraged her to taper off gradually, because of the risk of withdrawal symptoms. I also gave her 7.5 mg tablets of Doral as a sample for sleeping pills. I did not feel that she would benefit from long-term tranquilizers or sleeping pills, especially in light of her previous alcohol addiction.

One Year Later: After my initial evaluation with Irene, she consulted with three other psychiatrists. One year later, Irene returned to me with complaints of terrible anxiety, and a feeling that things were unreal. Her sense of initiative, motivation, and the joy of living were gone, and she was hard pressed to tell me whether her depression or her anxiety was worse. She told me she had developed a dread of aging and felt afraid of death. Although she still had thoughts of suicide, she continued to say that she would never kill herself. I noticed that she had less stamina than before, and she said she had experienced some medical complications since our last visit, including congestive heart failure.

Irene's health had gotten much worse in the last year. She had recently been medically admitted to a major local hospital because of severe confusion and anxiety, with late complications of aortic valve replacement.

When I readministered the Seventeen-item Hamilton Depression Rating Scale test to Irene, her score of 21 again bore out her report of feeling depressed most or all of the time. Irene told me she also spends a lot of time thinking about worrisome things, such as the feeling that she was no longer of any use and was unable to accomplish anything of value. She was losing interest in those things that had given her life meaning—her furniture business, decorating, and gardening—and was again feeling a wish to die, although she had made no suicide attempts or plans.

She showed no signs of psychomotor agitation or slowing, but she had experienced a definite loss of energy, although she was able to sleep well while taking trazodone. Physically, she did not feel well and described several symptoms, including a feeling of tension in her body, occasional palpitations and hot flashes, pain in her left hip and down the side of her left leg, and a swishing sound in her ears accompanied by some hearing difficulties. She didn't care much about eating but did make herself eat, although she had lost 5 pounds. She had no sex drive and reported that her depression was greater in the morning.

She was taking her heart and blood pressure medicines, estrogen, and antianxiety and antidepressant medications. She had failed to respond to Zoloft and Paxil, and was now on Prozac (all SSRIs, serotonin antidepressants).

Diagnosis and Treatment Recommendations: I diagnosed Irene with chronic major depression complicated by medical problems of leukemia and congestive heart failure.

Because she had failed to respond to trials lasting more than a month on two previous SSRI antidepressants, it made no sense to me to give her a prolonged trial on a third SSRI. I explained this to her and suggested that she go ahead and try Wellbutrin.

When we met about six weeks later, Irene and I had to conclude that the Wellbutrin had failed to provide her with any benefits, even when we had tried it with lithium augmentation. As a next step, I suggested she try an MAOI antidepressant, but Irene declined because of her fear of side effects. As an alternative strategy, she agreed to try Pamelor (nortriptyline) along with lithium.

Within three months, Irene was doing much better. Despite the fact that she was now on chemotherapy for her leukemia, she told me she was feeling quite well and that her doom-and-gloom feelings were gone. In mid-April, her cardiologist began to object to the Pamelor because of the risk of it causing irregular or weak heartbeat, so Irene and I decided to try her again on Prozac with Ritalin added. Her miserable feelings returned and we decided she would resume taking Pamelor.

When I saw Irene over the three-month period, she was doing quite well again. The Pamelor, along with a low dose of lithium, had made her feel good enough to do some interior decorating work, and Irene thanked me for the improvement in her mood and quality of life I had helped her to achieve. She was deeply touched when some friends planned a surprise party for her eighty-fifth birthday and eighty-one people showed up. Although she was concerned about failing her driving test at the Department of Motor Vehicles, she planned to protest its decision.

Conclusions: Irene clearly illustrates two basic principles of geriatric psychopharmacology. The first is, clinicians should never simply write off depression as being due to medical problems and age, and assume it is untreatable. In spite of the fact that Irene has two life-threatening illnesses (leukemia and congestive heart failure), the quality of her life improved dramatically on the right antidepressant. The second principle is that it is important for a clinician and a patient to keep trying. If one drug doesn't work, they should try others from different classes. Although Irene experienced no relief on SSRIs and Wellbutrin, no benefit from the stimulant drug Ritalin, and refused to take an MAOI, she finally had an excellent response to taking a tricyclic antidepressant (Pamelor) augmented by lithium.

Michael: A case of geriatric chronic major depression

Michael, an eighty-year-old architect, came to see me. Michael was in his second marriage of nineteen years and had three children who lived on the East Coast. Michael complained of persistent depression and said he was "psychiatrist shopping" in hopes of getting better. When I asked him for a history of his present illness, he told me he had felt down and low for most of his life. Five years ago, however, his emotional condition had worsened after he experienced a medical emergency where he almost blacked out and fell and hit his head. Although the fall caused a subdural hematoma, bleeding on the covering of the brain, it did not require surgery. He subsequently required a right carotid endarterectomy, an operation to unclog the artery in his neck, which was successfully accomplished at a local hospital. The surgery was simple, but Michael's failing health and sense of frailty came into play as he hit bottom, became depressed, and began seeing Dr. D.

Michael was a New York architect for forty-five years. Thirteen years ago, phasing into semiretirement, he came to

California where he became the part-time advisor of graduate studies at a local university. This job required that he go to his office every day from around nine to three, and sometimes his wife worked with him. Although he didn't officially practice in California, he did use his architectural training in his work.

Michael's medical history included the above-mentioned subdural hematoma and an endarterectomy. He also required a pacemaker to regulate his irregular heart rhythm. The pacemaker was inserted three or four years ago, and he has had no problems with it. Aside from these conditions, he has had his prostate gland removed and wears a hearing aid.

When I asked him what kind of medication he was on, Michael told me he took blood pressure medications, lithium, and Prozac.

When I asked Michael to describe his symptoms to me, he said he was irritable, didn't want to get out of bed in the morning, and had an "unusual feeling" in his stomach. His energy level was low, and he was not doing any exercise, but he attributed this to old age, even though he admitted that he had to force himself to do anything. He noticed that he had begun sleeping more than usual and was taking daytime naps. He had experienced no change in appetite, and his concentration was unaffected. He remained able to enjoy activities. Although he had not been sexually active over the past three years, he said that neither he nor his wife had any sexual drive. He said he enjoyed going to musical events and the theater. Even though he had thought about suicide, he said he did not have the "courage" to act on it.

When I asked Michael to help me to piece together the long-term course of his illness, he admitted he had experienced some periods of depression even prior to his accident five years ago, and that these times were becoming more and more numerous over the years. In spite of this, Michael seemed to feel quite good about his accomplishments. He felt he had been quite successful in his work and that he was still quick minded and a good problem solver.

I thought it might shed some light on his condition to understand what kind of work Michael did, so I asked him to describe a typical day to me. For approximately six hours each day, Michael sat in his office, where he basically answered phone calls and took care of letter writing. He was also responsible for writing a monthly newsletter. Recently, he had been assigned an office assistant, but he still did much of his work himself. After he came home from work, he spent his evenings watching television, visiting with friends, and occasionally going out to dinner. Although he was raised Jewish, he didn't have any current synagogue affiliation and only attended High Holy Day services.

When I asked Michael to tell me something about his family history, he said his father was an immigrant who was a furrier and then owned a drugstore. When the businesses did not go well, he committed suicide. Michael described his mother as more educated than his father, although she suffered from periods of hysteria. His brother, younger by three years, came home an invalid after World War II, but subsequently made a career as an attorney. Michael's sister, younger by ten years, suffered at times from depression for which she took antidepressants on and off.

Neither Michael's three children nor his two grandchildren had any psychiatric problems of which he was aware. He seemed to have a good relationship with his children, talking to them often on the phone and going to the East Coast to visit them about once a year.

In the past, Michael had tried some antidepressant medications. About one and a half years ago, he took Pamelor, which he said worked for awhile but stopped having any effect after a few months. He reported that he never got blood levels assessed to check if the dosage was ideal. Next, his doctor tried him on Prozac alone, at a dose of one tablet per day, but Michael said that he felt sedated on that dosage. When the Prozac was augmented with lithium in the spring of 1992, this combination had no effect on his depression and he initially felt even more sedated. The only other drug he was currently using was Ativan to help him sleep.

When I asked him if he had any marital issues, Michael said his marriage was going well. He also told me he had divorced his first wife to marry his present one, who was then a widow working for him as his secretary. Although his wife treated him well, he also said that he enjoyed being away from her sometimes for business meetings in Orlando because he enjoyed the challenge of his work.

Diagnosis and Treatment Recommendations: I found Michael's mental state to be very bright, alert, well oriented, and cooperative with no evidence of hallucinations, delusions, thought disorders, or psychomotor agitation or slowing. In spite of this, it was clear to me he was suffering from a chronic major depression, although he showed no evidence of psychotic features.

I explained to Michael that it would be both important and helpful to me if he would question his siblings in detail about any past medication trials they may have had to determine if any of the drugs they had taken were beneficial to them. I explained to him that we had several choices in terms of energizing antidepressants, but that because of his significant cardiac history, my recommendations would be as follows. First I suggested that we do a trial on Wellbutrin because this was among the safest for his heart of all the available antidepressants. My second choice would be a trial on desipramine, while monitoring his blood levels. If that failed, I would suggest he try a high dose of BuSpar. My fourth choice would be for Michael to take an energizing MAOI such as Parnate. All of these drugs shared the qualities of being nonsedating with very minimal heart toxicity. I explained to him that there was a very slight risk of seizures with Wellbutrin, but, in spite of this, he agreed to stop his Prozac and start taking Wellbutrin.

When I saw Michael two and a half weeks later, he was off the lithium, was taking 300 mg of Wellbutrin per day, and felt that "a miracle had happened." He told me he felt great, in spite of the fact that he had slight transient memory problems, and felt a little spacey, scatterbrained, and light-headed. He was talking and joking more with his wife and had gone on a business trip and thoroughly enjoyed it. Although he had developed a bad headache after a glass of wine, he said that drinking hard liquor was less likely to cause this. Michael had talked to his siblings about their medications and gathered as much information as he could. He said his brother was on Elavil, was not helped by it, and found Prozac even less helpful, and his sister had said she got beneficial results from a low dose of Sinequan and used Xanax for sleep.

Michael's wife came into my office during this session and commented on how much more talkative and interactive her husband had been in the last two and a half weeks. She said he had been waking up earlier, and that his general mood was more agreeable. Both asked me if I thought Michael needed psychotherapy. Since he was generally happy with life and not feeling the need for anything else, I said it was okay for him to just take the medications. I also suggested that we experiment with Wellbutrin at a slightly lower dose to try to decrease the side effects.

A month later, Michael was still doing very well. He had enjoyed going to a convention in Orlando that he and two assistants ran, had coped with hassles with his hotel there, and dealt with a new young president of his group who didn't respect his seniority and experience. Now he was back and ready for cataract surgery the next day. Michael felt that the three to four 75 mg tablets per day of Wellbutrin were working far better than the Prozac and lithium he had taken in the past. Although he did have some upset stomach and constipation, he felt those symptoms were much easier to live with than his depression. I suggested he continue with his current medications. He had a new hearing aid and a pacemaker, and joked about being kept alive and going strong by high-tech medicine and a busy life.

Nine months later when I saw him, Michael and his wife were weathering some difficulties in the marriage. His wife had told him she felt like an unappreciated housekeeper, and he felt she was constantly telling him what to do. Lately, nothing they had done together seemed to give them any pleasure. When he asked me for some insight, I said he seemed to have a fear of dependency, especially since he had experienced so many illnesses in the past year. I also pointed out to him that it was probably a real adjustment for him to no longer be in charge as the executive architect, since so many of his life interests in the past had been focused on his work, which had recently been terminated.

When I saw Michael the following spring, he had just come back from a cruise with his wife that he enjoyed very much, and a visit to friends and relatives in New York. Although he still complained of seeing too many doctors and having too many medical problems, he was pleased to have been hired as a consultant for a large architectural firm. His wife still complained that he didn't do enough to stay busy and active and healthy, and that their relationship didn't provide much emotional intimacy for her. In spite of all these things, Michael's depression remained under control through his medications.

Conclusion: Michael represents another example of why it is important to not give up on a medically ill elderly person, and to continue to try multiple medications until something useful and tolerable can be found. Once the proper medication is discovered, it can make a world of difference in the quality of an older person's life. Michael's case illustrates another important point in geriatric medicine: couples age very differently. An age difference that was unimportant nineteen years ago is now magnified by medical and psychiatric problems into a huge difference in activity levels that is a source of stress between husband and wife. Michael's wife wants to be far more socially and physically active than he does, and resents his naps in front of the television and his complaints about medical problems. Teaching Michael and his wife to accept each other's differences and express appreciation for their long-term loyalty and caretaking of one another is an important task of therapy.

Clare: Depression and ECT

Clare was a sixty-two-year-old Caucasian female who had never married. We met on December 1, 1994, when she came to her first interview with me, accompanied by her only daughter. Clare was a high school graduate with some limited college experience who had been employed most of her life as a customer service and secretarial worker. Last summer, she retired following the onset of a severe depressive episode that caused her to be hospitalized for two months at a Harvard teaching hospital. During that time, she received twenty-one ECT treatments.

When I asked Clare if she could give me some history on her present illness, she said the onset of her problems with depression came at age nineteen when she was engaged to a young man named John. He took off with another woman at their college and married her. After hearing that news, Clare had a terrible depression, during which she stayed in bed for two weeks. Her next depression occurred when her mother died in the mid-1960s when Clare was thirty-four. At that time, Clare was hospitalized and received six ECT treatments that seemed to help her, but she can't remember if she was given any kind of medication. The next time she was hospitalized for depression was about five years later. On this occasion, she received no ECT but was treated with Valium. Clare did well for about twenty years. She had no hospitalizations or long-term antidepressant treatments during that entire interval. When she became depressed again, however, she was hospitalized. It is significant to note that during the twenty years when she was free from depression, she was taking Valium on a long-term basis and then Xanax for about five years. Although she took the Xanax at variable dosages, she did take it almost daily. She never experienced any major withdrawal or abuse problems with either of these drugs, which I noted was unusual.

There were several stressful events in Clare's life that led to her current depression. She had a radical mastectomy for breast cancer with node involvement. Fortunately, she was told that she did not need radiation or chemotherapy and has had good follow-up visits with no recurrence of cancer, but she was also told that she would have to be on tamoxifen forever to avoid possible recurrence. Another tragedy that contributed to her current depression was the death five years ago of her boyfriend of ten years, with whom she had lived in a nonsexual relationship for about eight years. He died suddenly from a ruptured aneurysm, and she took his death very hard. She said he had never taken very good care of himself and drank too heavily.

Except for the eight years she spent living with her boyfriend, Clare had lived with her father for essentially all of her life. When her father, on whom she was very dependent, had a hip fracture and went to live with her sister, Clare could no longer stay with him because her sister was unwilling to have Clare share her home after her prolonged psychiatric hospitalization. For this reason, the week before I met her, Clare had been forced to leave Massachusetts and come to California to live with her daughter.

It was significant that Clare's father and sister refused to make a place for her at this time in her life. Clare's father was a poorly educated blue-collar man who never acknowledged or talked about depression, even though Clare's mother suffered from severe episodes. Clare's aunt also had depression problems and actually died at a psychiatric hospital. Ironically, Clare's sister has also had recurrent depressions. She had never had ECT treatments, but was doing well on desipramine. Clare's daughter has never had treatment for depression.

Clare seemed unsure when I asked her if she had ever engaged in any obsessive behaviors or thoughts, but she did acknowledge that she had certain compulsive behaviors. She said that at work she used to go over things she had done three to five times to make sure that they were correct. She would also sometimes feel she had to go back and check to make sure that she had turned off her appliances and locked her door to the point where her need for these behaviors would annoy her. I reassured her, telling her that it didn't sound as if she had a significant degree of obsessive-compulsive disorder. Clare also described having panic attacks, when she would suddenly become afraid something bad was going to happen. At such times, her symptoms included breathing faster, shortness of breath, sweating, an urgency to either urinate or have a bowel movement, and a tightness in her chest. Because of these anxiety attacks, she avoided going into movie theaters, because they were dark and the screen was so big, and driving into town and driving at night, although she did not have trouble taking airplanes or trains. She was unable to describe the frequency or duration of these attacks but did say that taking Xanax would sometimes help her to face these fears. Clare said she had never had any hallucinations, but she did confess that last summer, at the onset of her depression, she had been afraid of everything outside of her house. At the time, she sensed that strange things were going on, although she specifically denied seeing any visions or hearing voices.

Although Clare said that, in general, she felt normally high or euphoric, there were periods when she felt wonderful, much happier than normal, as if everything were in order. During these times, she felt no irritability or grandiosity but experienced other slight changes in her behavior. She required less sleep, dropping from her normal eight hours to only six hours; became more social and sexual; and began thinking faster, although not necessarily talking faster. Although she had always been a careful saver, her spending would increase slightly. Clare felt that others never noticed or felt she was too high during these periods. The reason for this, Clare felt, was that most of the time she did not engage in any behaviors that could be labeled as very impulsive, out of character, or troublemaking. For example, she never indulged in truly excessive spending. When I questioned her daughter, she certainly couldn't remember any times when her mother seemed in what she would consider an abnormally high state. Clare couldn't remember her sister or her mother ever having any full-blown manic episodes either.

There was no seasonal pattern to Clare's depression. When she did get depressed, she didn't want to eat, slept much longer, and had her sleep broken repeatedly by periods of wakening. Other symptoms included a lack of energy, concentration, and decision-making ability; feelings of inferiority to others; slow thinking and moving; loss of interest in life; and an inability to enjoy things. During such times she could not be cheered up but generally felt better in the evenings. The mornings were a "nightmare." At times she had thoughts of suicide, wishing that she were dead, but she never made an attempt, she said, because she is a "coward."

Although Clare felt that she drank too heavily while living with her boyfriend, she now drinks very rarely. She never used street drugs, and smoked only four cigarettes per day. She did not regularly exercise.

When I asked Clare what kinds of medication she was taking, she said she had been on 75 mg of Wellbutrin twice daily for almost two weeks. This drug had given her some severe side effects, especially nausea, and she wanted to discontinue taking it. She had also been on tamoxifen for a long while to prevent breast cancer recurrence. Other medications included one baby aspirin per day and an antinausea medication recommended by her inpatient physician. She also took Compazine to combat the nausea caused by the Wellbutrin without particular benefit.

When I asked Clare what other types of medications she had taken from September through December prior to her hospitalization, she listed Zoloft, trazodone, Prozac, and possibly Elavil. She had never taken desipramine, imipramine, doxepin, lithium, or MAO inhibitors.

When I spoke with her previous doctor at Massachusetts General Hospital, he described her condition as agitated major depression with some psychotic features and vague thoughts of people stalking her. He had also done a medical workup, including giving her an MRI and an EEG. As for medication trials, she had never received a full tricyclic trial, but had tried Thorazine and Haldol, which made her sedated without truly changing her thinking. She had received eight unilateral ECT treatments without any real benefit and fourteen more bilateral treatments that did not help. Her doctor said she had one episode of vomiting when she started on Wellbutrin, but that he questioned whether this response was related to the drug. He described her as a passive-dependent person with family conflicts, and confirmed her story that neither her sister nor her father wanted her to live with them. He did not think she was bipolar, and was not sure if her depression was really recurrent.

I thought Clare seemed alert, oriented, polite, cooperative, well dressed, and friendly. Her mood also appeared to be normal. She had some difficulty recalling the details of her illness, and occasionally her daughter filled these in for her. On her first visit, she seemed to have no psychomotor agitation or slowing, or any psychotic thought processes.

Diagnosis and Treatment Recommendations: I felt Clare was suffering from a major depression in partial remission, although there was some question as to whether she might have bipolar II illness. Since she very much wanted to get off the Wellbutrin, and since her sister had reportedly done well on desipramine, I asked Clare to try taking it. I told her to return in one week, and suggested she consider cognitive behavioral therapy to help her focus on her depression-causing thought patterns. I also suggested to Clare's daughter that she develop some very clear expectations regarding her mother's functioning while living with her. The daughter has been extremely involved in preparing for her mother's arrival, had attended support group meetings, and had gotten in touch with me on several occasions with permission from Clare. At the time, I had suggested that the daughter look into active retirement homes in her area as an alternative to having her mother living with her.

When I saw Clare a week later, she already appeared much brighter than she did on her last visit. She was speaking for herself instead of turning to her daughter, and was able to name and describe numerous retirement homes she and her daughter had visited and to remember the names of restaurants where she had eaten. She was taking 100 mg/day of desipramine with minimal complaints of side effects. Although she still suffered from nausea and headaches, she was unclear if these were from her prolonged ECT series or from her medication. She was sure, however, that she had less nausea on desipramine than on Wellbutrin. I hadn't yet done a blood level test on her, but felt confident enough from her response to suggest that she continue to gradually increase her dosage. Clare's daughter had called her outpatient psychiatrist, who confirmed that he had not done a trial of tricyclic antidepressants, such as the desipramine, that had worked well for her prior to her being given ECT. He also confirmed that Clare's sister was taking desipramine.

Clare was hoping to move into a retirement home and then to get some of her furniture and possessions from Massachusetts, as well as her car, so she would be able to drive locally. She hadn't yet become acquainted with the local area.

When I saw Clare two and a half months later, she told me her daughter had thrown away her Xanax, saying she did not want her mother to get readdicted. She did this in spite of knowing how nervous Clare was about her move from her daughter's home to the retirement community. This behavior seemed overcontrolling and intrusive.

When I saw Clare a week later, however, she seemed to be doing very well and getting to know her neighbors and the neighborhood around the retirement community, Leisure World, where she had just purchased a condominium. She was planning to take some courses at a local college, and perhaps work part-time. She was still taking 150 mg daily of the desipramine and tolerating it very well.

Conclusions: Clare represents a person who finds herself dealing with a staggering number of major adjustments all at the same time. She was facing breast cancer, her father's inability to have her live with him, a prolonged course of ECT, a move from the East Coast to the West Coast, and a very caring yet overcontrolling daughter who tried to run her life and make medication decisions for her, even when Clare was able to do these things for herself. One of the lessons here is that it is important to respect a person's autonomy whenever possible. Children should only make decisions for a parent when it is really essential and urgent that they do so.

The second issue this case illustrates is the importance of getting a medication history from family members. Although Clare's illness did have some psychotic features, it is very possible that an aggressive trial on desipramine would have prevented her from needing the ECT. I certainly hope that it will prevent her from needing it again!

Kate: Antidepressants and pregnancy in a woman with panic disorder

Kate was a thirty-nine-year-old woman who had been married ten years and had two children, aged four and seven. She had a bachelor's degree in English and had had a successful acting career. She was now a homemaker whose husband was a very prominent businessman. Kate was referred to me by her friend.

Kate told me that over the last twenty years, she had had six or seven surgical procedures for the removal of a painful benign occipital tumor following an auto accident in which she was involved. As a result of this accident, she was treated long term by a neurosurgeon who was familiar with panic disorder because he had relatives who had it. When he realized Kate was suffering from this condition, he began treating her for it. At various times, she was also treated with Tenormin and Dilantin to try to control blood flow to the tumor, but was unable to comfortably tolerate either of these medications.

When Kate began having panic attacks at age twenty, she thought she was going "nuts" because her mother had similar attacks, which the family labeled as "goofy spells." After Kate's second child was born, she had episodes of what she then thought was tachycardia, or fast heartbeat. After two or three emergency room visits, she was told she was actually having panic attacks. She subsequently went to a cardiologist who gave her several tests, including an echocardiogram to look for heart valve problems, Holter monitor to look for abnormal heart rhythms, and treadmill studies to look for adequacy of the heart blood supply. This doctor concurred with the diagnosis of panic attacks, but also told her she had a very mild mitral valve prolapse as well. The cardiologist prescribed Xanax at a dose of up to 3 mg/day. When she started on the Xanax, Kate said, her "whole life had changed." Many times in the past she had gone to business dinners with her husband where she felt she could not swallow. This and several other anxiety symptoms got much better after she started taking medications.

Later, however, she went through another episode of illness where she was sick for two months and lost forty-three pounds. She was finally diagnosed as needing her gallbladder removed, and experienced significant relief after the surgery. In the meantime, her neurosurgeon, who was about to retire, fully researched the subject of anxiety and placed her on Klonopin and Pamelor, with the understanding that he would monitor her Pamelor blood levels carefully. Over the last three months, she had been on 50 mg of Pamelor per day and had a blood level of 101 on her last test, which was about at the middle of the range. She took 0.5 mg of the Klonopin three times daily. Kate was very satisfied with these medications. She had no significant side effects with them and felt better than she had in years. She was generally in good health.

When she consulted with Dr. K. about her anxiety, this doctor suggested she get into twice-weekly individual psychotherapy sessions along with her medications. Kate felt this was totally unnecessary because her life so far had been very good and positive, with no major traumas, and she felt she didn't need the psychotherapy. At that point, she was referred to me for management of her medications.

She first tried to control her pain from the occipital tumor with biofeedback, hypnosis, acupuncture, and acupressure without significant relief, but did quite well on about one tablet per day of Tylenol with codeine.

Kate had never drunk any alcohol, smoked cigarettes, used street drugs, or had any periods of depressions or highs. She said she never experimented with any abusable substances because she didn't want to lose control of herself as she had seen others do at times. She had never had periods of anorexia or bulimia.

She and her husband were both in their first marriage. They had two children and were not planning any further pregnancies, although they were considering adopting a third child. Meanwhile, they were actively using birth control and Kate's husband was planning to have a vasectomy. Kate's husband had a very good job, and they were both quite happy that she was staying home raising the children. In general, their marriage was going very well for both.

When I asked Kate to tell me about her family medical history, she said her father was quite healthy, but that her mother suffered from panic attacks and high cholesterol. One brother, aged thirty-five, had cyclic mood swings and felt that people were against him and that the world owed him a living. He had been in psychotherapy, but only briefly.

Kate's diagnosis of panic attacks was substantiated when I gave her a *DSM* Panic Symptom checklist, which revealed she had twelve of the thirteen *DSM III-R* symptoms. At their worst, her panic attacks occurred almost daily. When one hit, she experienced a range of symptoms, including shortness of breath, smothering sensations, dizziness, unsteadiness, palpitations, tachycardia, trembling, sweating, choking, abdominal distress, a feeling that things are unreal, numbness, tingling, chest pain, and a fear of dying, going crazy, or being embarrassed by fainting. Kate was so frightened that she would have an attack in public that she avoided her husband's business dinners, airplanes, restaurants, and other places where she might need to eat in public.

In general, Kate was a very attractive, slender woman, who appeared younger than her stated age. During our sessions, she was alert, oriented, and cooperative with no evidence of hallucinations, delusions, or thought disorder.

Diagnosis and Recommended Treatment: I diagnosed Kate as having a panic disorder with agoraphobia, currently in good remission on medication. Since she appeared to be stable, doing extremely well, and quite pleased with her treatment outcome, I suggested she continue with her current regimen and come every month or two for a follow-up visit. I gave her a prescription for 25 mg of Pamelor, to be taken twice daily, and 0.5 mg of Klonopin, to be taken three times daily. I gave her one refill of the Klonopin, but suggested she try to gradually taper down from this dosage.

About ten months later, Kate was doing extremely well on 1.5 mg of Klonopin and 50 mg of Pamelor per day, even with her husband in a new job that necessitated his traveling a lot. She came in for a very routine medication check appointment and told me she and her husband were seeking a surrogate mother to carry a child for them. I was very surprised, as she seemed quite young and healthy and didn't have a history of any major problems in her prior pregnancies. She'd had a talk with her obstetrician, who said she should never get pregnant on her present medications. Her doctor cautioned her that the danger wasn't absolute, but that there was some risk of spontaneous abortion and cleft lip/palate when taking benzodiazepine tranquilizers. I told her that her medications presented only minimal risk in pregnancy. I suggested she consult with a specialist in drugs and their effects on pregnancy.

Four and a half months later, Kate was delighted to be pregnant and still on medications. She had made the decision to carry the child herself after consulting with a total of five doctors who specialized in drugs and their effects on pregnancy as well as a genetic counselor. She was considering monitoring the pregnancy with a chorionic villus sampling, and was planning on frequent ultrasound. Kate had been artificially inseminated with her husband's sperm after centrifugation to increase their chances of having a girl. A few months later, Kate and her husband were happily parenting and showing off their very healthy six-week-old daughter.

Conclusion: I have included Kate's case history here to address the issue of pregnancy while on psychoactive drugs. Lithium appears to be the worst offender, but even that belief is controversial now. Tricyclic antidepressants, SSRI antidepressants, benzodiazepine tranquilizers, and most other psychoactive drugs may slightly increase risk in pregnancy, but not to the degree that they must be absolutely prohibited if a woman really wants a baby and needs the medications to be able to function. The first doctor Kate consulted warned her in a very dogmatic manner, and probably had not reviewed the latest literature on antidepressants and tranquilizers in pregnancy. Actually, they are quite safe.

Morris: A case of seasonal affective disorder

On January 2, 1993, Morris, a forty-five-year-old, self-employed veterinarian who had never married, was referred to me by Dr. B. for consultation and a second opinion. For the past seven years, Morris had suffered from recurrent seasonal depression. When I asked him for a history of his present illness, he said his problems with depression began seven years previously when he had two episodes of depression that began in October or November and lasted for about three months each. Although two years passed without any recurrence of this condition, he experienced episodes of depression again for another three years, also beginning in October or November of each year. The later depressions had typically lasted for about three months, although the current one was resolved in about two months, probably due to treatment with Zoloft. Morris had never experienced depressions at any other time of the year, but said that October through December was a relatively slow season in his veterinary practice.

Morris had no problems with substance abuse and was a moderate drinker. Normally, he had about two glasses of wine or beer per night, but he did not drink at all when he was depressed. He used no street drugs and had never had any manic episodes. At the time I first met with him, he was taking Ativan at bedtime to get to sleep, a multivitamin, and about 100 mg of Zoloft each morning. He said the Zoloft had begun to help his depression after he had been on it for about five weeks.

When I asked Morris to fill me in on some family history, he said he came from a small European Jewish family that were Holocaust survivors. His mother was an anxious worrier and had depression problems, for which she had probably taken antidepressants in the past. Morris's father had never experienced any psychiatric problems, nor had his sister.

Morris noticed that his depressions often followed minor medical illnesses, such as sinus infections or worries about getting sick. During these periods, his sleeping patterns changed from initial insomnia, to total sleeplessness, to anxiety about whether he would be able to get to sleep, to later episodes of early morning awakenings. His total sleep time dropped from his normal seven and a half to eight and a half hours down to five or six hours. During these three-month depressions, he lost his appetite, experienced gastrointestinal upsets and loose stools, and typically dropped 15 or 20 pounds. His sex drive became nonexistent. His concentration was diminished and he would put off tasks until his mind was clear. Although his energy felt low, he continued working his normal four full days and two half days each week because his was a solo practice and there was no one else to take over when he was not there. Morris admitted one of the things currently bothering him was his struggle to make an adequate living in his veterinary practice.

When depressed, Morris also experienced decreased self-esteem but had no delusions of having committed a sin or being punished, and no auditory, visual, taste, touch, or smell hallucinations. Mood reactivity—responses to life events—is present, and he has occasional variations in mood, sometimes feeling better in the evening than in the morning. Although he usually enjoyed photography, playing with his computer, and socializing, all of these activities brought him much less joy during his depressions. He told me he normally enjoyed photography with wilderness and portraiture as themes and was involved in a computer bulletin board network for vets. He had suicidal thoughts, but never made any plans to end his life.

When I asked Morris to tell me about his current feelings, he described them as "no energy, no hope, no enjoyment, life is not good." He sometimes experienced some dizziness and didn't feel like being active. Sometimes he felt the need to go outside of his office just to get some light. He felt so antisocial at times that he avoided eating in a restaurant and would pick up fast food to eat in his car while he was stopped at a local park.

When I asked Morris to describe his social relationships, he said he was shy and didn't like being told what to do because his mother had been manipulative. He said his relationships with women were "not many and not long," and that he didn't do much to meet people although he had joined a dating service. He felt he wanted marriage and children, but his efforts to find a wife had been inconsistent. Singles events terrified him. He wasn't completely socially isolated, however, and did have some friends with whom he enjoyed going out to dinner or movies.

Diagnosis and Recommended Treatment: I diagnosed Morris with recurrent major depression and a definite seasonal affective disorder that was unipolar without any psychotic features. I asked him if he had ever taken lithium, Tegretol, Depakote, Wellbutrin, Tofranil, Norpramin, or bright light treatment, and he said no. Because he had already run the typical three-month course of his depression by the time he came to see me, I suggested he taper off the Zoloft he was taking by about 25 mg every two weeks. I also suggested he taper off the Ativan. I then asked him to obtain a bright light visor or box to use as a replacement for the drugs, and to begin using it at least a month before he expected his next episode of seasonal depression to begin. I told him if the light therapy did not work, that research conducted by the National Institute of Mental Health had shown that seasonal affective disorder improved after treatment with lithium and MAOIs. I told him that if he was not willing to accept the dietary restrictions of an MAOI, he might begin trying the bright light treatment well before his expected episode of depression. If necessary, he could then add Zoloft and possible lithium augmentation to this treatment to try and minimize the time he spent feeling depressed next year.

Nine Months Later: When I saw Morris the following fall, he was taking 100 mg of trazodone before bed to help him get a good night's sleep, but this drug made him feel sedated when he woke up in the morning. He was also using bright artificial light (BAL) therapy up to an hour each morning. His seasonal depression had started nine days earlier with his usual diarrhea, terminal insomnia, and a decrease in appetite, but the symptoms were milder than they usually were at this time of the year. Unimpressed by his response to Zoloft last year, and reluctant to take an MAOI, Morris decided to try using lithium augmentation with trazodone and the light therapy to attempt to make the intensity of his depression as mild as possible. He also felt he had probably experienced some hypomanic periods, accompanied by increased energy and an episode of impulse spending—he spent $3,000 for a new computer. His diagnosis now appeared to be bipolar II.

By the end of the year, Morris was doing adequately with the lithium, trazodone, and BAL therapy. Although he spoke of reading a new book by Dr. Rosenthal, who recommended SSRIs, Wellbutrin, desipramine, or an MAOI for seasonal depression, he still did not want to try any MAOIs. Morris felt he would probably get better soon, as this time of the year marked his normal recovery period. Work at his veterinary clinic was still slow.

Sure enough, by the beginning of February, Morris's mood had lifted and he had stopped taking lithium without any noticeable effects, although he decided to continue taking 50 to 100 mg of trazodone nightly for insomnia. He also expressed interest in wanting to do some dating.

Conclusion: Since Morris clearly has seasonal affective disorder, bright light was my treatment of choice. In such cases, numerous antidepressants might be helpful, but Morris has not been impressed with their effectiveness, saying that in his case they did nothing other than slightly decreasing the intensity of his symptoms and helping him to sleep.

Sam: A case of dysthymia

Sam, a twenty-eight-year-old single male, came to my office. He was living alone while being supported by his parents. Sam had been treated with medications and psychotherapy for several years by another psychiatrist who was now referring him to me for a second opinion.

When I asked Sam to tell me about himself, he said he felt both anxious and depressed, and that his problems had begun around the age of twenty-one. High school life had been good to him. He was having fun, meeting girls, getting good grades, and doing all right socially with friends. Although he got into an occasional fight in school, he managed to graduate with a 3.75 grade point average.

After high school, he went to the University of Southern California for one quarter as a premed student. There, he began using marijuana and alcohol, and often drove while under the influence. He left the premedical program and transferred to State College where he was frequently on the President's or Dean's List and got straight A s. In college, he had a long-term girlfriend named Nancy. When I asked him what attracted him to her, his initial response was, "I liked her feet," which later turned out to be a foot fetish. He said that she was a warm, nice person who was attractive. Unfortunately, she wanted marriage and he didn't. In fact, he informed me, he had "always cheated on girls" he was dating. Currently, he was involved once again with a girlfriend who wanted to get married while he didn't.

Sam said that the onset of his depression was after a minor auto accident and the breakup of his relationship with another girlfriend, Sue. He felt devastated about the breakup and said he had never gotten over it.

From the onset of his depression, Sam said, his symptoms had been a "mixed bag," including periods of anxiety in which he punched himself in the face, and times when he felt "bummed," pressured, and as if he were screaming. In spite of this, he denied any history of hallucinations, except for two occasions: one when he was using marijuana, and another when he experienced acute hallucinations when withdrawing from antidepressants (which is quite unusual).

From college he went on to law school, where he initially got poor grades. Although he felt he was going downhill psychologically, and was repeatedly placed on academic probation, he did manage to finish school and take the bar exam, although he feels he flunked it. He met his current girlfriend, Julie, while he was in his third year of law school. After his breakup with Sue at age twenty-one, he did not have a regular girlfriend for six or seven years. Sam described his current relationship as very erratic in that Julie caused him a lot of turmoil and aggravation and pressured him to get married, even though he had told her that he did not feel ready for this kind of commitment. In the meantime, he maintained numerous outside relationships because he felt that dating several women was very exciting, and said he was not ready to stop doing so. Sam described his current goals as taking a bar review course, passing the bar exam, and resuming his training and teaching as a second-degree black belt in karate.

When I asked Sam to tell me about his depression, he described several symptoms. He said his mood was very unstable, shifting rapidly from a very high state to a very depressed one. His said his sleeping patterns were normal and that he got an average of eight hours sleep per night, and that his appetite was good, especially around dinnertime. He also indicated that he sometimes binges on food. His weight had normally been 120 to 125 pounds when he was a runner, but five or ten years ago he started doing a lot of weight lifting and gained 20 pounds, weighing in at around 145. His sex drive was not very good with his girlfriend, but was fine in his outside relationships. Although his energy level was only 30 or 40 percent of what was normal for him, he said that his concentration was "okay." He had no problems making decisions. He did confess that he thought about suicide at various times, and had made a few halfhearted attempts. He had run his car engine in the garage with the door closed, slashed his wrists, and the previous week, closed his eyes while driving on the freeway. Sam's most lethal attempt had been made ten years ago when he took a room on a very high floor in a hotel and thought of jumping or overdosing. He did understand, however, that if he overdosed on any of his medications, his current doctor would no longer prescribe Xanax for him.

Sam admits he has had problems with drinking at times, but never any serious school, legal, or family problems. Although he had some stomach problems with alcohol, he had never vomited blood, or experienced any withdrawal symptoms, blackouts, or seizures after drinking.

Sam was taking 0.25 mg of Xanax, one or two times daily, as needed; and 5 mg of Valium, which he used very intermittently. He also took Tylenol, Parafon Forte, Naprosyn, and Donnatal sporadically, as he felt the need. When I asked him what his ideal medication would be, he told me one that would not cause him to gain weight and would help him to be happier in general.

When I asked him to tell me about his medical history, he said he had been told that he had degenerative disc disease, but was seeking a second opinion. At birth, he had an undescended testicle that was operated on. He had a "pre-ulcer" condition diagnosed after gastroscopy, although he has been hospitalized only once for stomach problems. He had allergies to dust, dogs, cats, and aspirin.

When I asked him about his family history, Sam said his mother had been in psychotherapy and was supposed to be taking a medication, perhaps Librium, he thought. He described his father, who was a physician, as someone who was extremely "together." None of Sam's three siblings had any known psychiatric problems, nor was he aware of any psychiatric hospitalizations, alcoholism, ECT, or suicides in any of his other relatives.

I was only able to get the vaguest history of Sam's medication trials. Although he was able to tell me that he had been tried on Elavil, Desyrel, and Navane, he was unable to describe the dose, duration, or his response to any of these drugs. He did recall, however, that he had never been tried on MAOIs, lithium, or BuSpar.

When I asked Sam to tell me about his personality over the long term, he described himself as "not happy." He also suffered from several anxiety symptoms, including feeling hyped up and anxious at times, and experienced such a high degree of frustration that he wanted to hit things, and punch and kick walls, cabinets, and doors. He felt these actions helped him to relieve some of his tension. Other symptoms he felt when anxious included difficult breathing, sweating, headaches, feeling hot, loss of concentration to the point where he lost things, fears that something bad would happen, and anxiety dreams.

Diagnosis and Comments: Sam presented a very confusing symptomatic history, which was very suggestive of a diagnosis of dysthymia. He certainly had some borderline personality disorder features, including chronic depression, anxiety, anger, and a pattern of unstable relationships. I have included this patient because he taught me a valuable lesson about psychopharmacology and psychotherapy during the seven years we worked together. In an effort to get him well, Sam and I tried SSRIs, Wellbutrin, MAOIs, Xanax, BuSpar, stimulants, and lithium. He finally told me, after a period in which he had been off medications for awhile and was involved in cognitive behavioral therapy (to which I had referred him), that he always felt worse when he took drugs, regardless of the type of antidepressant. I finally believed him, and he's done better ever since! Sam is now working full-time in real estate, using psychotherapy only occasionally to deal with stressful situations, and clearly says that he's "stressed and not depressed" in response to his life problems. Some people really don't benefit from psychiatric medicines, even though this is hard for their doctors to accept.

Jamie: Substance abuse and depression

Jamie is a thirty-one-year-old homemaker. She is in her first marriage of fifteen years and has three children, aged twelve, ten, and six. She is a high school graduate. Jamie said that she had felt depressed lately, only feeling good about one week out of the month. She was unable to function and didn't want to get out of bed or see people other than her children or her husband.

When I asked her to give me some history of her present illness, she said her depression had become unbearable over the last year. She had experienced monthly mood swings related to her menstrual cycle for one or two weeks a month from the age of thirteen, but over the past few months these changes in mood had begun to seriously interfere with her life. A year and a quarter earlier, she had seen Dr. H. for medications and Dr. S. for psychotherapy.

When I asked her to tell me about her medication history, she said she had tried taking a dose of 75 mg of nortriptyline two or three times during the day, along with 150 mg of the drug at bedtime, and an occasional dose of Ativan. This drug made her feel good, even "better than good," as if she could conquer the world. Although she felt that it made her too high, she didn't get into any trouble with it. She also took Klonopin, which helped her with her sleeping problems and panic attacks. She was on nortriptyline and Klonopin for about two months but never had a blood level taken.

Jamie had a history of alcohol problems. When she began drinking again, she complained of being tired in the mornings and unable to get up. At this point, Dr. H. recommended that she not stop her medicines, but stop drinking. Jamie said that Dr. H. would not provide medicines for her because excess alcohol makes antidepressants ineffective.

Although Jamie had been free of alcohol for two days, she readily admitted that she was an alcoholic who drank from one to two beers up to two bottles of champagne per day, and had been drinking excessively for about a year now. Part of her problem stemmed from a major trauma in her life, a therapeutic abortion she had two years ago during her second trimester for which she had never forgiven herself. The pregnancy was unplanned and both she and her husband had agreed she should have the abortion, and she was now using birth control pills regularly. An additional stressor was her mother's health problems, which had necessitated her living with Jamie for awhile. Her mother had undergone five spine surgeries in the past ten years, had a worker's compensation case that was recently settled, and had been recently tested at UCI Medical Center where she was discovered to have seizures of an unknown etiology.

Jamie said that her marriage was fine and that she and her husband had a good relationship. Her husband's job as a general manager at a car dealership was going well and he did not have any drinking problems.

When I asked Jamie if she had any other psychiatric problems, she told me she had experienced manic episodes while not taking antidepressants. These episodes lasted between one and two weeks. During these times, her mood was happy, her energy was very high, and her sex drive and sleeping patterns were normal, but she was unable to focus and found herself talking very fast, thinking nonstop, and trying to do too many things at one time. Although her spending patterns did not change, her use of the phone went way up and she would "call the whole world." During her manic periods, she didn't feel grandiose or change her style of dress, but she definitely felt more social. She didn't drive any faster, but she did do impulsive things that could potentially get her into trouble, such as seeing an old boyfriend, although she did not become sexually involved with him. She did not experience paranoia or hallucinations at this time, but she felt irritable and distractible, and would try to start a lot of different projects at once. Sometimes she would get a lot done, and sometimes she would merely run around in circles. Over the last year, she has had two or three episodes like this while off her medication.

When I asked Jamie how often she had been depressed in the last year, she said at least 70 percent of the time. She said she couldn't remember how often she had felt normal and had only experienced a few weeks when her mood was unusually good.

When I gave her the Seventeen-item Hamilton Depression Rating Scale, she had a score of 27. Jamie said she felt down 90 percent of the time, and experienced current depressive thoughts and feelings of guilt and punishment. She acknowledged that she is an alcoholic. Although she denied having any suicidal thoughts recently, she admitted she had taken overdoses of her medication in the past, but only to help her to sleep, not with the intent of killing herself. If she didn't drink, it took her thirty minutes to an hour to fall asleep. She often got up and cried during the night, and woke up one to three hours before she needed to get the children off to school. Jamie also sat and cried during the day. She hadn't been able to make herself do much homemaking, and the house was a wreck.

I observed that Jamie's physical movements and gestures were slightly slowed. She was tearful during the interview, and described a variety of symptoms, including tension, irritability, worry about small things, and physical symptoms of shaking, shortness of breath, dizziness, and feeling exhausted. She said her appetite was variable to nonexistent, her energy was zero, and her sex drive about 50 percent of normal. She was concerned about her health but not overly so, did not exercise regularly, and had no history of weight loss.

When I asked Jamie what the main reasons were behind her current depression, she listed the loss of having all her children in school, her abortion, and having to put a lot of energy into taking care of her mother during her visit. She did have a mild diurnal variation, feeling a little worse in the morning and better when her husband came home in the evening. She also told me she felt more depressed in the fall, and had felt better in the spring over the last two years. Other than thoughts about the abortion, she experienced no paranoia, and no obsessive-compulsive symptoms other than thoughts about her abortion. In spite of these feelings, she was able to enjoy activities and her mood was reactive to events.

Jamie said she had never had any legal or medical problems due to alcohol, but admitted she had driven while drunk and had periods where she stayed intoxicated all throughout the day. She also knew her drinking caused family problems—that it negatively affected her husband and children, and caused fights between her and her husband. In spite of her obvious problem, she denied ever having any withdrawal difficulties during the times she stopped drinking. The longest Jamie was ever without alcohol was about one month after her mother left. She has been in Alcoholics Anonymous, going twice a week at times. She had never been on Antabuse, a drug that blocks the metabolism of alcohol so that drinking would make her feel sick.

Aside from her drinking, Jamie had no other serious addictive habits. Although she did use marijuana anywhere from "rarely" to "daily," she did not smoke cigarettes or use "speed" or cocaine.

When I asked Jamie to tell me about her family history, she said her mother did not abuse alcohol, but had made suicide attempts and suffered from problems with depression, for which she took Prozac. The Prozac seemed to help her, but she got edgy on it. A maternal aunt said that Jamie's mother had manic depressive illness, and Jamie said her mother experienced high periods similar to those that she described in herself. Jamie's father did have alcohol problems but no depression. Of her siblings, two brothers and two sisters, only the youngest sister, aged fourteen, had drug problems. She had been hospitalized for depression but was not on medications.

When I asked Jamie to tell me about her past psychiatric medications, she said she had tried BuSpar for about two months with no effect, and Elavil with no benefit. She had never tried lithium, Tegretol, or Depakote. She did say her mother had done very well recently on Zoloft and Tegretol.

In spite of her difficulties with depression and alcoholism, Jamie had many positive qualities. Although she was tearful off and on throughout the interview, she was basically an attractive woman who looked her stated age. She was friendly, polite, and cooperative and showed no evidence of delusions, hallucinations, or thought disorders.

Diagnosis and Treatment Recommendations: I diagnosed Jamie with bipolar II depression (periods of major depression and also hypomanic episodes) and alcohol abuse. I explained to her the importance of complete abstinence from all addictive substances and encouraged her to attend Alcoholics Anonymous and to use Antabuse. Antabuse is a useful drug for alcoholic recovery because it blocks the metabolism of alcohol for up to two weeks after it is taken. Under these conditions, drinking alcohol makes the person experience a terrible headache, flushing, and nausea. I also recommended that Jamie begin Zoloft because her mother had done well with this, and gave her a prescription for it. In the meantime, I advised her to get a lithium lab workup to check for adequate thyroid and kidney functioning, to make sure there was no alcoholic liver damage, and to make sure she wasn't pregnant. If the tests were normal and she was not pregnant, we could potentially start her on lithium if she became too high while using the Zoloft. I requested her records from Dr. H., and Jamie agreed to continue her therapy with Dr. S.

For the next month and a half, Jamie seemed very pleased and proud of herself for staying on Antabuse and away from alcohol. She used Ativan and then Klonopin to taper off of the tranquilizers, and took 100 mg/day of Zoloft with a good response. She said she was now feeling better than she had in a long time.

When I saw her two months later, however, she said she had resumed drinking three weeks earlier in response to feeling insecure and criticized by her husband. At this time, I strongly recommended marital therapy.

A month and a half later, Jamie still had not begun to attend AA meetings, nor had she and her husband tried marital therapy. They were also now dealing with her husband's job loss, which had made therapy less financially accessible.

Conclusion: Alcoholism is a disease of denial. Jamie didn't think she needed complete sobriety to get better, yet her antidepressant only had a chance to work if she could get off the alcohol. She didn't believe she needed marital therapy and actually failed to show up at two appointments she had set up with a psychiatric social worker, yet she clearly had marital issues. She refused to become involved with AA, yet definitely had a very high relapse risk. The Antabuse was briefly helping her to maintain sobriety while she used it and the antidepressant was helping her mood, but without the long-term support of AA and a willingness to work on her marital issues, her chances of staying sober long term and overcoming the depression aren't nearly as good as they could be.

FAMILY ISSUES IN DEPRESSION

The Dynamics of Family Depression

Depression is a serious disorder that many people are burdened with every day and yet it is often left untreated. It can be as great a burden for the family as for the patient. Depression affects the family in a manner similar to other disorders, yet it also has some unique aspects that are important to discuss at this time.

When looking at the family dynamics of depression, it is important to understand the concept of secondary gain, which represents the emotional equivalent of a disability check. The person who is depressed might not consciously desire or even acknowledge the benefits of being ill; nevertheless, certain secondary gains might be present.

In some ways, depression may be the disorder where the secondary gains of the one who is ill lead to the most anger, resentment, and helplessness among family members. Due to lethargy, the person who is depressed is often unavailable to participate in household activities. When this happens, family members may begin to view the patient as passive-aggressive, feeling that he is avoiding certain activities in order to hurt others, to get back at someone, or to purposefully avoid doing tasks. Families often say one or more of the following to me when engaged in family therapy:

> "Why can't he just shake these off feelings?"
> "If she'd just get out of bed in the morning, she'd feel a lot better."

"He's doing this on purpose so that I have to carry all the load."
"She's getting back at me for being sick last year."
"He's taking out his anger at his mother for being inadequate on me."
"She just doesn't want to do anything with me."

Secondary gain issues include avoidance of tasks in which the depressed individual doesn't want to participate, being able to remain in denial about issues she feels are out of her control, and avoidance of being blamed for not doing something about her situation. Depression also allows her to suppress her rage rather than face her underlying issues.

Family members also have to face their own secondary gain issues that come from having a depressed family member. This dynamic may be evident in families where a key authority figure is depressed and unable to intervene, allowing other family members to be more free to do whatever they please. In such situations, adolescents may have no ground rules, may be coming and going as they please, and even engaging in dangerous behavior themselves. In one instance, the father sexually abused the children because the mother was too lethargic to deal with the children's complaints. In another situation, with a very depressed mother, the focus of the family was on her; hence, the father was let off the hook and does not have to deal with his own issues of inadequacy. If a child is depressed, it may give the depressed parent a way of masking his own depression and protect him from facing his own issues because he is so busy focusing on the child. This dynamic also works in the case of a depressed senior citizen whose condition takes the focus off her daughter-caregiver who is also severely depressed. If another family member is in dire need, some people can continue to function in spite of their own severe depression. Such individuals may even use someone else's need as a crutch to keep themselves going, whereas other depressed individuals cannot rise to even the most desperate occasions.

Enmeshment

There are numerous places throughout this book where I have talked about the concept of enmeshment. I'd like to explore this issue a bit further by describing a common scenario I found while working extensively with the families of adolescents at a psychiatric hospital. First, I need to point out that children often do not present the same types of symptoms of depression as do adults. Instead of being lethargic, for example, they may become hyperactive and often act out by using drugs, getting into trouble at school, refusing to do homework, stealing, getting involved in gang activity, making a serious suicide attempt, or even becoming homicidal. It was very common for an adolescent to be brought into the hospital where I worked with some or all of these symptoms. Family therapy was a major focus for adolescents at our hospital and, in fact, I do not feel that children or adolescents can be effectively treated without family therapy being a major part of the process. When an adolescent presented with depression, family therapy usually revealed that the person in the primary caregiver role (usually the mother) was also severely depressed. Sometimes her depression was hidden and other times it was very obvious. In many cases, once this situation was discovered and the mother received treatment for her depression, she became more emotionally available to her family and the child's depression disappeared. In other cases, both mother and child required treatment with medication, individual therapy, and family therapy.

One family I worked with extensively is a good example of the issues of enmeshment and how depression may be shared among family members. David, a seventeen-year-old who lived with his mother Janice, father Dave, and his twenty-year-old sister Susan, was brought into the hospital after attempting to commit suicide. His father had found David hanging from the rafters in the garage, luckily only a moment after David chose to take his life, and was able to perform CPR to revive his son. Frequently, the chosen form of suicide gives clues as to what the problem in the family is that might lead to such an act of extreme desperation. Sure enough, during a family session, David said that he felt "choked to death" by his father, who was so angry inside that he bullied family members to the point of being afraid to speak out about their pain, sadness, anger, and needs. The therapy went on to reveal that Janice, too, felt "choked" and was experiencing a severe major depression, along with frequent thoughts of killing herself.

It was very difficult at first for Dave, the father, to hear this. In fact, during a very moving session he tried to threaten me to keep the family from talking about their feelings. Despite his bullying behavior, when gently pushed to listen, he suddenly began to weep as he realized that his family needed to talk. Once the old "don't talk" rule was broken, Dave also began to speak about his fears, feelings of inadequacy, and sadness that the children were becoming adults and would soon be leaving home. Janice was relieved to have her depression out in the open and immediately agreed to meet with a psychiatrist and begin an antidepressant. Once the medication relieved her symptoms, and we had a few more family sessions that reinforced the new family rule to talk openly about feelings, Dave began to feel more adequate as a father and husband and David began to feel less depressed, to the point where he finally did not require any medication himself. I mention this family not only as an example of how rigid family rules can lead to very severe consequences, but also of how family members can work together to set a new course for the whole family.

Another example of how a family dynamic of depression is often played out can be seen in a description of the Alexander family. Sally is a single-parent mom with three children, Jennifer, who is sixteen, Danny, fourteen, and Amber, ten. Herbert, the father, is largely unavailable and is, in fact, a chronic liar who has stolen jewelry from Sally in the past when picking up the children for a rare visitation. Sally has major depression with occasional thoughts of suicide. Her parents were killed in a plane crash six years ago, and she has not been able to resolve her grief about this, leading to a great deal of irritability on her part. Sally often depends on her children to make her feel loved and cared for as her parents once did. Unfortunately, they are incapable of fulfilling this role because kids are kids and cannot fill such a void. Sally's biggest complaint is that the children do not do chores regularly. She is convinced she will feel more loved if the children pick up after themselves.

Due to depression, however, Sally is unable to follow through with teaching the children how to do certain things, nor is she consistent about the consequences when they don't do their chores. These inconsistencies place both Sally and the children in a double-bind, no-win situation. At these junctures, Sally then projects her anger onto the children. Jennifer becomes depressed herself as she tries to please Sally, yet nothing she does can satisfy her mother because the void is one the children cannot possibly fill. Danny acts out by doing daredevil behaviors—in a sense, he unconsciously acts out Sally's suicidal fantasies. These stunts leave Sally feeling even more empty and angry as she fears losing him. Amber plays the role of the only one who appears to meet her mother's needs by bringing Sally sodas and checking in on her. This behavior worked until one day Sally recognized that her daughter was doing these things to hide the fact she had been acting out like her father—lying, manipulating, and stealing. When she realized this, Sally was left feeling more inadequate than ever.

Treatment for Sally included medication and family therapy, which helped her to begin truly believing that she is very important to her children. Once she was able to set rules and teach them skills to become more independent, she was able to be in charge of the family again. Sally's work and motivation in family therapy, as well as the use of an antidepressant, lessened her depression. In addition, Jennifer's depression was relieved and Danny's daredevil behavior decreased. This allowed Sally to focus on the behavior problems now evident in Amber, which needed much attention. She was also able to begin focusing on her own grief process, which was now beginning to flow more effectively.

Enmeshment and Blaming Others

Blaming others (projection) is a common issue in depression and happens when the person who is depressed blames everything on the partner or other family members. Projection may block the depressed person from seeing the help that others around her are trying to give. It renders family members, as well as the one with depression, helpless. This helplessness leads to even greater depression and may eventually cause depression in those around her. This vicious cycle can only be relieved when treatment is obtained and family members are willing to do their part to stop accepting each other's projections and work on their own issues around depression and loss. If these issues are not addressed, the caregiver will "burn out" trying to fix the other person.

Taboo Enmeshment

Another important aspect of depression is the enmeshment that commonly occurs when two people in the family get paired up unofficially as a team that resembles a taboo relationship. This situation usually involves a parent-child dyad where both individuals become close in such a way that the spouse is excluded. In such situations, it is as if the child and parent are married, and the spouse may be treated as if he or she is the child or outsider of the dyad. This sort of relationship can develop in circumstances where, for example, one of the parents travels a lot or lives away from home for periods of time. It can also occur even when both spouses are present on a regular basis.

On an unconscious level, all three family members collude in the creation of this relationship, and it usually reflects some sort of intimacy problem within the marriage. For example, this sort of collusion may occur when there is divorce and the child goes to live with one parent. Soon they are teamed up.

I worked with a family that illustrated this dynamic. Ralph and Tina were married and had two adolescent children, Jeff, sixteen, and Rachel, thirteen. Ralph worked as a sales representative and was often away from home for two to three weeks per month. In his absence, Jeff and his mother Tina spent long hours together talking about Tina's problems in her marriage, their dreams and hopes in life, and problems Tina had in raising her daughter Rachel. The closer the two became, the more excluded Ralph, the father, felt and the more angry and competitive he became with his son Jeff. On the other hand, he also felt relief that Jeff was assuming this role because he knew that Tina was lonely. It let him off the hook of being her confidant and having to address the problems in the marriage.

As time went on, Ralph became more angry and distant, and Tina and Jeff became like a married couple. Since it is "taboo" for mother and son to be "married," it wasn't long before Jeff started acting out. He continuously threatened his father when he was home in order to keep his position as the acting "husband." On the other hand, because it felt "weird" to be "married" to his mother, Jeff became outraged at her. He was also outraged at Ralph for not taking care of his wife. He was further placed in a double bind because his mother was his "wife" and he might have sexual feelings toward her that would be unacceptable, and so would lead to aggressive feelings toward her.

The outcome was that both Tina and Jeff developed major depression. After much work in family therapy, which included a symbolic "divorce" of Jeff and Tina, a "remarriage" of Ralph and Tina, and psychopharmacological treatment of Tina, eventually the parents and children resumed their normal roles.

CREATING FAMILY "CONTRACTS": ONE ENMESHMENT SOLUTION

These sorts of unhealthy family dynamics, once altered, can greatly assist in the relief of depression among family members. When a person is severely depressed, however, he may initially be unable to participate actively with the family in changing the various dynamics. It is important to include the depressed individual in the family sessions and to have changes occurring in his behavior during this phase of his depression, but his recovery may also require that family members address the symptoms of their own depression directly.

When a person is depressed, it is important that she keep to a daily routine so that she does not succumb to the depression. The severely depressed person is often unable to do this alone, which in turn requires family members to work with her to get her motivated to attend to life. This places the family in the dilemma of measuring what the affected person can do realistically and how much help she needs, without treating her like a baby or enabling her so that she doesn't have to take responsibility for her own life.

To this end, it is helpful for family members to create a behavioral contract with the depressed person, outlining what he will be expected to do each day. This agreement should take into consideration what that person is capable of at the time, setting realistic goals stating what he would like to be able to do by week two, week three, and so on. Often these goals need to be reset at the beginning of each new week because the medicine will also be kicking in along the way over the first one to four weeks at a rate that varies for each person.

When setting up these goals, it is a good idea to have a time schedule laid out for each day, much like an appointment calendar. An example of one such calendar for a very depressed man is:

7:00 A.M.	Wake up
7:15 A.M.	Twenty-minute morning walk with dog
8:00 A.M.	Shower and dress
9:00 A.M.	Breakfast
10:00 A.M.	Water the yard
11:00 A.M.	Call wife at work to check in and discuss progress of contract
12:00 noon	Lunch (eat at least two-thirds of sack lunch prepared by wife)
1:00 P.M.	Afternoon; twenty-minute walk or errand (for example, buy groceries)
2:00 P.M.	Watch television for one hour

A contract of this type will help set expectations for the depressed individual, preventing him from lying in bed all day and succumbing to his lethargy. A few weeks after beginning the antidepressant, this agreement will gradually become more complex, adding items such as beginning to look for a job or returning to work. To ensure maximum effectiveness, it is important to include the person with depression in each step of this contract. It is also important to remember that when working with a depressed person, you are dealing with someone who usually feels hopeless about life ever returning to normal. For this reason, it is vital to keep the contract within a range that is achievable yet challenging.

It is also essential to keep in mind the availability of family members to enforce the contract. Using the example above, the depressed man may not be able to get out of bed on his own, making it important for his wife to make sure that he is up and ready to go before she leaves for work. She may also need to call him every hour to make sure he has achieved each task along the way. Or it may be necessary to ask a neighbor to check in hourly. It is important for family members to acknowledge whether they are able to engage fully in such a contract. If they aren't, hospitalization or day treatment might be necessary. Family burnout or suicidal thoughts on the part of the depressed individual may also signal the need for more intensive treatment.

Another factor to include in the behavioral contract is taking the medication as prescribed by the doctor. This may require monitoring because of the risk of overdose or the tendency of some individuals to avoid taking their medication. It may also be necessary to monitor a person's use of alcohol and street drugs, substances often abused by people who are depressed because of the initial high they receive when ingesting them. The belief that these substances make one feel "better" is a myth, because their actual effect is usually to increase depression. An equally important area that often needs to be monitored is food intake, since people who are depressed often either overeat or do not eat enough to sustain them.

DEPRESSION AMONG THE ELDERLY OR THE TERMINALLY ILL

Dealing with depression in an elderly person or a person who is terminally ill involves other important issues that need to be addressed. First of all, any of the dynamics discussed above can be present in these situations, but then become exaggerated. In diagnosing depression in these cases, it is important to first rule out medical problems that might be directly causing the depression, or medications that might have a side effect of depression. The natural grief process that occurs when one is ill is also different from major depression. Major depression includes a prolonged sense of hopelessness and helplessness that usually doesn't accompany normal grief.

An important strategy with the elderly or the terminally ill is to empower those persons to take control of their lives in any way they still can. An ill or elderly person usually has to depend on others more than usual, which might leave the person with a sense of loss. For some, giving up their independence is very difficult. Others respond by choosing to give up doing everything, becoming too dependent. The task of the family member becomes that of gently pushing the person to do as much as he realistically can, while at the same time assisting him to learn to accept help in the areas where he can no longer take control. It is important to include the elderly and the terminally ill in decisions about their care and to explain their condition to them openly. It is also important for them to be included in family decision making, so that their sense of purpose in the family remains intact. Clear, concise, and open communication enables these individuals to participate in family discussions, as well as helping them to understand their medical issues.

COPING WITH SUICIDE THREATS AND ATTEMPTS

Dealing with suicidal threats is also a very difficult situation for the family of a depressed person. These may come in the form of verbal threats that feel manipulative at times or may be actual suicide attempts or other self-destructive behaviors. Suicidality is not to be taken lightly, even if it feels manipulative or is chronic behavior. When someone makes suicidal threats, it is important to involve a mental health professional to both determine if hospitalization is necessary and to work toward resolution of the issues that surround the wish to die.

Different families react differently to suicidal behavior. Enmeshed families usually respond by becoming confused, frightened by unpredictability, and mistrustful of the member who attempts suicide. Families who are disengaged—the polar opposite of enmeshed—often downplay, ignore, or overlook the suicide attempt. Any attempt to kill oneself is a symptom of a process that involves the entire family. Understanding suicidal behavior can become quite complex and is often a problem that requires intensive family therapy to resolve the family dynamics involved in its creation.

Sometimes the suicidal individual is playing out someone else's role in the family, someone with whom she is in an unconscious suicide pact. In other words, there may be another person in the family who is very depressed and has suicidal fantasies, but would never act them out or even consciously acknowledge she had them. In such a situation, she projects these unwanted feelings onto the other depressed family member, who then acts them out. It is important to note that this projection is not done intentionally and is almost always unconscious on the part of both people.

There are times, however, when it appears to an outsider "as if" one person is purposefully encouraging another to commit suicide. For example, a woman feels suicidal and has spoken of shooting herself, and her husband "accidentally" leaves his gun cabinet unlocked. On an unconscious level, this kind of dynamic can involve many different factors. In some such cases, the depressed person might know a disturbing secret about another family member, who may then actually develop a fantasy that the person will die so that the secret will not be discovered by others. Other times, an individual may try to commit suicide in imitation of an earlier attempt by someone else in the family. Some families with a history of depression also have a history of other extended family members committing suicide, pointing to suicide as a viable option to escape the pain of depression. Depression can also lead to suicide when a person feels neglected and unnoticed, such as an individual who is quiet and never asks for anything. Such a person is often virtually forgotten about, as if he were invisible; therefore, he may feel obliged to "disappear" through death.

The situations described above are very serious dynamics that are hard for families to look at, just as it is hard to imagine that your loved one would kill him- or herself. Once these issues are addressed fully, families are able to move on to a healthier relationship that eventually excludes wondering if your loved one will kill herself next week.

Suicidal behavior usually requires inpatient treatment with intensive family therapy. Unfortunately, this kind of treatment is now being limited by insurance companies to very brief stays, necessitating that a majority of the work be done on an outpatient basis. A behavioral contract with a family member who is suicidal needs to be negotiated carefully and should outline the expectations of each family member. A family safety watch might be a useful item to include in this contract. Such a watch might include removing all weapons from the home, or placing all medications or consumable substances in a locked cabinet. In some cases where the person cannot yet be trusted, there is a need for a twenty-four-hour face-to-face vigil. As mentioned above, it may also be necessary to carefully monitor all medications to prevent the possibility of an overdose or the avoidance of taking medication. Since the use of alcohol or street drugs increases the risk of suicide due to decreased inhibitions, these substances might need to be eliminated.

FAMILY MEMBERS MUST WORK TOGETHER

It is vitally important for the entire family to be involved in the treatment of a depressed person. Working together, the family can assist in bringing about resolution to what may have seemed like a hopeless situation. It is important that the family members learn to monitor the depressed person in a manner that does not infantilize him, but assists by bringing him to a functional and healthy place. In addition, each family member can learn to change their own behaviors and unconscious processes that might be contributing to the problem.

CHAPTER *8*

BIPOLAR AFFECTIVE DISORDER (MANIC DEPRESSIVE ILLNESS)

Drugs discussed:
Eskalith, Lithobid (lithium), Tegretol, Depakote, Lamictal, Neurontin, Zyprexa, Klonopin

Bipolar affective disorder is the new name for manic depressive illness. It involves both periods of depression and mania or hypomania. Hypomania is a mild version of mania. In order to receive this diagnosis, a person must have had at least one manic or hypomanic episode, but may not have necessarily had a depressive episode. Eventually, most individuals with mania will have depressions as well. The diagnosis assumes that substance abuse or medical problems are not the cause of the difficulties.

The diagnostic criteria for a manic episode include a distinct period of elevated, expansive, or irritable mood for at least a week or requiring hospitalization to prevent disastrous consequences. In addition, three symptoms are required (four if mood is only irritable). These include grandiosity, decreased sleep, talkativeness, flight of ideas or thoughts racing, distractibility, increased activity in social, work, or sexual spheres, agitation, and excessive pleasurable activity with potential painful consequences (impulsivity). By definition, a hypomanic episode is milder, without the impairment in function and without any psychotic features. A bipolar patient who has a history of mania and major depression is diagnosed as bipolar I. An individual who has a history of only hypomania plus major depression is diagnosed as bipolar II.

An individual who has had hypomania alternating with periods of chronic mild depression for over two years is diagnosed as *cyclothymic*. Individuals who have a very regular seasonal onset of their depressions and hypomanic or manic periods are considered *seasonal subtype* of either major depression or bipolar illness. Occasionally and perhaps with growing frequency, we are recognizing that individuals may have both manic and depressive symptoms at the same time lasting for more than a week; such individuals are described as being in a mixed episode. This mixed episode is potentially very lethal because it involves extremely depressed or irritable mood combined with the driven, frenetic energy and insomnia of mania.

The natural history of bipolar affective disorder is that it is almost always a recurrent disorder. There are very few cases in which an individual who has had a manic episode will not go on to have either depressions or other manic episodes. The age of onset of the first illness in bipolar affective disorder has been gradually going down. This might be related to an increased prevalence of stimulant abuse or perhaps to greater genetic loading of the illness in families. A first onset of a manic episode after age forty-five in an individual with no family history of bipolar affective disorder is quite uncommon and suggests that a vigorous medical workup for organic causes of a mood disorder should be pursued. The first onset of mania in a teenager is not at all uncommon but must be distinguished from a period of cocaine or other stimulant abuse. The most reliable way to differentiate these possibilities is to obtain a urine toxicology screen immediately on hospital admission or when manic behavior appears during the outpatient appointment. Typically, the lifetime course of bipolar affective disorder reveals episodes with environmental triggers and long periods between episodes early in the person's life; over many years, the episodes tend to become more autonomous (coming on spontaneously "out of the blue") and more frequent. Cycle length (from the start of one episode to the start of the next) may go from two to five years early in the illness and then level out with a common periodicity of about one year. Individuals with four or more episodes of depression or mania yearly are called rapid cyclers.

Often, persons with bipolar affective disorder give a lifetime history of being very successful, creative, hard-working, high achievers at times when they are normal or slightly high. When very high, they may do impulsive things such as overspending (leading to huge bills or bankruptcy), having brief sexual affairs, gambling, shoplifting, moving across the country, and telling off friends and coworkers in nasty language. When depressed, they are often remorseful and tell coworkers that they suffer from burnout and need to take a leave of absence from the job and its pressures. They may withdraw from social engagements and stop doing the activities they once loved because these are no longer pleasurable.

The treatment of bipolar affective disorder is best discussed in three separate parts: the treatment of an acute manic episode, the treatment of an acute bipolar depression, and long-term maintenance.

ACUTE MANIA

Lithium has long been the drug of choice for the treatment of an acute manic episode for many reasons: it is effective in at least two-thirds of the individuals who take it, it is generally very tolerable, and it can often prevent future cycling into other episodes of depression or mania. Lithium often takes one to two weeks to show its effectiveness in a manic episode; often, the hospitalized manic patient requires more behavioral control, so short-term adjunctive strategies are often used. These include the use of antipsychotic drugs for psychotic features and agitation. Such drugs as Haldol, Prolixin, Navane, and Thorazine are very unpopular with patients because they cause emotional blunting and slowing down, and are used in very high doses during the treatment of mania to provide a chemical straitjacket. These drugs carry the risks of neuroleptic malignant syndrome and tardive dyskinesia, and they may cause individuals to "crash" from their manic episode into a period of depression. For all of these reasons, neuroleptics are avoided when possible and alternatives are preferred. The newer atypical antipsychotics such as Zyprexa (olanzepine) are more tolerable to patients, and the manufacturers are currently doing clinical trials to seek FDA approval for their use in mania.

Klonopin (clonazepam) is a high-potency benzodiazepine in the minor tranquilizer family but officially approved by the FDA for the treatment of seizure disorders. Klonopin has the advantages of being a very highly sedating drug that can restore sleep and control the withdrawal from alcohol or other sedative hypnotics, and that has a very rapid onset of action if used in appropriately high doses, typically from 4 to 16 mg daily in an acute manic episode. Sometimes the similar drug Ativan (lorazepam) is used instead of Klonopin because an injectable form is available. It is common for people in a manic episode to try to slow themselves down and get some sleep by using alcohol or other drugs (often marijuana), thus complicating the situation.

Some people with mania do not respond well to lithium, and these tend to be individuals who have dysphoric or mixed-state mania, rapid cycling with four or more episodes of mania or depression per year, or history of lithium maintenance "breakthrough" episodes. A "breakthrough" episode is one that occurs while a patient is taking his regular medicine, is at a therapeutic blood level, is not abusing street drugs, and gets sick despite doing all these things as he should. For these individuals, the anticonvulsants Depakote (divalproex sodium) and Tegretol (carbamazepine) are valuable adjuncts to, or replacements for, lithium therapy of an acute manic episode. Depakote is FDA approved for this use, but

Tegretol is not. The newer anticonvulsants Neurontin (gabapentin) and Lamictal (lamotrigine) are rapidly gaining popularity based on case reports of their successful use in bipolar affective disorder, but as of late 1998, there is a notable lack of large-scale controlled clinical trials in the research literature. These are in progress and hopefully the place of these new drugs in the treatment of bipolar affective disorder will soon be clarified.

ACUTE BIPOLAR DEPRESSION

An individual with a history of bipolar illness who is presenting now with depression may be treated in any of several different ways. There is no clear best way to treat this individual. The biggest risk of treating bipolar depression with an antidepressant is the risk of inducing cycling out of the depression straight into a manic episode. Bipolar patients who are maintained on long-term tricyclic antidepressants may go from very rare episodes of their mood disorder to rapid cycling (four or more episodes per year) or even continuous cycling between depression and mania. It appears that cycling from depression into a manic episode is less frequent with Wellbutrin (bupropion), Paxil (paroxetine), and the MAO inhibitor, Parnate (tranylcypromine) than it is for the tricyclic antidepressant drugs. Thus, these three antidepressants appear to be the drugs of choice for treating severe depression in a bipolar patient. There have been studies showing lithium to be equivalent to the antidepressants and ECT to be superior to the tricyclic antidepressants in the treatment of bipolar depression. Sometimes Tegretol and Depakote are used in the context of bipolar depression with rapid cycling. Once again, the roles of the new anticonvulsants Lamictal and Neurontin appear promising but are not yet proven in bipolar depression. Often, the initial treatment of depression in bipolar affective disorder involves a mood stabilizer (lithium or an anticonvulsant) and then the addition of an antidepressant if the depression does not begin to clear after a few weeks.

LONG-TERM MAINTENANCE TREATMENT

An individual with bipolar affective disorder is at risk for recurrence of his episodes. There are some very clear and obvious risk factors that are well worth knowing about, as these are highly preventable. Alcohol and cocaine abuse, amphetamines, barbiturates, opiates, reserpine, beta-blocker blood pressure medicines, and other blood pressure medications that act on the brain are all risk factors for cycling for people with mood disorders. Sleep deprivation is another substantial risk factor for mood cycling and may occur in the context of travel across several time zones or in the context of severe stress. Endocrine problems, especially hypothyroidism, or steroid administration may worsen the course of mood disorders.

LITHIUM

The primary drug for the long-term treatment of and prevention of mood cycling has been lithium. The problem with lithium is its ineffectiveness for about 30 percent of patients who try it, often due to their having rapid cycling illness with four or more episodes of depression or mania per year. The other problems of lithium include long-term weight gain, slowing thyroid function with possibility of developing a goiter, and decreased concentrating capacity of the kidneys. This can lead to large urine output with the annoyance of frequent urination. This can be readily treated with a diuretic; however, the lithium dose will then need to be adjusted downward. The major drug interactions of lithium are with non-steroidal anti-inflammatories such as Aleve (naproxen) and Motrin (ibuprofen). These are risky because both are available as over-the-counter drugs and both can raise lithium levels substantially. An individual taking lithium may take aspirin or acetaminophen without any problem. The other major drug interactions of lithium are with diuretics and ACE inhibitor blood pressure medicines, which can raise lithium levels.

For those individuals who have breakthrough episodes while taking lithium, a series of questions need to be asked: Did the breakthrough occur because the drug was stopped? because the level was too low? because hypothyroidism was developing gradually? because antidepressants were being added to the lithium? or because of illicit substance abuse? Lithium, like most drugs, is not effective if it is not taken regularly. A major review of lithium discontinuation by a researcher, Suppe, a few years ago showed that rapid, rather than gradual, discontinuation of lithium put the individual at very high risk of depressive or manic episodes in the following several months. Gelenberg's study on lithium levels showed that levels of approximately 0.8 or more are better than lower levels for long-term maintenance. Hypothyroidism is frequently associated with the development of rapid cycling in individuals who are taking lithium and is very readily corrected by the addition of small doses of thyroid hormone (Synthroid, Levoxyl, levothyroxine). The antidepressants are best avoided long term because of the risk of causing a switch from depression to mania or rapid cycling. If they are needed, the drugs mentioned earlier for the acute treatment of bipolar depression (such as Wellbutrin or Paxil) appear to be best. Substance abuse, especially stimulants, alcohol, and sedative hypnotics, are major offenders for worsening the course of bipolar affective disorder. Rapid cycling may occur from the beginning of the illness or develop after several years of bipolar illness and is a significant marker for lithium nonresponsiveness.

In those individuals who have breakthrough episodes while on lithium and who do not have the above problems in the lithium treatment, the anticonvulsants are especially useful. Depakote appears to be a first-choice drug and has recently won FDA approval for the treatment of mania. Tegretol has been used even longer by psychiatrists and also appears to be an effective anticycling drug. The choice between these can be difficult, and sometimes an individual will respond quite nicely to one of these but not the other. Tegretol carries some risks of sedation and it also induces liver enzymes that metabolize other drugs, including birth control pills. This makes the birth control pills less effective in preventing pregnancy. Tegretol can also cause bone marrow suppression so that the body cannot fight off infections. Depakote can cause nausea, weight gain, hair loss, and tremor but tends to be less sedating than Tegretol. Both of these drugs require blood sampling every week initially to every month or two during long-term treatment to determine therapeutic blood levels of the drugs as well as to look for very rare but potentially dangerous side effects such as bone marrow or liver toxicity.

PSYCHOTHERAPY AND DEPRESSION

It would be unreasonable to discuss the pharmacology of manic depressive illness without a word about psychotherapy issues. The psychology of manic depression and its impact on the family is extremely important. This illness carries with it a high risk of divorce, often because the spouse of the manic depressive sees the depression episodes as periods of genuine illness and sees the manic episodes as periods of reckless excesses, anger, and striking back by running up huge bills, having extramarital affairs, and being emotionally abusive. It is very common for the individual with manic depressive illness to say that when she is genuinely upset about something her family members will ask, "Are you taking your medicine?" rather than acknowledging the legitimacy of the emotional issue. This can be very frustrating and dehumanizing for the person who has genuine issues to discuss with the family and yet every feeling is viewed as a potential sign of illness.

The most common psychological issue in manic depressive illness is denial of its lifelong recurrent nature and the need for lifelong treatment. Recent studies of the kindling effect tend to show that with every episode of manic depressive illness, the next episode is likely to come sooner, so that typical episodes at the beginning of the illness may occur at three- to five-year intervals, and after a few episodes, they may occur at once-yearly intervals or more frequently.

The challenge of "picking up the pieces" of a life thrown into chaos by mood swings can feel overwhelming. Often the cost of the mood swings is bankruptcies, divorces, and job losses to the point where a very creative, bright, successful individual is virtually alone and penniless in the world and truly has to start over in building a life for himself.

The importance of having a family and outside support system as stress buffers, avoiding abusable substances, avoiding periods of sleep deprivation, and maintaining a lifelong relationship with a psychiatrist who is capable of responding when the patient is going into a manic or depressive episode cannot be overemphasized.

Mary: Bipolar I affective disorder (with mania)

Mary is a twenty-two-year-old, single female with an associate's degree in business administration. She is currently living with her parents. Mary stated that she was referred because "things are not getting better." She recently felt suicidal.

Mary had the onset of problems when she had a knee injury while skiing approximately ten years ago. This led to Mary becoming depressed and staying in bed for days on end, not doing anything and feeling worthless. She was talking and writing slowly, and her parents were actually writing her school papers. She developed a fear of speaking in front of her speech class. She gained about 10 pounds, and lost her interest in competitive swimming. She slept a lot, up to about eleven and a half hours per night. She had decreased energy, decreased sex drive, and decreased concentration. She did not have any psychotic symptoms such as thoughts of sin, evil, guilt, or punishment, nor did she have auditory, visual, taste, touch, or smell hallucinations or paranoia. She began psychotherapy for the depression and within a few months was improving and swimming again. She lost weight, got her energy back, had normal mood, had normal sleep of about seven hours, and her speech was back to normal. Two years ago, on her twentieth birthday, she recalls feeling normal. For the next three months, she was participating in competitive swimming, feeling good about herself, and had a boyfriend for a few months. Then, just two months later, she found she couldn't sleep because she had "so much energy" and her mood was "hyper." Initially, her mother thought she was doing great because she got a passport to travel and was buying clothes. Her father became concerned that she spent a thousand dollars on clothes, knowing this was very out of character for her. She had grown up in a family that was not very religious and she suddenly "got religion" and became a fundamentalist Christian.

A lot of unusual behavior for Mary began occurring over the following several weeks. She attempted to buy a business; it was unclear to me if this was a realistic possibility or a grandiose plan. She felt high, and more talkative, social, and sexual. She sold her car without forethought, and very suddenly became paranoid, feeling that someone was out to kill her. She became afraid of a teacher at school, as well as her boyfriend. She felt extremely high with "runner's rush" just before becoming paranoid. She couldn't stop swimming and told her parents that it kept her going. She was taking twenty units of college credit and working part-time. She lost her sense of proportion. At that point, she was admitted to a private psychiatric hospital. Her doctor started her on Haldol because she was "in a dream stage." She feared that the world was going to explode with fire.

She came back to reality after her hospitalization. As often happens after a manic episode, she became depressed and this lasted for over six months.

The depression worsened at a three-month midpoint while she was taking a logic class. She was unable to complete an exam due to blurry vision from her medications. For the last three months, she had stayed in bed a lot, getting up only two hours before going to work at her part-time waitress job, and then would return to bed as soon as she returned home. She describes her mood over the past two months as down. She states that her energy is "none" and she can't concentrate well.

She still has sexual interest. She participated in some activities but found no enjoyment in them. She has gained 5 or 10 pounds.

She developed suicidal ideation very recently and ran her car in the garage. She expected to die, but was found by a neighbor. She has had thoughts of overdosing or shooting herself. She has stayed in bed, feeling that she can't fit in or talk to anybody. She indicated that she had similar suicidal ideation during her depression last summer, but made no attempt to act on it.

She has remained on Haldol at a dose that has been decreased down to 2 mg daily and she indicates she has been on Prozac for about a month without any benefit.

She denies any drug or alcohol abuse as precipitants for either the present depression or the previous depression or manic episode.

She states that the paranoid ideation was gone shortly after she left the hospital. She did have ideas of reference, feeling that the radio and television were talking about her when she was just out of the hospital, but denied any special content to messages about her. She denied experiencing mind control, mind reading, thought diffusion, or auditory, visual, taste, touch, or smell hallucinations.

Mary had a significant family history of psychiatric problems. Mary's sister has bulimia and is not currently being treated with medicines or therapy. Her mother was present at the initial meeting and indicated that she experienced post-partum depression after Mary's birth, but not after the birth of her two other daughters. She related the post-partum depression to her husband's transfer of his job. She indicated that her own father wrote her letters from Europe telling her to work hard and this would help her get over the depression so she did not seek treatment. Her mother spontaneously stated that at times "I feel so good that I could touch the sky, it's so great to be alive. I am grateful to have such an experience." The highs are experienced only by herself and have not been apparent to her husband; they have been very brief and not accompanied by impulsive or out-of-character behavior. The mother also indicated that she has had depressions lasting over a month, when younger and living in Europe. They were clearly worse during the winter and better in the spring and summer, and less intense once the family moved to California and she began to work with children in day care. Thus, Mary's mother appeared to have bipolar II disorder (depressions and hypomania, with a seasonal component) that had not been treated.

Mary has never been on lithium, Tegretol, tricyclic antidepressants, or Wellbutrin. The referring doctor has worked with the family on occasion and found Mary's mother to be somewhat overprotective and a workaholic. The family attempts to deny significant mental illness in any members. Mary has two siblings, one who is a compulsive overeater and another who is bulimic. Her doctor indicated that Mary has told her of lack of motivation, problems concentrating, and feeling that her brain is damaged, that she has weird body sensations and thought broadcasting. The doctor has noted psychotic symptoms independent of the mood disorder.

Initial Diagnosis and Treatment Plan: I found Mary to have bipolar affective disorder, currently depressed but with a history of mania with psychotic features. The differential diagnosis includes the possibility of schizoaffective disorder. The difference between bipolar affective disorder with psychotic features and schizoaffective disorder is a subtle one; in the latter, psychotic features (hallucinations or delusions) are present at times when the patient is not in a depressive or manic episode. Usually a mood stabilizer is used for both, but the use of an antipsychotic may be time limited with bipolar affective disorder and long term with schizoaffective disorder.

I indicated very strongly to the patient that she should maintain hope of recovery as a sustaining force in resisting the suicidal ideation. I told her there were many pharmacological treatments that had not yet been tried. Her parents were very appreciative of this and indicated they had some preference that I assume her treatment because of these statements. I also indicated to them my recommendation that the Prozac be stopped, the Haldol be tapered off gradually if possible, and the patient be started on a course of lithium, possibly augmented by Wellbutrin or an MAOI. The parents indicated their concern that the patient did not seem to be forming a close relationship with Dr. S. I suggested that they work with the referring psychiatrist, however, for the acute hospital stabilization phase. I indicated that I would provide a copy of this consultation to her.

Revised Treatment Plan: Two months later, Mary returned. She was last seen while in the midst of severe depression and was hospitalized for ten days shortly after I had met with her. She started taking Lithobid and Wellbutrin. She started school and is currently taking twelve units of college classes. She feels back to normal, in terms of being out of the depression, but she does not have much enthusiasm for studying. She said if she had a choice, she would rather be working in or owning a corporation. She indicates she is doing well in most of her classes, but writing is really difficult for her. She says many of her friends are attending school out of this area. She does not currently have a boyfriend, but she would like to have one. She feels down on herself and insecure because of her weight gain, her lack of self-confidence, having acne, for eating junk food, and for sitting and watching television. She says it is hard for her to interact with people sometimes.

Mary states that she is not happy and does not know what she really wants to do long term. When asked about goals of therapy, Mary indicated she wants to work on increasing her self-esteem. I stated that my goals are medication maintenance and not committing suicide, which is still on her mind. We decided to meet every other week. She agreed to follow through with homework assignments discussed in her sessions. My expectations of Mary are that she come to all appointments, take her medications as prescribed, not use abusable drugs, stay alive, and work on goals for herself. She requested prescriptions for her routine maintenance medications which are Lithobid 300 mg, two tablets twice daily, and Wellbutrin 75 mg, one tablet twice daily.

After three years of working together, Mary paged me for an emergency callback, and accused me of needing a psychiatrist, that she was firing me, and she didn't need lithium anymore. She was belligerent with her family members, which was out of character when her mood was stabilized, so they took her to UCI Medical Center for an evaluation for admission.

Two weeks later, Mary again came to see me. She had been hospitalized for a manic episode, and at the time of admission had a lithium level of 0.2, indicating that she had not been taking her medicine. She was angry about having been placed into restraint and seclusion for behavioral control, and was even angrier when her father came into the session and said that she had seemed to be hallucinating at home. She said she was the youngest child in the family and the parents were reluctant to let her break away and were overcontrolling. Mary's father was concerned that she had spent $500 in the first few days out of the hospital and had taken away her credit card and bankbook. Her father went on to say she was pretending to use sign language, rearranged the kitchen during the middle of the night, and called her boyfriend and was hostile toward him on the phone at 6:00 A.M.

Rehospitalization occurred two days later, when the father brought Mary in for an appointment and she refused to come into my office. She stood in the parking lot gesturing with her hands and speaking in a disorganized manner, and was found by the police after wandering away. She was scared, angry, and labile, and looked around as if she were hearing voices. The initial plan in the hospital was to evaluate for medical causes of mania and aggressively pursue medication stabilization.

Conclusion: Mary had done quite well on a long-term maintenance schedule of lithium and Wellbutrin. What happened? On her first admission, the lithium level was very low so she may have stopped taking it regularly. It turned out that the routine admission labs held the clue to what the patient admitted only much later. She was taking diet pills obtained from a friend. The lab report on her urine showed amphetamine. This manic episode might not have happened if she had not been using stimulants. The risk is far too high in bipolar patients to even consider using stimulants for weight loss!

Lisa: Bipolar affective disorder, manic cycling into depression

Lisa is a forty-one-year-old married female. She lives with her husband and daughter, who recently graduated eighth grade, and two stepchildren. She works in sales. She was brought to the emergency room on my insistence after her husband had called me stating that Lisa had a loaded gun and was out on the street waving it around. He told me she had exclaimed that she thought the gun was a beer and she was going to put it in her mouth.

Lisa had a two-day history of having an unusual amount of energy; little need for sleep; acting crazy; demonstrating pressured speech, grandiosity, and explosive behavior coupled with ideas of reference; lability; and irritability. She reportedly felt like things were moving around, disappearing, and being switched on her.

Lisa reportedly has a history of very similar brief psychotic episodes occurring annually for about twenty-five or thirty years. She was once prescribed lithium by a psychiatrist but stopped it after just a couple of doses.

Lisa's developmental history is significant in that she grew up in Europe until age eight, then came to the United States with her parents and one sibling. She had a difficult time adjusting to her new peers and in adolescence began acting out. She left home at age fifteen when she became pregnant, and subsequently got married. That pregnancy resulted in the birth of a daughter, who is a severely mentally retarded, chronically institutionalized child. Her first marriage was very miserable and lasted for four years.

Shortly thereafter, Lisa remarried. In that marriage, she and her husband have had one daughter together. Her husband had two children from his first marriage. Her daughter just graduated eighth grade and is about to start a private school. The other children are ages twenty-two and nineteen and still live at home.

Lisa has an annual period where she has a breakdown around July fourth, plus or minus a couple of weeks. This has gone on annually since she was a child. The date is the anniversary of learning she was pregnant with her first daughter. It is also the anniversary of having her parents forget her birthday in mid-July when she was ten years old. There is also an episode that occurred at this time of year when she was about seven years old. She and another child were wading in the ocean near her father. They were pulled under by the currents and her father chose to save her friend, and someone else—a stranger—saved her from the water. She was upset that her father chose to save the friend, although the father was positioned closer to the friend. She states that each year around this time she has the feeling that she has done and seen it all, and becomes tired of life.

Lisa told me that her current episode, which began a couple of days earlier, is the worst she has experienced and is the only one for which she has been psychiatrically hospitalized.

Lisa has quite a history of depression, lasting from two days up to six months or even one year. The depressions were obvious at around age thirty, though severe acting out during adolescence may be a marker that depression began at that time. She was treated with psychotherapy repeatedly until she "got bored" with the therapy and terminated. Prozac was prescribed by her general practitioner for about one year and although it worked, she disliked taking it and stopped it on her own.

Lisa has often felt that the pain of life was greater than the pleasure. She feels unappreciated by her husband, that he is chronically stressed over money problems, and that financially she would be just as well off if she were separated and working on her own. She has been in marital therapy at times and finds it works when they are engaged in the therapy process and making an effort. She is now thinking she would like to get back into therapy for a year to see if things can truly improve between the two of them, and if not she would consider filing for a separation in order to try to get her husband to appreciate her more.

Many people with bipolar affective disorder have a family history of mood disorder or substance abuse; Lisa had both in her family. Her father was a heavy drinker who stopped drinking for fifteen years and later resumed it. Her dad had very difficult long-term depressions, which began after she ran away from home at age fifteen. Her mother is also described as a heavy chronic drinker and depressed.

Lisa indicates she is sometimes self-destructive and drives her new car 140 mph on the freeway when there is no traffic. She states she would like to do skydiving but her husband won't let her.

At the time of admission to the hospital, Lisa was described as grandiose, pressured, euphoric, and irritable with ideas of reference. At the time of my evaluation, she displayed none of these but rather was tearful and sad and described a lot of pain around the anniversary issues and the parenting and marital issues.

Diagnosis and Treatment Plans: Lisa has bipolar affective disorder, most recently manic but now cycling down into depression. It is unclear whether this should appropriately be labeled a seasonal affective disorder or a recurrent anniversary reaction. She also has hypothyroidism, which is being treated. My treatment plan was as follows.

First, Lisa was sent to the emergency room at UCI Medical Center where she was placed on a seventy-two-hour legal hold for her protection. I warned her that this was to be a "cooling-off period" after her potentially dangerous behavior the night before. I then suggested that Lisa start on Depakote because she had refused to take lithium in the past; she was agreeable to trying this medication.

Conclusions: A manic episode may be part of a seasonal affective disorder or a psychologically driven anniversary reaction. In this case, it's hard to tell the difference. Lisa clearly had an annual period of severe illness to the point of dangerously irrational behavior and had never been willing to accept preventive treatment before. After a long discussion, we decided that using an antimanic drug such as Depakote or lithium beginning a few weeks before her usual time of illness made a lot of sense and she agreed to do this. It will be up to Lisa to follow through with treatment, and it will benefit her to become involved in ongoing psychotherapy. A psychotherapist knowledgeable about bipolar disorder will be able to help her learn to identify times of vulnerability before they become full-blown manic episodes requiring hospitalization.

Dan: Bipolar affective disorder, mixed state (both manic and depressive features)

Dan is a fifty-seven-year-old married male. Dan was brought in by his wife for agitated behavior, depression, and intimidating her.

Dan has a twenty-year history of bipolar affective disorder, with three psychiatric hospitalizations. He had been treated with lithium until nine years ago when he opted to discontinue it. His wife, Jan, told me there has been no history of substance abuse and no history of significant depression or mania over the last nine years while he has been off psychiatric medications. Fourteen years ago he had a severe episode in which he bought a $50,000 motor home on credit and stood in front of traffic and got deeply into pyramid investment schemes.

It is readily apparent that he is in an episode now that is precipitated by the death of his mother three weeks prior to admission to the hospital, and the death of his father last week. His wife indicated she had observed several symptoms, including sweaty hands, fluttering eyes, not sleeping, decreased appetite, talking erratically, crying, being unable to go to work, problems concentrating, and waking up his wife with erratic and irrational statements.

Jan reported that Dan had no major medical problems but does smoke cigarettes. Family history shows a strong genetic loading for bipolar affective disorder; his father, brother, and cousins have all had bipolar affective disorder.

My examination of Dan on the morning after admission revealed that he was alert, polite, and cooperative. He was in the seclusion room due to his agitated behavior, but he was not in restraints. He requested to get up and walk through the seclusion room but was in no way threatening. Dan was wondering why he was in the hospital. He stated he has had a rough time and that the death of both parents was unexpected.

He seemed unaware of being extremely agitated and combative the night before.

At the time of the interview, Dan did not understand why he was in the hospital. He felt his mood as appropriately upset at the loss of his parents. He denies any suicidal or homicidal ideation. He denies any hallucinations. There is no evidence of delusions. His orientation was such that he knew he was in a psychiatric hospital but did not know which one. He gave the date as it was six days prior.

Diagnosis and Treatment Plan: Dan appears to have had a mixed state with both manic and depressive features, as part of his bipolar affective disorder, and is now showing some symptom resolution on medication.

Dan has bipolar affective disorder with a strong familial component and a very long cycle length. He presented as highly agitated, combative, and disorganized, and had rapid improvement after a good night's sleep with Ativan and Haldol in the hospital. His episode was triggered either directly by the stress of losing both parents or by the resulting sleep deprivation. He was agreeable to using a mood stabilizer for a few months after these stressful events. He was reluctant to accept long-term medications.

Like most people who have infrequent episodes of illness, Dan was reluctant to commit to long-term medication maintenance, yet this is usually recommended to prevent further episodes.

Subsequent outpatient therapy revealed he had an ongoing mild depression. He was dealing with long-standing boredom in running his small grocery store, deciding to sell it, and wondering what to do to keep himself busy as his wife pursued her full-time work. He had a long-term difficulty with obesity, smoking, and lacking anything to get enthused about in life besides his sons. He remained on medications in an effort to minimize the long-term depression. Four years after his hospitalization, he is doing very well with lithium and Paxil.

Karen: Bipolar affective disorder with seasonal affective disorder subtype

Karen is a twenty-seven-year-old single female living alone, with no children. She works as a fund-raiser who is involved in writing grants and public speaking for a nonprofit agency.

She told me on her first visit that she had been taking Tegretol due to a history of mania. She was seeking a new psychiatrist since her previous doctor was a two-hour drive away from her home.

Karen provided a concise history of mania, having developed her first manic episode two and a half years earlier. At that time, she didn't sleep for three nights, she didn't eat, and she was confused. She wanted to go into a hospital and she was actually briefly admitted to a series of several hospitals. She was treated with lithium and neuroleptics without success. These were stopped and she was switched to Tegretol with a good response. She also engaged in psychotherapy with Dr. C. She began Tegretol at a dose of eight tablets daily and within six months had tapered it down to no medication, and stopped all aftercare.

Karen then began getting depressed, and saw Dr. C. again and restarted the medication. She most typically takes three to six tablets per day of Tegretol 200 mg. She indicates there have been periods when she pushes up the medication dosage when she begins feeling she is having symptoms.

Karen recognizes when she is becoming manic. Her early symptoms are feeling that it is tough to go to sleep, it becomes difficult to concentrate, and she feels more aggressive. Her severe symptoms include not sleeping or eating, feeling confused, feeling paranoid, being irritable, having racing thoughts, talking a lot, an increased sex drive, feeling more social than usual, having more energy, and being more distractible and very confused. She does not experience hallucinations, excessive laughing or joking, spending sprees, or activities that would get her into trouble.

On the other hand, Karen has had seasonal depressions essentially every year since she was in high school in New Hampshire, typically starting in November. She spontaneously stated, "I hibernate in winter." During this time, she does not go out, is socially withdrawn, and feels less self-confident. She does not notice a change in her sex drive, but people with whom she is involved in relationships tire of her social isolation. This has led to breaking up with boyfriends over the years. Her winter depressions are as intense in California as they were in New Hampshire.

Last December, while in a depressive episode, Karen went to the Caribbean with her mother and found she felt much better within a couple of days of getting there. The depressions leave her feeling anxious and less self-confident, and disturb her usual eight-hour sleep cycle in that she requires up to twelve or fifteen hours of sleep. She does not overeat and does manage to continue her usual exercise regime. She has never been suicidal, been hospitalized, or missed a lot of work because of the depressions.

Karen has had migraine headaches since about junior high school. She occasionally takes aspirin with codeine, Nuprin, or Valium for these. They occur about once a month. She has very severe ones about every three months for which she sometimes requires an injection of Demerol in an emergency room.

Karen does not smoke cigarettes, does not drink alcohol due to getting headaches from it, and does not use any street drugs.

As is often the case, Karen has a strong family history of mood disorder. Her father has been hospitalized a couple of times for depression. He has made a suicide attempt, which resulted in his receiving ECT; he has been well without any treatment over the last six years. To the best of her knowledge, he has never been manic. Her mother has had no psychiatric problems. She has three brothers: one is depressed at times but never treated; her older brother is a pathologic gambler; her younger brother has no psychiatric distress. She is not aware of any definite psychiatric history in second-degree relatives, although one aunt might have had mania. (Note that pathologic gamblers are often self-treating depression or acting out manic impulses; bipolar affective disorder was the most common psychiatric diagnosis in one study of pathologic gamblers.)

Karen described herself as ambitious, intelligent, fun loving, sociable, and conservative. She enjoys movies, going out to dinner, and playing tennis.

Diagnosis and Treatment Plan: Karen has bipolar affective disorder, currently euthymic (definite seasonal affective disorder), and migraine headaches. She will continue on her current Tegretol six tablets daily.

Three years later, Karen moved back to Palm Springs. She began seeing a new doctor who placed her on Zoloft at 100 mg/day along with Tegretol. She has obtained a bright artificial light visor to use during winter depressions and found it helpful. She is doing well. She described Zoloft as a "miracle drug," feeling it helped tremendously to relieve the depression and prevented most migraine headaches. Eventually, she discontinued the Tegretol and remained on Zoloft alone.

A couple of years later, Karen's brothers called me concerned that she was getting manic again. She was hospitalized as she had become combative, anxious, scared, and stressed, and was fearing that relatives would harm her ill uncle. I had a discussion with the doctor treating her in the hospital, and he confirmed the brothers' concerns. Out of necessity, the doctor had given her oral and long-acting depot Haldol, which led to problematic side effects. The goal was to get her back onto Tegretol to control mania. She remained in the hospital for approximately three weeks to obtain stabilization.

Conclusion: Karen, like many with bipolar affective disorder, has experienced major life disruption with a manic episode.

She tolerated the chronic mild depression that she experienced while on Tegretol and had no manic episodes while taking it. She felt much better on an SSRI antidepressant and was able to discard the Tegretol for a couple of years before another manic episode came back and disrupted her life eight years after the original episode. We will never know if that episode would have occurred if she had stayed on the Tegretol as a mood stabilizer. Her current doctor won't really know if readding the antidepressant to her Tegretol will increase her risk of another manic episode or will simply raise her baseline mood level back to normal. These are very difficult judgment calls and require close collaboration of patient and doctor in making decisions that carry risks no matter which direction they are made.

Laura: Bipolar affective disorder II (major depressions and hypomania)

Laura is a thirty-year-old single woman working as an elementary special education teacher.

Laura stated that she wants a psychiatrist to work with her because she has previously been treated on Prozac for nine months, prescribed by her internist, who told her it was to be used on a time-limited basis and that she should discontinue it. After having been off it for seven months, she went down to Mexico to get the drug and restarted it on her own. She knew, however, this type of medication needs to be monitored by a medical doctor.

Laura had experienced depression problems since she was a teenager and had her first really severe depression four years earlier after the breakup of a long-term relationship. During this severe depression, she was feeling like she was hitting bottom; she was losing weight, felt lethargic, fearful, and tearful; and felt that every problem seemed bigger than it was. Prior to that time, she had never had depression interfering with her work and school and had never been on any medications.

This first severe episode followed a period of living with a man who was twenty years older, who was underemployed and working at menial jobs. He had multiple addictions, including alcohol, and probably had bipolar affective disorder. This was the first and only relationship in which she was very seriously involved with a man. At the time she got involved with him at age twenty, she had little sense of self-identity. She would get wrapped up in his emotions and the roller-coaster ride of his manic depressive illness. She felt needed as long as she was taking care of him and mothering him. If she had good self-esteem, she would have left much earlier.

When she completed her teaching credential and was offered a job, she wanted to get married. When he refused, she began recognizing that he was not right for her and decided to move near the job she was about to begin. Although this was a positive step for her, it still left her devastated and lonely and triggered a depressive episode.

Laura grew up in Southern California with her father, who is also a teacher, and mother, who is a homemaker. She has two older brothers. She had a perception that her family valued self-sufficiency, though she complained that her father always treats her like his little girl. It seems she got a lot of mixed messages from her family. There was some inappropriate sexual exploration with older brothers, but she feels she has been able to work that through with them since she has become an adult. She was a good student in junior high and high school and was active in student politics, athletics, and cheerleading. She also did well in college, and won an award for a project she did with her students while student teaching.

Laura came from a very stoic European family, with many relatives demonstrating symptoms of various mood disorders. Two uncles committed suicide, a maternal grandfather was alcoholic, the father was depressed and extremely self-controlled;

the only emotion he ever expressed was anger. She said that her mother is "like me," up for everyone else, but with a sense of tremendous loneliness, despair, and feeling that she has sacrificed a lot in her marriage. Furthermore, her mother had a history of blacking out with drinking and her father was alcoholic, which led to her decision to become a nondrinker. Laura's two older brothers also demonstrate some symptoms that might indicate depression or even hypomania.

Laura had never been on any other antidepressants prior to trying Prozac. During the initial trial of Prozac, she had a side effect of headaches for the first week or so, but these went away. The Prozac helped her to experience more self-confidence, feel that she could count on her emotional state being steady, and feel better about breaking up with her boyfriend. She found herself crying less, and eating better. She began improving within two weeks and had a full response at one to two months. She was on the Prozac for nine months and felt that one 20 mg pill per day was a fully adequate dose. She was taken off it at her doctor's request and then she went back on it on her own seven months later, having purchased it in Mexico. She briefly tried it at two pills per day and had severe nausea and headaches while on that dose. She states that while on the higher dosage she felt like a "cold fish," detached, and though she gets her job done, she has little empathy or emotional response to others. She has some slight emotional reactivity, but it is less than it has been in the past. She often goes for about three months doing well and then for no apparent reason goes into a crying spell for perhaps a week. Though she says it feels like an emotional release, it disrupts her life. During these periods, she is also anxious, irritable, tense, and on edge; she overworks and experiences less need for sleep, restless sleep, an increased sex drive, and increased creativity. She thinks faster and makes cruel sarcastic comments, but fortunately she does not go on spending sprees. Her energy is about 20 percent above normal and she exercises slightly more than normal. Her friends often comment that she is on edge, negative, quick to judge, sarcastic, and feels everybody hates her because of these episodes of irritable hypomania.

Laura is concerned about her sexual response. She indicates that off of Prozac she was orgasmic with masturbation or intercourse, but on Prozac is not orgasmic in either way. This may become more of a problem for her when she gets involved in a serious relationship. Laura is dating but currently has no serious relationships. She feels less vulnerable this way as she has realized that she used to seek love or self-esteem through sex.

Laura said that off of Prozac she is depressed 60 percent of the time, normal 20 percent, and high 20 percent. On Prozac she is depressed 20 percent, normal 60 percent, and high 20 percent of the time.

Laura described herself as a quiet, hardworking person who did not know herself and had low self-esteem, but now she speaks her own mind with confidence and takes care of herself first.

Diagnosis and Treatment Plan: Laura has bipolar affective disorder, type II (major depressions and hypomania). I asked her to have routine screening labs including blood chemistry, complete blood count, thyroid functions, HIV, syphilis screening, and urinalysis. I also suggested that she try Prozac, one pill every other day, to decrease the sexual dysfunction. If that did not adequately relieve this side effect, then she would go off Prozac for a few days and try Wellbutrin at 100 mg two to three times daily.

Laura decided to go on Wellbutrin 100 mg three times daily, which relieved the sexual dysfunction. She did complain of occasional word-finding difficulty, but had much better emotional responsiveness than when taking Prozac.

Just a year later, Laura began having one-week periods of hypomania (with irritability at times) alternating with two to three weeks of depression and only a few days normal in between, so I recommended tapering off Wellbutrin and starting lithium.

Within a few weeks on lithium, she stated feeling quiet and calm, free of negative thoughts and feelings, and with a stable mood. She complains of feeling bored at times since she was accustomed to living a high-energy lifestyle, and now spends more time relaxing at home. I discussed my concerns with Laura that often people go off the medications because they prefer feeling high, but that this can have devastating effects.

Contrary to my recommendation, Laura went off medications on her own for two to three months and felt much more depressed. She complained she was cycling on her antidepressant, had been bloated often, and had gained a lot of weight on lithium, which is why she discontinued it. She now knew it was not a good idea to discontinue her medicine without discussing it with her doctor. She requested that I restart her on the lithium at a very low dose.

A year later, Laura was doing very well. The depressions were easily controlled by increasing the Wellbutrin from 300 to 450 mg/day and occasionally adding in lithium. She was on her summer break, dating several men, running, and very pleased with her state of mind.

By the following spring, we reduced the Wellbutrin to 300 mg/day. Laura's mood was very stable, she felt enthusiastic, and was working hard. She preferred Wellbutrin much more than lithium long term.

Conclusions: Laura, like Karen, felt better on an antidepressant than on a mood stabilizer. She had rapid brief cycles and she came to realize that she could control these with minor antidepressant dose adjustments and using lithium on an occasional as-needed basis. This isn't officially recommended in any textbook, but it appeared to work quite nicely for her. She illustrates another major point: Patients sometimes feel that an SSRI antidepressant such as Prozac makes them much less in touch with their emotions and this can be helpful (feeling less overreactive and rejection sensitive) or harmful (less able to relate emotionally to another person) subjectively. The sexual dysfunction was a major motivator for changing from Prozac to Wellbutrin, but the emotional disconnectedness was another reason; both improved with the change in antidepressant. Another factor to underline is that it is very important to communicate with your doctor about medication changes you wish to make so that the changes can be appropriately monitored.

FAMILY DYNAMICS IN BIPOLAR DISORDER

I have spent a great deal of my career working with people who have bipolar disorder, with a special emphasis on working with them in the context of family therapy. Since bipolar disorder runs in families, it is not unusual for there to be more than one member affected, so extensive family therapy is often indicated. It can be helpful at times to include extended family members in addition to family of origin or immediate family. Most likely, there is a variety of dynamics that often have been present for quite a long time before the illness surfaced and may have even been handed down through the generations. Bear in mind that the person affected with bipolar disorder may play any role in the family such as parent, child, sibling, spouse, aunt, uncle, and so on, but the following dynamics are often present regardless of position.

ENMESHMENT IN FAMILIES WITH BIPOLAR AFFECTIVE DISORDER

Enmeshment, a concept discussed in chapter 7, is present when family members speak for each other, not allowing people to have their own voices. It also occurs when one person displays an emotion and others begin to take on that emotion even though they were feeling fine before. This can lead to family members feeling they have to suppress emotions to keep others from feeling what they feel. Another way enmeshment is displayed is when one member continually does things for another, rendering that person helpless to perform tasks that are age appropriate—often this is done unconsciously to keep that person from being able to grow up and move out into her own life. Another way this can appear is when people within the family system become a pair that is psychologically unhealthy; for example, when a mother and son are aligned in such a way that they seem like husband and wife and the father is excluded from their dyad. In my experience, it is no surprise when one of the members that make up this unhealthy dyad is the one with bipolar disorder. Also, it does not have to be obvious to nevertheless have a great effect on the one with bipolar disorder as well as the family system as a whole. An example of this more covert situation is when the mother continually talks and worries with her husband about the son with bipolar disorder to the exclusion of developing a marital relationship that is based on the couple's own issues independent of the son.

Families with enmeshment are challenged to learn a new way to be close that encourages growth, self-expression, and acceptance of members as individuals with their own unique thoughts, feelings, and choices to make in life. Enmeshed family systems can be dangerous if these issues are not addressed. I have often seen this entanglement unintentionally set up the person with bipolar disorder (who has been trying to individuate from the family) to stop taking his medication when another family member begins to feel abandoned. Enmeshment also rears its ugly head when family members collude with the person with bipolar disorder to remain manic so as to take the focus off another family member who is masking symptoms of the disorder. Again, enmeshment is most often very covert and difficult to see, especially when you are the one participating in this within your family. Enmeshment requires a juggling act when the identified person needs to become individuated, yet is too manic or depressed and is rendered more dependent by the very nature of the illness. This creates a double bind where you are "damned if you do" encourage individuation and "damned if you don't." This concept of a double bind is discussed more thoroughly in chapter 9 on schizophrenia. It usually requires work in family therapy to create a new way of being close that isn't focused around the illness.

I first met Jeff when he was fifteen years old. His parents were divorced, and he lived with his mother, Shirley. His father, Ben, lived nearby and saw Jeff regularly. Shirley's father and brother both had bipolar affective disorder, which taught her to have a high tolerance for bizarre behavior. This resulted in Jeff being manic for several months before being brought in for treatment. He was referred to me by the psychiatrist who had just put Jeff on medication. Jeff and Shirley were very enmeshed and seemed more like a husband and wife than son and mother in several respects. Jeff called his mother Shirley. Jeff had no sense of autonomy, and Shirley waited on him hand and foot despite working at a very demanding job. Jeff emotionally supported Shirley by listening to her talking about her very stressful job. It occurred to me that Jeff was not engaging in the normal developmental task of adolescence, which involves becoming gradually more independent of one's parents and developing a strong sense of self. I observed that Jeff and Shirley were so enmeshed that this was contributing to the psychotic behavior as well. Psychosis is the ultimate loss of a sense of self, and the very coddling behavior that was going on between them only served to make matters worse. Immediately I began working with Shirley to stop relying on Jeff for her emotional support and to begin relying on her peers. I also worked with the two of them to plan specific age-appropriate tasks for Jeff to take on around the house and for his personal care, such as cleaning his room and making his lunch. Gradually, over the next few weeks, not only did the medicine kick in and reduce the psychotic symptoms, but Jeff felt a higher level of self-esteem and sense of autonomy. It was the combination of medicine and psychotherapy that helped him return to a more normal place. I worked with the family over the long term as Jeff had very severe bipolar affective disorder that was unrelenting even with the best of care. In this regard, I was able to observe that when Shirley and Jeff returned to the old enmeshment, his psychosis worsened; when they moved out to a more individual stance, his psychosis improved.

DENIAL OF THE ILLNESS

Denial of the symptoms that are going on in a family member can be a problem for both the family and the person with bipolar disorder. Oftentimes, families have a high tolerance for manic behavior. In other words, they have grown accustomed to chaos in the household because other family members may be hysterical and also act out in impulsive, aggressive, or sexual ways. In addition, other family members may have traits of bipolar disorder that are untreated so when they see another family member gradually increasing the same behavior into mania, they are not able or willing to acknowledge it for fear it will make them have to look at their own behavior. Enmeshment again plays a role here, as it is possible for one person to have the role of expressing feelings for other people in the family, and indeed it is most often the one with bipolar disorder. When one person carries the emotions in the family, of course others are allowed an illusion that they are not filled with the emotion. Anger, sadness, guilt, fear, anxiety, and so on can be assigned to one family member to express, but a particular feeling may really belong to another member who is reluctant to own his feelings so he sets off another to express it. This can be dangerous for anyone, but especially for the person affected with the illness. When family members can learn to own and express their own feelings in appropriate ways, the one person with the greatest symptomatology will be better relieved. This will lead to the person with the illness to be less likely to be in denial about her problem and hence, decreases the risk of poor medication compliance and relapse of episodes.

REALISTIC EXPECTATIONS ARE IMPORTANT

While many people with bipolar disorder function well in society and even hold prominent positions in the community, many others cannot. A common family retort to mania is that it is self-centered, pleasure oriented, thoughtless, spiteful, and impulsive. It *appears* that the manic person makes an active choice to engage in such behavior. The family may view the depressed person who is crying, lying in bed, refusing to eat or overeating, and not engaging in productive activities as being lazy, overemotional, weak, and not whole. When the person becomes angry about something or expresses a feeling that is not acceptable to the family, he may be accused of being manic or irritable or depressed rather than being respected for having legitimate feelings. Confusion in the individual is common and can at times be misconstrued by others as poor listening skills or inattention. For the person who is a more vulnerable carrier of bipolar disorder, it seems that the slightest amount of stress can increase hypomania, which can eventually lead him into a full-blown manic episode or set off a severe bout of depression. It becomes a balancing act for the affected person, the family, and the therapist to determine realistic expectations and to be able to be fluid in shifting expectations as needed. In other words, it is important that there be expectations of the patient to function to his greatest capacity, but not beyond, and to understand that "greatest capacity" may change as the patient cycles through episodes.

Juggling becomes one's way of dealing with various issues when the person with bipolar disorder becomes or appears to be manipulative. Mostly, the job of the patient is to learn to be honest and truthful with herself about how much she can actually perform in day-to-day life and how much she is wanting others to cater to her. This is not always as easy as it seems because the person may have a very distorted view of herself that in the moment is her reality. For example, I work with a woman, Beth, who is a rapid cycler between mania, hypomania, and depression. She is among the most fragile of people with bipolar disorder. Her moods often cycle within a few minutes and may even overlap. She is very careful about taking her medicines but still has major difficulties and is totally disabled. Beth is often helpless and cannot perform simple tasks such as going grocery shopping. In the past, she was manipulative in that she longs to be taken care of by her mother, who is too elderly to do so. But at times, she has pushed herself to take part in certain activities and promptly decompensated by either becoming depressed or hypomanic. Often our task together is to decipher her difference between acting helpless and truly being unable to undertake a task.

It is also the job of the family to address ways they enable the person to behave inappropriately. Beth's mother is also very dependent on her. When Beth is doing well and going out with friends, her mother will take to bed, not doing anything to help herself. This forces Beth to step in and do more than is reasonable for a very fragile person, which then causes Beth to decompensate. Beth begins engaging in crazy behavior and becomes homebound eventually so that her mother is not left alone.

Some patients become so self-focused and grandiose that they feel all others around them should cater to them, and even may appear to set themselves up to be taken care of by not taking their medication properly. This leads to them becoming manic. A double bind is created whereby if family members don't cater to the individual, she may become more crazy, yet they are reinforcing the patient to become ill. This can make family members feel as if they are jumping through hoops to keep the patient grounded. This can obviously create so much stress on the family members that they cannot continue this behavior very long. The thing family members can do, however, is to look at their own conduct that may be establishing or maintaining this type of behavior. It's much like the codependence that occurs in families of alcoholics. In some extreme cases where manipulation cannot be worked through in family therapy, the person may need to be removed from the family, much like setting boundaries on an alcoholic—you still love them, but you lovingly refuse to allow them to take advantage by setting appropriate limits with the hope they will eventually behave in a healthy and responsible way. For the alcoholic, this would be to stop drinking, and for the person with bipolar disorder, this would be to take his medication properly and work to master certain life tasks, including maintaining mood stability.

People with bipolar disorder have substantially higher divorce rates than people who have depression alone. Depression usually elicits caretaking by families, whereas mania elicits anger among family members. It is not unusual for the person with mania to do embarrassing things at public gatherings, to become paranoid that others are out to get him or his spouse is cheating on him, to squander the family resources, to abuse drugs and alcohol, to engage in life-threatening behavior, and to even place the family in risky situations. These behaviors are usually manifested when there is noncompliance with medications and in instances where there is denial that there is a need for treatment. When the person with bipolar disorder won't accept treatment and the behavior is severe enough, divorce may seem like the only solution.

It is important to discuss the issue of alcohol and drugs. Some people with bipolar disorder utilize substances to decrease their symptoms. Cocaine and amphetamines are sometimes used for their transient antidepressant effects. Alcohol is sometimes employed as a sedative and to induce sleep. Substances appear to be helpful in the beginning, but as is often the case, they prove to be more harmful later. It is important for families to look at their codependent behavior and begin to make alterations as well as assess their own consumption of substances.

I have tried to simplify issues that can be very complex and intertwined within a family system and can run across several generations. The person identified as having bipolar disorder is not the only one with a problem. All family members need to work on themselves in regard to how they are a part of the problem, too. Likewise, each person can be a part of the solution. In fact, when you can see that by changing your own behavior in a positive way you can shift things positively for another person in the family, you have more control over a difficult situation than when you push for the identified patient to make all the changes. I also have observed many times that the prognosis is greatly improved, even for the most disturbed person with bipolar disorder, when the family is motivated to participate in treatment and their own self-growth.

CHAPTER 9

SCHIZOPHRENIA

■ **DRUGS DISCUSSED:**
Haldol, Prolixin, Stelazine, Thorazine, Navane, Clozaril, Seroquel, Zyprexa, Risperdal, Cogentin, Artane, Akineton

Schizophrenia can be a devastating disorder with acute psychotic symptoms that totally disrupt normal communications and interactions with the world, and chronic residual symptoms that often rob individuals of their drive, ambition, socialization, and enjoyment of life. The diagnosis of psychotic disorders in the spectrum of *schizophrenia, schizophreniform,* and *brief psychotic disorder* requires, first and foremost, the presence of psychosis. Psychosis is defined as the presence of hallucinations, delusions, or thought disorder. Hallucinations are sensory experiences not shared by others, typically voices, but sometimes visions, smells, tastes, or unusual touch sensations. Most typically, voices are making negative, nasty, critical, hostile comments, but the voices may also be arguing with each other or carrying on a running commentary describing what the person is doing or thinking. (Smell, taste, or touch hallucinations always suggest the need for a medical-neurological evaluation as these are rare in schizophrenia but common in medical problems.)

Delusions are firmly held, fixed, false beliefs that are not part of the person's cultural or religious background. Sometimes these beliefs are spoken of casually. Usually they are held with a strong sense of conviction, a sense of their central importance in the person's life, and often a sense that the person has special importance or is in special danger or has changes occurring in their body. Specific delusions may include thought broadcasting (others know one's thoughts without speaking them), thought withdrawal (leaving the mind blank or empty), or thought insertion (thoughts are put into the mind that don't belong to the person experiencing them). Delusions are sometimes plausible to the listener (for example, the FBI really might be following someone who is involved in criminal activities), but at other times seem patently absurd (for example, satellites are broadcasting special messages to a receiver implanted in the person's head). Thought disorder is more difficult to define, but the listener is generally aware that what he's hearing doesn't make sense, doesn't flow logically from basic assumption to conclusion, is disjointed, or veers off the topic of a question or conversation. Thinking may be disorganized, rambling, and leading nowhere, or there may simply be very few thoughts and a sense of nothing going on in the person's mind.

The time course of these psychotic symptoms leads toward the diagnosis of brief psychotic disorder (less than one month), schizophreniform (one to six months), or schizophrenia (greater than six months) if the symptoms are not part of a substance-induced or mood disorder or due to a medical problem.

SCHIZOPHRENIA

The definition of schizophrenia is the most rigid in this spectrum as it is the most chronic and debilitating of the three disorders. The six-month period must include a time with the above acute psychotic symptoms plus a total duration of all symptoms of at least six months. The period before the full-blown psychotic symptoms appear often involves withdrawal from people and the world and tremendous anxiety. The postpsychotic period may involve residual symptoms that do not respond as completely to medications as do the acute psychotic symptoms.

The prodromal (early illness) and residual (long-term) symptoms include the "prepsychotic" symptoms of peculiar behavior, odd beliefs, and unusual perceptions; the "negative" symptoms of social isolation, blunted affect, and lack of initiative; and the important and obvious decline in role functioning (as a student, worker, parent, and so on).

The symptoms of schizophrenia are sometimes grouped into positive and negative ones. Recently, cognitive symptoms also have been appreciated. The positive symptoms are hallucinations, delusions, and thought disorder. Negative symptoms include affective flattening (lack of facial expression, eye contact, gestures), alogia (poverty of speech or increased latency or thought blocking), apathy (low energy and poor hygiene), anhedonia-asociality (loss of interest and pleasure in recreation, sex, relationships with others), attentional impairment (for example, at work), and a general lack of goal-directed behavior.

The positive symptoms typically respond well to medications, both the classical or typical drugs such as Haldol, Prolixin, and Thorazine, and the new atypical drugs such as Clozaril, Risperdal, Zyprexa, and Seroquel. The negative symptoms may not respond at all to the older typical medications, but often improve with the new atypical drugs. Cognitive (intellectual) functioning may worsen with the typical neuroleptics, especially if drugs to control muscular side effects of stiffness or restlessness such as Cogentin or Artane are added. Cognitive functioning may actually improve with the new atypical drugs.

THE DEVELOPMENT OF SCHIZOPHRENIA

The worldwide lifetime prevalence of schizophrenia is about 1 percent, and estimates in the United States range from 0.6 to 1.9 percent of the adult population. The course of illness has changed since the availability of medications, with about 70 percent of patients responding positively to them, but only 5 percent showing full and complete recovery to their pre-illness state. The unfortunate lesson of working in an acute care psychiatric hospital is how frequently people who do respond to medications stop taking them or take street drugs that cause relapses. The life expectancy of an individual with schizophrenia is slightly reduced and the suicide risk is about ten times that of the normal population. These facts make lifetime follow-up, with monitoring for medical illnesses, depression, substance abuse, demoralization, and actual suicidal ideas and plans, essential for treating this illness.

Typically, the illness begins in the late teens or early twenties just as the person is preparing to leave home and enter college, often at a point where family and patient have great expectations and life plans, and suddenly must begin dealing with a lifelong illness.

The causes of schizophrenia remain unknown, but there appear to be genetic risks; abnormal brain structure and function (on CAT, MRI, and PET studies) all clearly show this to be a very biologically based illness. CAT and MRI studies of brain anatomy are useful in ruling out brain tumors (a rare cause of psychosis) and may show enlargement of the fluid-filled ventricles in the brain in schizophrenics. Unfortunately, PET brain imaging studies that visualize brain regional metabolic activity or receptor density remain research tools rather than clinical ones because the abnormalities demonstrated in schizophrenia don't really help much in choosing a treatment approach. *Major tranquilizer* and *minor tranquilizer* are two very important terms in understanding drugs used to treat schizophrenia and anxiety.

MAJOR TRANQUILIZERS

Major tranquilizer, neuroleptic, and *antipsychotic* are essentially interchangeable terms and refer to a group of drugs that have true antipsychotic effects to decrease hallucinations, delusions, and disorganized thinking. These drugs are not addicting, not abusable, and certainly can't be sold on the street because they are not subjectively pleasant to take. Examples include older typical drugs such as Haldol, Prolixin, Stelazine, Navane, Moban, Loxitane, Mellaril, Thorazine, and newer atypical drugs such as Risperdal, Seroquel, Zyprexa, and Clozaril. The newer atypical drugs cause far less unpleasant muscle stiffness and restlessness, are less emotionally "numbing," and are much less subjectively difficult to take than the older-generation drugs. They also appear to have much lower risk of long-term movement disorders. These drugs are used in the treatment of brief psychosis, schizophreniform, and schizophrenic disorders, and sometimes are used in the treatment of mania or psychotic major depression short term. They are essentially never used in the treatment of anxiety disorders.

Minor Tranquilizers

The minor tranquilizers include the benzodiazepines, meprobamate, and barbiturates. Meprobamate and barbiturates are obsolete from a psychiatrist's perspective, though still used in anesthesia and treatment of some epileptics. The benzodiazepines are potentially addicting, abusable, and salable on the street for their subjective "high" state; they are used for the treatment of anxiety or insomnia. They are occasionally used briefly in the initial hospital treatment of a schizophrenic patient who is agitated and not sleeping, but they have no long-term beneficial effect on psychotic symptoms.

Antipsychotic Selection

The choice among antipsychotic drugs is based on several criteria, but I've often told my residents in training that the most important one is what the patient is willing to take. Because these drugs can cause unpleasant feelings of stiffness, restlessness, sedation, or sexual dysfunction, many patients stop taking them shortly after leaving the hospital. Thus, avoiding side effects and respecting patient wishes to use or not use certain drugs are of major importance.

Among the typical antipsychotics, there is a spectrum from those that are low potency (requiring high milligram per day dose) with sedation as a major side effect to high-potency nonsedating drugs that have greater frequency of muscular side effects (stiffness or restlessness). Low-potency sedating drugs, typically used in the 300 to 800 mg/day range, include Thorazine (chlorpromazine), and Mellaril (thioridazine). Medium-potency drugs, typically used in the 50 to 200 mg/day range, include Moban (molindone) and Loxitane (loxapine). High-potency drugs, typically used in the 5 to 50 mg/day range, include Haldol (haloperidol), Stelazine (trifluoperazine), Prolixin (fluphenazine), Navane (thioxanthene), and Trilafon (perphenazine).

Several studies have looked carefully at the issue of dose of these drugs and examined the role of rapid tranquilization using very high dose at the start of hospital treatment of an acutely ill patient. Typically, these studies have failed to find any benefit in outcome when doses of over about 10 mg/day of Haldol or 800 mg/day of Thorazine (or its equivalent) are used. Haldol is a very safe drug for rapid tranquilization (the use of a drug as a "chemical straight-jacket" for an agitated violent patient) and it was quite common ten years ago to treat patients with 40 to 80 mg/day in the hospital; now we are realizing that we may be increasing the side effects tremendously without increasing the therapeutic response by such high dosing. Higher dose does not translate into faster or more complete antipsychotic response. Most patients can do well with a Haldol dose of 5 to 20 mg/day, or Thorazine dose of 300 to 800 mg/day. If sedation is required to control combative behavior or severe insomnia at the start of treatment, a few days of giving Ativan or Klonopin may be a very tolerable alternative to pushing to high dose of the antipsychotic medication.

Among these drugs, Haldol is one with a reasonably well-established therapeutic window for plasma levels of about 3 to 22 mg per ml. Patients generally show better response when blood levels are in this range. Other antipsychotics have many metabolites and poorly defined therapeutic blood levels.

Depot neuroleptics (long-acting injections) are available for those patients who clearly benefit from medication but are reluctant to take it on a daily basis. Prolixin Decanoate has a typical duration of action of two weeks after an intramuscular injection, and Haldol Decanoate typically lasts for four weeks after an injection. The use of these drugs is sometimes very helpful in eliminating the power struggle between patient and caregivers over whether the medication is being taken.

Side effects of the typical neuroleptics may include neuromuscular, endocrine, sexual, and weight problems. Neuromuscular side effects include acute dystonia (muscle spasms) and Parkinsonian stiffness or slowness, both of which are readily relieved by Cogentin, Artane, or Symmetrel. Akathisia, or the sense of restless muscles, skin and muscles itching to move, and inability to sit still, may be relieved by a low dose of Inderal (propranolol) or a benzodiazepine such as Valium or Ativan. Tardive dyskinesia is a delayed-onset movement disorder associated with chronic use of major tranquilizers, with risk factors frequently listed as including total duration and dose of drug, female gender, old age, mood disorder (rather than schizophrenia), and dental problems. Because it is essentially untreatable, the key is prevention by using the lowest possible dose of the major tranquilizer possible long term. It typically presents as involuntary, repetitive, rhythmic, purposeless movements of the mouth, tongue, and cheek in an individual who has taken an antipsychotic for several years.

Endocrine side effects are a direct result of dopamine blockade by the major tranquilizers and include breast enlargement and milk production, irregular or no menstrual periods, and loss of sexual drive or responsiveness. Weight gain is common with these drugs, with the exception of Moban and perhaps Loxitane.

Atypical antipsychotics include Risperdal, Zyprexa, Seroquel, and Clozaril. Risperdal appears to be effective against positive and negative symptoms of schizophrenia and to have minimal neurological side effects at a dose of 6 mg/day or less. Its dose-response curve in research studies showed optimal response in large patient groups at 6 mg/day, with no additional benefit statistically at doses up to 16 mg/day. Many clinicians using it now find that doses in the

1 to 4 mg/day range are fully adequate to treat outpatients with psychotic symptoms and that this drug has a remarkably benign side effect profile compared to the standard antipsychotics. Zyprexa has the advantage of no effect on prolactin, so that it does not interfere with menstruation or cause breast enlargement or milk production. It is the atypical antipsychotic with the greatest similarity of actions to Clozaril, and it may have some mood-stabilizing effect in bipolar affective disorder. It shares with Clozaril a significant risk of weight gain.

Clozaril has a very special place in the treatment of schizophrenia for those who have failed to respond to two or more other antipsychotics or who have developed intolerable side effects or tardive dyskinesia. Because Clozaril has a risk of agranulocytosis (knocking out the bone marrow's ability to make white blood cells that are essential to fighting off infections), blood counts must be done weekly in anyone who is taking this drug. After six months, the risk of this problem is decreased and the blood counts may be done every other week. Clozaril carries a higher risk of seizures than other antipsychotics and is often associated with sedation and weight gain. Nonetheless, this is a breakthrough drug because it can substantially improve symptoms and quality of life in about one-third to one-half of patients who haven't responded to anything else. The response may take several months to develop, so patience is truly required. Clozaril does not appear to cause the neurologic side effects of the standard antipsychotics and may not cause tardive dyskinesia.

ALTERNATIVES AND ADJUNCTIVE TREATMENTS

Sometimes families become desperate when standard treatments don't work. It is important to realize that several treatments that sound promising have been tried and failed to demonstrate effectiveness. These include megavitamins, gluten-free and additive-free diets, hemodialysis, and acupuncture. Drugs that sometimes have a secondary role when combined with standard antipsychotics include lithium, carbamazepine, or propranolol for control of aggression. (Carbamazepine may cause the antipsychotic blood levels to decrease so this must be followed carefully.) Antidepressants may sometimes help with social withdrawal and depression. Luvox should not be used with Clozaril because of the risk of dangerously elevating the Clozaril blood level.

NEUROLEPTIC MALIGNANT SYNDROME

A very rare side effect of neuroleptics is the sudden onset of high fever, severe muscle rigidity, confusion, and unstable vital signs. Typically, the person is sweating and breathing rapidly. This is a potentially life-threatening medical emergency and must be treated as such in a hospital intensive care setting.

PSYCHOSOCIAL TREATMENTS

Two forms of psychosocial treatment have actually been shown to reduce relapse risk of schizophrenics in a way that is very synergistic with medications. Family therapy to deal with high expressed emotion situations in which critical comments, infantilizing, and emotional overinvolvement stress the patient has a significant impact on long-term outcome. Social skills training to teach coping strategies and socialization skills and to form therapeutic alliances and encourage communication about medication effects may also decrease relapse rate.

Sheila: Chronic schizophrenia

I began seeing Sheila about four years ago. Sheila is a thirty-seven-year-old single female who lives alone and works on the night shift as a security guard.

She came to the initial interview with her mother. Sheila's mother was very concerned about her daughter. She said that even as far back as kindergarten and grade school she was concerned that Sheila was somewhat shy and socially withdrawn. Sheila states she hears voices and feels agitated on medicines.

Sheila told me she was psychiatrically well up to a year and a half earlier when she had the sudden onset of auditory hallucinations. Sheila was hearing voices in a variety of situations. In addition, she did not want to turn on the bathroom lights because she felt she was being watched by cameras. She went to the emergency room three or four times over the next couple of weeks and was given injectable medications. The only obvious stressor was that her neighbors had had a loud argument.

There was no major medical illness, street drug abuse, depression, or mania prior to the onset of the voices. The voices were given names by Sheila: "Jessie," "James," and "Amy." The voices never said anything good even though they called her "Sweetness." There was a sense of her actions being controlled by voices telling her what to do or not do. The voices came from inside her head. They did not argue. They did, however, have running commentary on her actions and thoughts throughout the day. The voices never told her to hurt herself. There were no ideas of reference (feelings of being talked about) from the radio, TV, or newspaper. There was no thought control, thought insertion, or thought withdrawal. There was a sense of her mind being read by others, but she could not explain how this would occur.

Sheila has had depression, which always followed once the voices worsened. The depression would last for one to three weeks. During that time, she didn't feel like doing anything, her energy was low, her sleep was increased from nine hours up to twelve hours a day, her appetite and weight were increased, her concentration was poor, and decision making was difficult, but there was no suicidal ideation.

There were no other significant medical or psychiatric problems, such as manic episodes, obsessions, compulsions, panic attacks, or eating disorder, nor were there any seizures or history of significant head injury. She had occasional headaches throughout her adult life.

Sheila is an extremely light drinker. She does not use any street drugs and does not use cigarettes. She walks a great deal as part of her job as a security guard. She has always been in good physical health and has no family history of mental illness.

Sheila would like a medicine that would decrease the voices and agitation. She clearly indicates that Mellaril is better than Risperdal for the voices.

Sheila's typical day involves sleeping a great deal—up to twelve hours a day—taking a walk, watching TV, having very little social activity, and often sleeping most of the weekend. She has not dated anyone for three or four years.

Diagnosis and Treatment Plan: Sheila has chronic schizophrenia. I gave her a prescription for Mellaril 50 mg to take between 100 and 200 mg daily with the suggestion that she start at 150 mg, as a regular dose. I also gave her propranolol 20 mg three times daily as needed for restlessness. As an alternative to that, diazepam 2 mg may be used for restlessness. I suggested that she experiment with the diazepam and the propranolol to see which works best for her in controlling the restlessness.

When I met with Sheila a month later, the restlessness was well controlled with a dose reduction of Mellaril to 50 to 100 mg/day and use of Valium (diazepam) which she found better than Inderal (propranolol).

Conclusions: It is important to note the history of negative symptoms with shyness and social withdrawal dating back to childhood and the adult lifestyle of oversleeping, having no social life, not completing college, living alone, and choosing a job that doesn't require interaction with other people, which is common among those with schizophrenia. Sheila was experiencing side effects to the antipsychotic drug that were causing her significant distress that was very easily managed by minimizing the antipsychotic dose and adding in a very low dose of a minor tranquilizer to control the restlessness. This was easily remedied, but had Sheila failed to tell me about these problems, she might have eventually gone off the medication altogether; that would have surely brought back the voices.

Bob: Chronic schizophrenia with stuttering

I originally saw Bob eight years ago. Bob is a twenty-four-year-old unemployed male living with his parents. He was brought to the interview by his father on urgent referral by another psychiatrist.

Bob stated he has seen a psychoanalytically oriented psychotherapist for two months. The doctor started asking about sex and masturbation, which are very routine areas of inquiry, and this made him extremely nervous.

Bob states he became shaky, depressed, anxious, and down on himself and wanted to shoot himself because he began talking with his therapist about masturbation. He indicates that over the last five years before coming to see me, he has not been working, and has gone out only rarely with friends. He attended community college sporadically. He realizes he has no direction in life. He thinks "bizarre things." He gets "high" when he wears bright jackets. He changes clothing to imagine himself being superior. He describes a fantasy world inside himself. He sees people on bikes flying to new planets. He feels afraid to date because it would be a totally new experience for him and "I haven't grown up." He feels he has made very little progress in two months of psychotherapy "because things have gotten out of hand looking inside" of himself. He describes fantasizing and drifting off into a world of his own and being lost in thought at times. He worries about what is good and bad. He worries about what he is doing and what he should be doing. He has insomnia.

His father indicates Bob has had a learning and speech disability since childhood. Bob was in psychotherapy in high school but not since that time. Bob states that in high school he began therapy because his thoughts were incomplete. He had very strange feelings. He also indicated that in high school he heard a talk about suicide which led him to consider it as an option. He then took a Tylenol overdose. He was not placed on psychiatric medicines at any point.

In the last couple of months, he has experienced deeper depression and suicidal concerns, and has been nonfunctional. Bob appeared very disorganized in his speech and was very anxious, but denied auditory, visual, taste, touch, and smell hallucinations. He does have feelings that strangers are talking about him. He feels people are watching him, especially when he masturbates. He feels that people comment and make fun of him. He denies ideas of reference from the radio or TV. He describes some compulsive symptoms; for example, he bought paint to use on a model he was making. When he had paint left over, he felt he had to make more models to use up the paint. He reports that he can't think what's best for him anymore. He has difficulty organizing, getting out his ideas, and making choices. He has thought about taking his own life.

Bob denied substance abuse. There was no family history of psychiatric problems. Bob would like a medicine that would help him think more clearly and understand people's behavior, and he'd like to be capable of true success.

Diagnosis and Treatment Plan: In light of Bob's very poor social and work functioning over the long term, the differential diagnosis certainly includes chronic schizophrenia and stuttering, as well as the possibility of mild mental retardation. I requested records of psychological testing and past treatment to help elucidate this. Indeed, the testing indicated lifelong social isolation and dependence on parents with little history of relationships outside the home. There was no work history.

His IQ is borderline normal. Significant strength was on block design, where he did above average. The Rorschach ink-blot test showed constant overload, rationalization, regression, and unusual responses throughout the record. He views himself as a failure. His family was viewed as supportive, but there was some tension around issues of individuation. The tests were suggestive of multiple symptoms such as depression, anxiety, obsessions, rumination, and chronic social withdrawal. The testing summarized that he was suffering from severe depression and disordered thinking. This was the psychologist's way of saying he had schizophrenia.

The summary of treatment by Dr. S., who had treated him in high school, noted Bob had learning difficulties, speech dysfunction, immature social adaptation, and obsessive-compulsive traits. Dream material indicated fears of violence, depression, and anxiety. There is enthusiasm about music, astronomy, and martial arts. There was some suicidal ideation toward the end of treatment. At termination, he continued with learning disorder, depressive traits, and social immaturity, but no signs of psychotic process. Dr. S. mostly focused on emotionally supporting Bob.

Because of the overwhelming anxiety with disorganized thinking, I gave Bob a prescription for Navane 2 mg to increase from one to four daily. I also gave him Cogentin 1 mg to use twice daily if needed for muscle stiffness.

By the end of the month, Bob had increased the Navane gradually to 14 mg/day, and was given Valium for anxiety to take in an occasional low dose, but he was still having difficulty with stuttering. He still prefers his fantasy life and isolation to dealing with the outside world, yet is able to work in a speech therapy class and use his father's encouragement to go out into society and have simple interactions with people. Bob's father says that his thought processes are more disentangled and that Bob is in contact with the real world more now since being on medication.

Conclusion: This individual enjoyed solitary pursuits such as building models, astral photography, bodybuilding, and riding a motorcycle, but socialization was extremely difficult because of the anxiety associated with his underlying schizophrenia and his stuttering. He preferred to remain in his make-believe world of fantasy and fun; I often joked half-seriously with him that being a costumed character at Disneyland might be an ideal job for him to take advantage of his gymnastic talent and love of brightly-colored costumes. With great patience, medications were fine-tuned over several years, and he was nudged along daily by his father to develop the social skills that he needed so desperately. He began by asking for what he wanted in a fast-food restaurant and buying movie tickets for himself because these actions allowed him to experience an immediate reward for his efforts. Unfortunately, during treatment his mother died and he realized that his father was aging, which caused him a great deal of distress since he was so dependent on his father for everyday survival and companionship.

The treatment goal was to help Bob catch up to where a normal person of his age would be: able to take care of himself and obtain the basics for survival during periods when his father left the area for a few days on business trips. My goals for him included getting a job that would require some superficial people interaction, but he made it clear that he was in no hurry for this. He was equally reluctant to become involved in any social groups that might help him make a few new friends and correct the emotionally traumatic experience of having others ridicule his stuttering in high school. After eight years of working with him and his father, he is able to go to the gym and work out by himself, and will exchange brief greetings with others there; he enjoys riding his motorcycle and learning computer-aided drafting, but he is still not working or socially involved with others. He has not gone on a date or made any new friends throughout the time I have known him.

Carla: Chronic paranoid schizophrenia

Carla is a thirty-six-year-old, never married female who is living with her parents. She has a high school diploma, and works in a local hospital as an aide. She is referred by her psychologist, Dr. A., who accompanied her to the interview.

Carla states she has depression and paranoia about what other people say and do. Carla describes ongoing problems since high school. She began to hear voices around tenth grade, saying sexual things and accusing her of prostitution with men, which she never did. Eventually, those voices went away. In eleventh grade, she began hearing voices that related to a sexual fantasy and thought there were guys talking outside her window, but realized it was only in her head. She found herself looking for hidden speakers in her house. She thought a cute guy was attracted to her. She sometimes received "special messages" in the newspaper and thought there was a camera planted in the bathroom mirror, and she sometimes had a thought and then heard her thought spoken on the radio.

One issue is obsessing over a man she met at an AA dance five years ago whom she had gone out with on a date, talked to, and visited a few times but with whom she had not been sexually involved. She indicates that since this time she has felt he was talking through other people or sending messages to her through other people. She also describes the onset in the twelfth grade of the phobia of having her head shaking out of control and her body twitching and people watching her. She also describes a discomfort in facing people and feeling watched, self-conscious, and judged. She indicates that around the time of her birth date, she was watching television and the characters began teasing her about her sexuality. She felt they were taking television cameras into her bedroom. She has felt that she has been teased since she was a child about her sexuality. She is still a virgin. She states that she gets messages that "they" are watching her when she masturbates. At work, she feels other people know that she is thinking a certain way, that they study her and have cameras on her. She has felt that others could read her mind since high school.

Carla has four siblings and she is the only one in the family still living at home with her parents. She has never lived independently.

Carla's father was an alcoholic and has been sober for twenty-four years. Her father is active in AA and her mother attends Al-Anon. Her sister is a recovering drug addict. Carla describes herself as shy and ornery for the most part. She complains of feeling aggravated and agitated lately.

Depression Symptoms: Carla describes being depressed since her last birthday, when she thought a guy was interested in her. When she realized this was not the case, she began feeling angry, worried, and lonely. Her appetite was fine, weight was up 7 or 8 pounds, and her sleep was normal. She didn't feel like doing much. She did not enjoy her usual activities, and has had some suicide ideation but never a plan or attempt. She did have a desire to hurt people verbally.

Her therapist said Carla has had some relief by expressing anger verbally in therapy sessions. She felt they had a positive therapeutic relationship. Their main focus lately was dealing with Carla's sense of loneliness, desire for a boyfriend, and fears of social situations.

Medication History: According to Carla's therapist, she was previously treated about eleven years ago for paranoia, hearing voices, and extreme self-consciousness. She was treated initially with Vistaril and then Mellaril at an unknown dose, which was helpful for a differential diagnosis of social phobia versus generalized anxiety disorder versus paranoid personality. Social phobia would explain the fear of twitching or doing other embarrassing things in a social setting. Generalized anxiety disorder would explain chronic anxiety. Paranoid personality would explain a sense of people spying on her. None of these, however, would fully explain the voices that she had been experiencing.

A year into the initial treatment with her first psychiatrist, Prozac was added, and soon thereafter, the Mellaril was stopped. This had some benefit in helping with depression, but it did not help the phobias. Carla was hoping for a medication that would decrease the thoughts about her phobia and feeling she can't control her body.

Carla was polite, alert, oriented, cooperative, casually dressed, and obese. She had a very clear-cut history of hallucinations, paranoid ideation about people spying on her, and a sense that others could read her mind. She is not psychomotor agitated or retarded.

Differential Diagnosis: The patient presents with some symptoms of social phobia and erotomania; however, these occur in the context of long-standing paranoid delusions as well as intermittent auditory hallucinations. The simplest and most comprehensive diagnosis is that of chronic paranoid schizophrenia.

I feel it is beneficial for Carla to continue her supportive individual outpatient psychotherapy with Dr. A. I gave her a prescription for Loxitane and also one for Moban. I indicated to her that I wanted her to try each of these medicines in low dose for at least a couple of weeks to determine if either one would be both helpful and tolerable in terms of her very fearful reactions to the world around her. I indicated to her that these medicines were chosen because they are very unlikely to induce weight gain, unlike most other antipsychotics.

By a year or so later, Carla has remained paranoid over the long term, and has been unwilling to take adequate doses of Mellaril, Moban, Loxitane, or Risperdal to control this. She felt things in my office were arranged to give her messages or torture her, still gets paranoid when watching some TV shows, and feels people are spying on her in her bedroom and at work. She's had medical leaves from work signed for by her psychologist, has been advised by me and her psychologist to take neuroleptics long term but refused to do so, and has only been willing to take Zoloft, which she feels is of some help for depression.

Conclusion: The therapist who had seen Carla for six months hadn't made the diagnosis of paranoid schizophrenia, and in fact, had treated the patient as if she had severe anxiety and would benefit from psychotherapy for this. Supportive therapy was subjectively helpful but didn't work to eliminate psychotic symptoms (delusions), which can't be eliminated without medicines. Insight was completely lacking in this unfortunate patient. She remained miserable, unwilling to acknowledge that she needed the antipsychotic medication, and always feeling the world around her was a very hostile place.

Unfortunately, schizophrenia (like mania and substance abuse) often involves a loss of insight into the fact that one is ill. Carla's refusal to take the medicines that might help her is a terribly common and frustrating problem for psychiatrists dealing with paranoid patients, who want to get the psychiatrist to "see it my way" and ally with them in viewing the world as a dangerous, hostile place.

Ben: The man whose mother made me a king

I will report this case in detail because it illustrates several points. One is that family therapy is sometimes much better than individual therapy, especially when the identified patient doesn't acknowledge any need for treatment, yet the family sees him suffering and terribly nonfunctional. The second is that recovery and rehabilitation from the devastating effects of schizophrenia is a family affair; it can't happen without family participation if the patient is living with his family. The third point is the importance of long-term medication trials and the special role of Clozaril in treating the patient who is only partially responsive to other conventional medicines.

Ben was first seen about four years ago. Ben is a twenty-five-year-old, single Caucasian male. He dropped out of college due to what he called a nervous breakdown. He is unemployed and living with his father, Bill. He rarely sees his mother and stepfather due to a falling out. Ben was not happy to be seeing a new doctor and reports that he was "forced" to do so by his father.

Ben has a history of substance abuse, but has been clean for the last five to six years. He primarily used marijuana, but he also used LSD and psychedelic mushrooms as well as cocaine a few times. He had one car accident and was found to be in possession of illegal substances. He spent six months in jail, which led to his sobriety.

Ben has seen numerous mental health professionals over the last five years. He was hospitalized twice within the first six months after his first episode, and has been on various psychiatric medicines, including Haldol, Prozac, and Norpramin (desipramine). Ben tells me that his first hospitalization was on recommendation of a psychologist because he couldn't control his mind, he couldn't sleep or eat, he was screaming uncontrollably, his thoughts were not clear, and his mood was erratic. He denied hearing voices, but he felt his old friends were badgering him, though Ben does not really have any friends.

For the next few years, he described his life as being a "living hell." He stated he tried Prozac for one year at 40 mg/day with no benefit. He tried desipramine with levels being checked for about six to twelve months with no benefit. He managed to stay out of the hospital for the most part until just a couple of weeks before coming in for our initial meeting.

Prior to this hospitalization, he was placed on Klonopin for a few days, but had too short a trial to evaluate that because he experienced another episode. Ben had become outraged that he was having such difficulty with life, and felt things were going wrong with his body and mind and that he was losing control. Ben's current medication is Risperdal 3 mg at bedtime, Desyrel at an unknown dose, Zoloft 100 mg/day, and Ativan 0.5 mg twice daily. He has been physically healthy except for an appendectomy.

Other Psychiatric Symptoms: Ben states he has had depression for at least six years continuously, with it never being fully gone. He has gained 20 pounds recently. He doesn't sleep well, sometimes not at all, and other times just a few hours. He feels he is always thinking. He usually has low energy. When asked about his sex drive, he said he has not had sex in a long time. He is not socializing or dating. His last romantic relationship was in high school. His only fun and leisure activities are playing golf and going to movies with his father. His typical day involves sitting around the house not doing anything and not working. He states that he hasn't felt stable enough to work in a long time.

He denies any manic episodes, any obsession or compulsions, anorexia, bulimia, seizures, or head injury. He denies any history of homicidal or suicidal ideation.

The patient states his stepfather is messing with his mind, trying to hurt him, and driving him crazy. He says he has strange sensations in his anus and he attributes this to his stepfather. Ben feels that others "mess around" with his mind. He denies ideas of reference from the radio or TV. He denies feeling his actions are controlled, although he thinks people are trying to make his life difficult.

Ben's goals at the time of the initial evaluation were to get a job and to be able to become independent of his father. Ben, however, does not feel that either a psychologist or psychiatrist can help him. Ben showed little insight into his illness.

Ben has a maternal uncle with the diagnosis of paranoid schizophrenia. The uncle murdered someone fifteen years earlier, and was in a hospital for the criminally insane.

Diagnosis and Treatment Plan: Ben is a chronic paranoid schizophrenic. He was doing well on the medications he had been given in the hospital (Risperdal 3 mg at bedtime, Desyrel unknown dose, Zoloft 100 mg/day, Ativan 0.5 mg daily). I did suggest that we stop the Ativan, since this is an abusable drug, in light of his history of drug abuse.

A month later, Ben brought in his mother and father to our meeting. He wanted to discontinue medications and psychotherapy. He again stated that he just wanted to get a job, and make up with his mother with whom he was estranged. He has no idea how his parents could help him to achieve those goals. Ben saw both his parents as being intrusive, demanding, and controlling in asking things of him he didn't feel he wanted to do. He commented that his parents had spent $30,000 on psychotherapy for him but he wished they would have just spent it giving him a place to live and money to support himself. He indicated he was very jealous of his mother and stepfather for having received a major legal settlement. He wanted them to support him financially. His mother felt very overwhelmed, since she did not understand her son's illness nor his anger at her. Having the parents present for this session allowed me the opportunity to explain the nature of Ben's illness and emphasize the necessity for keeping appointments and for taking the medicines regularly as prescribed. When the parents were able to understand this, I asked them to be thinking about possibly assisting him in certain ways in exchange for following through with the treatment plan. We planned to engage in bimonthly family therapy.

To my surprise, Ben's mother called me several times before our next meeting. She was terrified of having her son labeled as schizophrenic and wanted me to change the diagnosis. I went over the criteria with her, hoping she would understand.

In our next meeting, Ben asserted himself to express the things he needed to help him get on his feet. He also asserted himself in telling me he did not want to talk about the voices going on in his head. I helped him to talk directly to his parents about the areas of his life where he felt they were intrusive. The purpose of this was to help Ben develop a sense of self.

Prior to the next family session, Ben's mother invited him over for a visit for a couple of days. He accepted the invitation, but only stayed for a few hours. He has felt very uncomfortable ever since that happened. I could see he was becoming agitated as we focused on this subject. I worked with Ben to assert himself about his discomfort. Ben indicated that the voices were less bothersome, but that he is feeling worse since the visit with his mother. He could not acknowledge that it was a positive step, but instead felt it was impulsive. His mother, on the other hand, was delighted that he came for even a short period of time. She became emotional as she spoke about wanting her son to be comfortable back in her life. His father was thinking practically and wanted to discuss the concrete things Ben needed to get his life going in a positive direction. It took some urging to get Ben to talk directly to his parents rather than to speak as if they were not there about what kind of help they could give him and what he needed to get started in life. Though it was difficult for him, with encouragement Ben expressed a desire to either go back to college or get a job. He asked if his parents would help financially.

I wanted to help Ben feel he was in charge of the rate of change in his life in terms of rebuilding the relationship with his mom, going back to school, or entering vocational rehab. I also made a point of praising him for the efforts he had made rather than criticizing him for what he had not done. We again addressed the issue of medication compliance. Ben agreed to continue Risperdal and Zoloft.

My goal over the next several sessions was to help Ben be more assertive with his family, and to take more charge over getting his life together. Another goal was to teach the family to be more clear and concise and less emotionally expressive, since this led to confusion for Ben. Finally, I wanted the family to be less critical of Ben, and to employ forms of positive reinforcement for his attempts to get his life in order as well as for complying with treatment. I wanted the family to learn to praise Ben for even small steps toward his goal.

With these objectives in mind, Ben's mother was able to work through her guilt feelings that she had caused her son's problems by divorcing his father. This guilt caused a great deal of distress for everyone concerned, especially Ben, who would become more anxious as she mourned. She was beginning to understand that it was to the advantage of the family for her to work through her issues elsewhere, and learn to be more straightforward and clear with Ben. Ben's father began catching himself when he would begin on a critical note with Ben. I also worked with Ben to state directly his ideas, and with the parents to respond appropriately. Again, they needed to be clear with him what they would do to help him, as well as what they expected from him in return.

Even with the changes that were starting to occur within the family, Ben's mother cringed when Ben asked me point-blank if he had schizophrenia. She knew I would be nothing else but straight with Ben. I told him, "Yes, you do." I made it very clear that it was of a different type than Ben's uncle. Ben's mother displayed her fantasy that Ben could live a normal life if he just got the right therapy. The more she tried to deny the severity of Ben's illness, the more agitated he became.

Despite my efforts and some forward movement, Ben began to deteriorate over the next few weeks. He was unable to see any of the positive changes that had been occurring. He began complaining of vague, diffuse pains that he blamed on the visit to his mother and stepfather. He had begun ruminating over past failures and the loss of the last seven years due to illness. The voices were back and were arguing with him and he was yelling back at them. An increase in the Risperdal to one and a half tabs twice a day did not seem to make much difference. He showed very little initiative and had no energy. He spent a good deal of time pacing and being very bored.

We discussed the possibility of trying Clozaril. Ben's father was receptive to the idea since he had previously heard about it. Ben, however, was reluctant at this point.

Ben went for a second opinion to Scripps Institute in San Diego, where he had a complete neurological workup. Scripps confirmed the diagnosis of schizophrenia and Clozaril was again mentioned as a possible direction. He still refused, but was placed on BuSpar and Moban. He was still having breakthrough symptoms when he returned to see me so we switched to Loxitane to try for a better response. Unfortunately, he felt it slowed him down, leaving him feeling tired and drugged. He chose to discontinue it despite the fact that it helped the voices go away, he was able to go on an occasional outing with his mother, and he was able to actively look for a college program that suited him. We then changed to Navane, up to three 10 mg capsules daily. Navane decreased the voices significantly, but the body sensations and discomfort continued.

Ben was once again restless with his treatment and sought out a psychotherapist in Los Angeles. The therapist asked him to come three times per week for individual therapy despite the fact that Ben was not insight oriented, and that he had to drive over an hour to get to the appointments. This therapist was of the opinion that medications should only be used on a short-term basis, and that long-term individual psychotherapy would be the answer to Ben's problem. Furthermore, he did not agree with my diagnosis of schizophrenia. This was just the information that both Ben and his family wanted to hear. Fortunately, however, Ben did not discontinue taking the Navane. As I suspected, it wasn't long before Ben stopped seeing the therapist. Ben was terrified of developing a close relationship with anyone, and seeing the psychotherapist three times per week overwhelmed him.

I held back my frustration as I discovered the therapist had undone so much that we had worked toward in the family sessions. Once again, I set out to teach Ben and his family about why I chose the diagnosis of schizophrenia. I spoke about the facts that though some therapists have a different point of view, most mental health professionals recognize that schizophrenia requires treatment with medication on a long-term basis and often on a lifelong basis. I also expressed that most therapists acknowledge that supportive psychotherapy is extremely helpful, while psychoanalysis does not prove to be beneficial. I pointed out the positive gains the family members had made in their relationships with Ben. I could certainly understand why they wanted to deny the severity of their son's problem, but I know from experience that denial leads to deterioration. Deterioration leads to devastation if not stopped. I suggested the family members become involved with the Alliance for the Mentally Ill (AMI) so that they could meet other families and learn of their experiences, as well as get support for themselves. After a few family sessions, and attending the AMI support group, finally I began to break through their denial.

It was clear that it was time to start looking at Clozaril as an option since we still had not made progress in ameliorating Ben's symptoms. The family talked to several people at AMI and learned of Clozaril's helpfulness in difficult cases. While it has very positive results, it also has several potential side effects that must be carefully monitored. I explained to the family that Clozaril has a slight risk of seizure, of suppressing bone marrow, and of causing weight gain, and that it carries the necessity for a weekly blood count, but may be the very best medication hope for getting a really complete response and decreasing the hallucinations and paranoia. Both Ben and his parents were in agreement to begin Clozaril.

After a few weeks on Clozaril, Ben had moved into a rental cottage his mother owned, had signed up for a couple of classes at a local community college, and was thinking of goals for the next year. He had made an application to a four-year college as well and was eager to hear from it. His parents, however, were concerned that if he became more independent he might make some of the same mistakes he had made in the past. His mother was critical of him, and she expressed that she would not support him if he chose to use drugs. I asked him whether he felt any of the therapists were making any difference and he said that he didn't really think that therapy and talking about things made any difference in his condition. I asked him if he felt the medicines were making any difference and he indicated he is having a good response on the Clozaril 25 mg, two tablets twice daily, and is willing to stay on that. He has been sleeping better since he has been on Clozaril and the voices are at a very tolerable level, as are the body sensations.

Despite the clear progress, his mother continued to badger him. I certainly could understand his mother's concern, but thought perhaps there might be a better way of discussing this that would not alienate Ben. I reminded her of this, and she reluctantly began to change her tone. She asked Ben to agree to make changes toward independence one step at a time. I validated his mother's request. I pointed out to him the advantage of staying locally at least for the next year. He would have his parents around to provide emotional support and help for him. I would also be available to him. He had tried many psychiatrists in the past, and it seemed that we connected well enough for treatment to be effective. Again, with several family sessions, we were able to come to some agreement, which allowed Ben to become more and more independent while still having his parents available for support. Getting to some agreement required Ben's mother to set some boundaries around what she was willing to support financially, while at the same time allowing Ben autonomy to make some choices about his life. She also negotiated a plan so that Ben could become responsible for himself by working for one of her businesses in order to pay rent for the cottage.

Ben's mother indicated it was the fear of Ben not liking her that got in the way of setting expectations when he moved into the cottage and through most of his life. Also, his mother and father often undermined each other's efforts in setting limits. What they were learning is that this is harmful to Ben in the long run and does not support Ben to become more independent.

A couple of weeks later, Ben came in saying he doesn't think his medicine is doing him any good nor does he see any real change, and he doesn't really want psychotherapy. His mother was pushing him to do individual therapy, as she was getting tired of coming to the sessions. I was amazed that it seemed we were back at square one again. I spoke to the family again about denial. I knew I would have to do this over and over again. It seemed that as Ben got better, his family could go back into denial about the seriousness of his illness.

Ben's family members worked over the next few months and genuinely made a great deal of progress, though we went in and out of the denial phase of their grief of Ben having schizophrenia and requiring long-term treatment.

It was time to review our treatment goals. I pointed out that we had gone from a phase of Ben and the family being terrified by Ben's mental illness, his talking to voices and needing to be hospitalized, to a point where Ben could be friends with his mother, stepfather, and father. He was now doing fun things and talking with them. His parents were learning to be like coaches in providing guidance, leadership, and direction for him in terms of launching him into independent adulthood. We all agreed that treatment was certainly on the right track. Ben was still on Clozaril but at 400 mg/day. He was still hearing voices at times, but they were easier to ignore. We set goals to help Ben continue working toward individuation.

Within six more months, Ben was painting the cottage where he is living. He is also going to work for his stepfather doing some painting this summer. He would be willing to consider applying to a local four-year college or continuing at community college in case he can't get into a four-year school. His mother indicated she feels that all members are functioning very well as a family, and she indicated she really enjoys being with Ben as he works on sanding and painting the rental house in which he is living. Ben's father indicated that he and Ben planned to do some hiking together. Both parents indicated they are feeling that they are functioning well together and that they are able to talk about things and have an honest relationship.

The next step was to help Ben put together a budget to cover all his basic living expenses. Ben was now receiving Social Security income due to his illness. Everyone agreed this would further Ben's individuation.

In just one year since our initial session together, Ben was moving to his own apartment. He was preparing to go to a four-year college. He was living within his means with minimal financial help from his parents. This proved, however, to be very stressful for Ben since so much was happening at once. I worked with Ben to take measures to decrease his stress as much as possible. We also discussed the need to follow up with our visits even when he was feeling good to provide support and monitoring. I explained that even though the medications are working, there is the potential for breakthrough symptoms when stress is paramount.

Jumping ahead some three years since the onset of treatment, Ben is still doing well. He is attending college, socializing a little with peers, continues to have a good relationship with his parents, and is planning a vacation with his sister. Ben's mother is a recognized sculptor and gave me a sculpture of a king's crown. I display it prominently in my office. I explain to others repeatedly the crown is the gift from the mother of a man who stopped screaming at his voices and was able to rejoin his loving family and participate in the world, despite his protests that there was nothing wrong and he really didn't need psychiatric medicine or family psychotherapy.

It is easy to see the dynamics that materialized in this family. These dynamics are not uncommon in families where schizophrenia is the culprit.

FAMILY ISSUES IN SCHIZOPHRENIA

The Entire Family Is Affected

The person affected with schizophrenia can be in the role of parent, sibling, child, spouse, or extended family member. Regardless of which member is the one identified as having the illness, it can cause a great deal of distress for the entire family. It is not unlike the situation when there is mental retardation or other severe handicaps, where parents give so much time to the ill one and siblings feel left out. Siblings may also feel pressured to be perfect in order to not bring any more problems into the family, leaving them little room to be expressive, creative, and real. Similarly, children who have parents with schizophrenia usually become the "parentified child" who is now in the role of caretaker and forced to look after the parent, rather than be in the healthy relationship of parent looking out for the child. The child is then unable to be free to develop at a normal rate and be a carefree child with the security that her needs will be met by her parents. If the ill member is a spouse, expectations and dreams of how the relationship would be create a great sense of loss. For example, the person affected by the illness may have been the primary wage earner, leaving the partner needing to seek new training or education to become more employable to support the family.

Every person in the family becomes the "affected" person in a sense, as schizophrenia leads to embarrassment and confusion in all members. There is such a major loss that is created for the family. The change in relationship with the loved one with schizophrenia may have the impact of a death in the family. That person will never be the same. He may not be able to live up to the dreams the family had for him. Indeed, he may not be able to grow to be an independently functioning adult. All of these factors alter the course of the family forever. This can manifest itself as family members long to be like "other" families; they begin to feel guilty that they have been spared from being the one with the illness, and they may even develop a fear of becoming ill themselves.

There are many things the family can do to improve the course of the illness for both the individual with schizophrenia and other family members. One is to gain understanding of the illness. I highly recommend that families become engaged in a support group, at the very least in the early stages of diagnosis. The Alliance for the Mentally Ill (AMI) has chapters throughout the United States and can serve as an excellent support system and resource. I also recommend that families read about the illness; an excellent book that I suggest to families is *Surviving Schizophrenia* by E. Fuller Torrey.

COMMUNICATION

Communication plays a major role in dealing effectively with schizophrenia in the family. There are basic rules of thumb in dealing with a person with schizophrenia. There are certain dynamics that operate within the family system as a whole that most often require participation in family therapy to shift to a more positive way of functioning. First, I will address the dynamics that are present within the entire system. When these dynamics are shifted into a more productive way of communicating, one can see a difference in both the family members and the person identified with schizophrenia. The psychiatric literature is full of evidence regarding what has been called the "schizophrenogenic" family system, but I will put forth here in layperson's terms what I have directly experienced in working with numerous such families. Often, family members communicate with what I call "crazy talk." In this situation, people talk at the same time, overriding others so they cannot finish their thoughts or statements. It also becomes difficult when no one can agree on simple things; one family member will see a color as black, and another will see it as charcoal, and another will argue it is gray. The schizophrenic family member finds reality a confusing mass of rubber bands twisted together in a ball that has to be unraveled. This ball of twisted rubber bands plays itself out as communication filled with double binds, leaving the recipients of this communication "damned if they do and damned if they don't."

There are other communication skills that are helpful for family members to learn and use as new ways of dealing with the person with schizophrenia. It is important to communicate both verbally and nonverbally a sense of hope while giving up the expectation of a cure. The person must be treated naturally without condescension. Communications need to be brief, concise, adult statements given while looking directly at the person. One thing should be requested at a time. Arguments are futile and lead to more confusion for all. Clear rules are essential. You must work toward being patient at all times. It is vital that you don't try to argue a person out of her delusional beliefs. It is best to acknowledge the validity of the person's feelings about something without accepting her interpretation of them. For example, if the person feels there are things hidden in every dumpster she sees that she believes are contaminating her, acknowledge her reality and validate the outer reality—"I know you have reason to believe there are things hidden in that dumpster that might harm you, but I think the reason has to do with the fact your brain is playing tricks on you because of your illness." Don't use humor or sarcasm when dealing with delusions. In addition, help the person to limit expressions of delusional thinking to times when she is with trusted family members rather than with strangers.

NEGATIVE EFFECTS OF CRITICISM

Other family characteristics common to families with schizophrenia are overly critical members filled with hostility, as well as overinvolved members who overidentify with the ill person and become intrusive. These families are also often highly expressive of emotions. As with bipolar disorder, I have seen the person with schizophrenia become more delusional in this type of communication scene as it occurs; likewise, I have also seen a decrease in delusions as the family works to cease this crazy talk.

A very important note with regard to relapse prevention is this: It has been found that contact with a highly critical family after hospital discharge greatly increases the chance of relapse and subsequent rehospitalization; on the other hand, if the family is understanding and supportive, there is a lower relapse rate. This has been termed in the literature as *expressed emotion,* which is a modifiable issue in families. Again, this most often requires the assistance of an experienced family therapist who is not hesitant to point out this style of communication and who can avoid being sucked into the confusion. It also necessitates a family that is willing to keep working at it without giving up. Most important, it is essential that family members work through their guilt and begin to see themselves as a part of the solution rather than blaming themselves. It is my observation that families who do this type of work fare much better in dealing with the ill family member as well as being better able to manage their own stress. There is less relapse. There may even be less potential for younger children to be affected by the illness (this might be an interesting area for research).

As described in relationship to bipolar disorder, enmeshment plays an important role in keeping the system acting in old ways that are no longer tolerable, since they create too much distress in the person identified with schizophrenia. Certain circumstances create a double bind in terms of shifting enmeshment within the family system, such as when schizophrenia strikes an adolescent or young adult. The normal developmental task at this time includes moving away from home, perhaps going away to college, beginning a career, falling in love, and so on—the parent is left with the question, "How can I encourage my child to become more independent when he is now sick?" It is only natural for families to want to care for a disabled young adult child as they would a sick child of ten. Yes, alterations from the normal expectations of this person are necessary, but a modified version of encouraging independence is absolutely a must. Developing a balance of caretaking and encouraging independence is a very important goal of family therapy.

EMOTIONAL ALOOFNESS REQUIRES PATIENCE

Emotional aloofness is a major symptom of schizophrenia and it needs to be respected and not taken personally by family members. There are times when social withdrawal will occur, and this also requires respect. The family can learn through family therapy to determine if the person is using this as a coping mechanism to deal with his internal chaos or if this is a sign of deterioration. It can be difficult for families who are new to the illness and who are naturally fearful of what this means when they have not yet identified the signs and symptoms of the patient's process. These families are still in a state of shock at the "loss" of their loved ones. Furthermore, it is important to see the person as human and not to blame all his bad habits on the illness—expectations of the person should be reasonable, such as the need to bathe regularly, keep the living area reasonably clean, attend therapy, and take prescribed medication. Many times, people with schizophrenia remain silent even when you are speaking to them. It is important to continue to talk to them because they often need to remain in your presence, and it's not unusual to discover at another time that what you said to them was heard and was important to them.

HELPFUL HINTS

There are other tips that will be helpful in dealing with a person with schizophrenia. The person will do best with a predictable and realistic daily routine, including a good diet, exercise, hobbies, self-help group or day treatment, chores or some other sort of reasonable expectation, and some socialization. It is important to learn the signs and symptoms that occur *before* relapse. Unfortunately, this may mean the person goes through a few episodes before a pattern can be identified. Family members as well as the patient can learn what stressors increase symptoms and can avoid or modify them. It is important to note that she may have ups and downs for no apparent reason, however. In addition, family members may experience their own emotional distress just prior to an episode. This is probably attributable to enmeshment, where a rumbling of feelings in one member can set off a rumbling in another. If enmeshment can be harnessed and tamed, it can actually be transformed into intuition that is of great value in assisting the ill person. Secondary gain for both the family and the patient has been explained in detail in chapter 7 on depression. In short, there may be unconscious reasons that the family does not want the person to be at his best, such as a fear of independence or exposure of family problems and secrets. Even the person with schizophrenia may stop taking his medication in order to keep the status quo in the family.

When the judgment and insight of a person with schizophrenia becomes impaired, it brings up legal issues. A person can be placed in a psychiatric hospital against his will if he is a danger to himself, a danger to others, or is gravely disabled, which means he cannot provide food, clothing, or shelter for himself due to a severe mental disorder. The details of legal holds vary slightly from state to state. As an example, in California the person is initially placed on a short-term hold for up to seventy-two hours. This can be increased to a fourteen-day hold if the person continues to meet the above criteria. A conservatorship becomes necessary when it is clear that a person needs to receive treatment involuntarily or requires protective hospitalization for a longer period.

Contracts are also helpful in setting limits around issues of medication compliance, violence, substance abuse, and poor follow-through with house rules and expectations. If a decision is made to have the person with schizophrenia remain at home, a contract with clear expectations can be laid out so he knows exactly what is acceptable and what is not. The contract also makes it clear to the family when to tell the patient he can no longer live there. It cannot be emphasized enough that the family can play a role in enforcing the use of medication as well as undermining medication compliance.

In closing, family members can be part of the problem or they can be part of the solution. There is much documentation of the value of the family being actively involved in treatment. Also, families that become involved in support groups and become educated about schizophrenia fare much better than families who remain in chronic crisis as to how to deal with their loved ones.

A BEHAVIORAL CONTRACT FOR THE SCHIZOPHRENIC FAMILY MEMBER LIVING AT HOME

The schizophrenic person and his family need to have a very clearly defined set of rules if hospitalization is to be minimized and out-of-home placement is to be avoided. In our experience, it is important to have a contract that spells out expectations and consequences in detail as a condition of the ill family member living at home. We have provided a sample of the issues that we often see families facing. Important issues are:

1. Agreement to see a psychiatrist regularly and take prescribed medications. If there is a problem with medications, call and talk with the doctor.
2. Agreement to not use street drugs or alcohol.
3. Agreement to household adult responsibilities, such as paying rent and doing some regular chores (cleaning room, taking out trash, and so on). Participation in family dinners at least three times a week.
4. Agreement to "quiet hours" during which other family members can have peace and quiet to sleep.
5. Agreement to notify the family when planning to be out of the home late or overnight.
6. Agreement on personal hygiene standards for bathing and changing clothes.
7. Agreement on where or if smoking is allowed inside or outside the house.
8. Agreement to participate in some out-of-the-house activities at least two to three times a week (volunteer work, school classes, part-time job, socialization and support group, church, twelve-step group) to help develop friendships and avoid isolation.
9. Agreement that property will not be damaged.
10. Agreement to hospitalization if the family and/or doctor feel that it is necessary to control dangerous behavior.
11. The family agrees to provide housing and food, transportation (or bus fare) to planned activities and therapies, and to avoid hostile criticism.
12. The consequences of complying with the above contract will include a weekly reward, such as a financial bonus (rebate of part of the rent), a special meal out, or the use of the family

car. The consequences of violating the contract once in a month will be a warning; twice will lead to a two-week notice to follow rules strictly or move out.

A discussion of these basics of living together can go a long way toward setting the stage for success. Violation of these rules must have very well-specified consequences that everyone knows in advance.

CHAPTER **10**

ALCOHOL AND DRUG ABUSE

DRUGS DISCUSSED:
Antabuse, Trexan, Zyban (Wellbutrin)

ALCOHOLISM

Alcohol is one of the most commonly abused substances in this country because of its ready availability and its ability to provide very short-term relief of anxiety and insomnia. The diagnostic criteria for alcohol dependence include a maladaptive pattern of alcohol use with tolerance, involving the need for increased amounts to get the desired effect or the production of a much smaller effect by the same amounts that used to be consumed. In addition, there is withdrawal when alcohol is stopped abruptly and so alcohol is taken to avoid this. It is taken in a larger amount than intended over a prolonged period of time. Usually, attempts to cut down or control alcohol use are unsuccessful. A great deal of time is spent using, obtaining, or recovering from the alcohol and its effects, and this begins to interfere with major obligations at work, school, or home. Alcohol is used in situations where there are physical hazards, such as driving or operating machinery. The person begins to give up important social, occupational, and recreational activities to spend more time drinking. Complications develop, with legal problems such as drunk driving arrests, fighting, and automobile accidents, and the person continues drinking despite adverse consequences. Thus, alcohol dependence is a very severe pattern of chronic use leading to major life problems. Alcohol abuse represents a milder form of the problem, in which recurrent alcohol use interferes with role obligations, causes interpersonal or legal problems, causes a person to give up social, occupational, or recreational activities, and it may involve intoxication during hazardous activities such as driving.

The major complications of alcoholism are loss of job, loss of social relationships, and major medical problems including liver damage (cirrhosis), motor vehicle accidents, and damage to the heart, stomach, and pancreas which may be terminal. Dementia may result from very chronic alcoholism with its accompanying malnutrition and head injuries from falls.

There appears to be a significant genetic component to alcoholism, as demonstrated by both adoption and twin studies. Serotonin might be related to alcohol dependence; there are some preliminary studies which show that serotonin reuptake inhibitor antidepressants may decrease drinking in alcoholics.

The treatment of alcoholism by psychiatrists has not been impressively successful, and many Alcoholics Anonymous groups are strongly against psychiatric treatment because members have been prescribed benzodiazepine minor tranquilizers (which were addicting) while they continued to drink. Nonetheless, psychiatric treatment has several potential options for the alcoholic individual.

First is assistance with "drying out." It is pointless to try to treat depression or anxiety in an individual who is actively drinking. Usually the alcoholic who is having major life complications from drinking sooner or later will "hit bottom" and decide the time has come to stop drinking. Alcohol withdrawal can be a very serious and complex process with confusion, delirium, and even seizures occurring during abrupt alcohol withdrawal. Often, alcohol withdrawal is done in a hospital and the individual is given multiple vitamins (to treat chronic nutritional deficiencies) as well as minor tranquilizers such as Librium, Valium, Ativan, or Serax in order to ease withdrawal symptoms and prevent severe delirium or seizures. Drying out is just the beginning in terms of recovery from alcoholism.

The next critical step for the alcoholic is to enter a psychosocial rehabilitation program, such as Alcoholics Anonymous (AA), that is geared to long-term changes, to providing intensive personal support, and to obtaining the goal of long-term sobriety and accepting that alcoholism is a lifelong illness that will require a lifelong effort for recovery. Alcoholism is a disease of denial, and often the alcoholic feels he will be able to drink "just a little," or stay sober without a support program; the voices of experienced others in AA soon confront this self-deceit.

The pharmacologic treatment of the recovering alcoholic has been controversial at times. Basically, many alcoholics discover to their dismay that once they have become sober for a few months, life is not good and enjoyable and, in fact, they may be suffering from severe depression or anxiety. After one or two months of complete sobriety, I believe serious consideration should be given to providing such an individual with nonaddicting medications to treat the depression or anxiety which she may be experiencing. An individual with a personal and possibly a family history of recurrent major depression or panic disorder might be treated with a selective serotonin reuptake inhibitor. The person with chronic generalized anxiety may be well treated with the nonaddicting drug BuSpar. Some individuals have a personal and/or family history of bipolar affective disorder, and lithium (or an anticonvulsant such as Tegretol or Depakote) may be helpful for them. There is some older literature to suggest that lithium improves the chances of long-term sobriety in alcoholics even in the absence of a mood disorder, but this conclusion is controversial.

A second major strategy in treating alcoholism is based on the assumption that alcohol produces its euphoric effect through endogenous opiates or endorphins. By providing a medication that blocks the effects of endorphins, the alcohol-induced high is substantially decreased and the craving for alcohol is also decreased. This strategy has been implemented with naltrexone (Revia) and appears to help alcoholics resist the urge to drink.

An older approach to preventing return to drinking is the use of disulfiram (Antabuse), a drug that blocks the metabolism of alcohol and leads the alcoholic who drinks to build up toxic levels of acetaldehyde. This toxic metabolite causes nausea, sweating, flushing, and a throbbing headache, and makes the person feel extremely ill. Antabuse can be used on a voluntary basis when an individual is agreeable to showing himself and his family that he is making the commitment to not drink. It is sometimes used under court order, in which case the drug is taken under supervision of a probation officer, nurse, or pharmacist. The effect of Antabuse in blocking alcohol metabolism lasts for about a week or two, so an individual who is on Antabuse but decides he wants to resume drinking will often simply stop taking the medication; he will find that he can drink one or two weeks later without any adverse reaction. Antabuse may be used short term at high-risk periods in a person's life. I have asked patients to take it for a week or two prior to going into a difficult situation such as a college or family reunion, where old drinking memories or uncomfortable feelings may be stirred up. The use of Antabuse during these times of high relapse risk is a form of "insurance" that the commitment to sobriety will not be lost.

TRANQUILIZER ABUSE

Alcohol, barbiturates (including headache medicines such as Fiorinal or Fioricet), benzodiazepines, meprobamate (Miltown), and numerous other tranquilizers and sleeping pills can be abused by an individual who takes very high doses, obtains prescriptions from many sources, buys the drugs on the street, or mixes them with each other or with alcohol. Barbiturates may be obtained over the counter in Mexico and other countries. The withdrawal syndrome from abruptly discontinuing tranquilizers and sleeping pills can be very similar to that of withdrawal from alcohol and the treatment is essentially the same. A benzodiazepine minor tranquilizer (for example, Librium, Ativan, Valium, or Serax) is given until the point where the patient who is in withdrawal is becoming comfortable and relaxed; then the dose is tapered off gradually in a planned way over the following few weeks. Because withdrawal from minor tranquilizers is always elective and never an emergency, it is worth taking a few weeks to go through a gradual process so that the risk of sudden withdrawal and seizures can be minimized. As with alcoholics, the importance of psychosocial support, a twelve-step program, and alternative psychologic and biologic treatments for the anxiety or depression that may emerge during abstinence are quite important.

One severe form of alcohol and tranquilizer withdrawal that is very preventable occurs when a person enters a hospital for a medical problem and doesn't tell the doctor the truth about his substance use. Suddenly, a few days after admission for an injury or even an elective operation, the person is confused, anxious, and extremely uncomfortable, perhaps even in a delirium or having a seizure, until the diagnosis is made and appropriate medication is given. It is extremely important to tell your doctor about both prescribed and nonprescribed drug use when being hospitalized and cut off from normal supplies of drugs and alcohol, even if you don't think that anything bad will happen if you don't take the drugs or alcohol for a few days.

STIMULANT ABUSE

Cocaine, amphetamine, and Ritalin may all be used for their stimulant and euphoric effect. Stimulant abuse may initially begin with an attempt to get increased energy, to get a short-acting antidepressant mood-lifting effect, to lose weight, or to feel more sexual. With continued use more and more craving develops, and with the more frequent use of higher doses, the cocaine or other stimulant abuser will begin to get paranoid, irritable, and violent and may even hallucinate. Treatment of this syndrome is often best done in a controlled setting or hospital where the individual doesn't have access to medication. The use of low-dose antipsychotic drugs to control agitation and paranoia is not unusual. During the period of coming down from stimulant abuse, depression, sleepiness, and ravenous appetite are common. The antidepressant desipramine or the anti-Parkinson's drug amantadine may sometimes be used to decrease cocaine craving. Tegretol (carbamazepine) has been tried in attempts to decrease craving. Unfortunately, no good controlled data supports these drugs as being highly effective in decreasing craving and relapse into stimulant abuse. Attempts to prevent relapse are mainly focused on a twelve-step program.

OPIATE ABUSE

The opiates include prescribed drugs such as codeine, Percodan, Vicodin, Demerol, Dilaudid, and morphine, as well as street drugs such as heroin. Opiate addiction may be highly variable in its presentation, based on whether an individual is obtaining prescribed drugs from physicians and using them orally or is obtaining heroin from street sources and injecting it. The individual who injects is at much higher risk for developing complications from shared needles such as hepatitis, syphilis, and AIDS. Opiate withdrawal is a miserable experience but is actually far less medically hazardous than withdrawal from alcohol or tranquilizers. Opiate withdrawal may be made far more tolerable in one of two ways. The first or classical approach is to offer the individual a cross-tolerant, similar drug to the one from which she is withdrawing, but to choose a drug with a much longer duration of action. This is the basis for methadone opiate withdrawal, and can only be done in licensed detoxification centers. Some individuals may choose to switch from street drugs to methadone and then enter a long-term methadone maintenance program in which the drug is provided orally on a daily basis. Thus, the narcotic addiction persists but the source becomes a legitimate medical one and the route of administration is oral. The risk of infections and criminal activities are greatly decreased.

The newer approach to opiate withdrawal is to give a blood pressure medicine, Catapres (clonidine), which prevents most of the physiologic withdrawal symptoms that make opiate withdrawal so uncomfortable. This can be done on an outpatient or inpatient basis. A radical approach to ultrafast detoxification is to place the patient under general anesthesia and then flood the opiate receptors with a strong opiate antagonist, leading to prompt withdrawal without conscious awareness or discomfort. This approach requires an intensive-care hospital setting.

A strategy for preventing return to opiate abuse is to block the opiate receptors using a long-acting oral drug that prevents the opiates from having their euphoric effect. Naltrexone (Trexan, Revia) was used for this purpose long before it was used to decrease alcohol craving in alcoholics. Narcotics Anonymous is an essential part of long-term recovery.

NICOTINE ADDICTION

Although tobacco use is seldom a presenting reason for seeking psychiatric treatment, it is certainly a major public health hazard and is responsible for many unnecessary deaths from cancer and heart attack. Nicotine is highly addicting and is clearly a psychoactive drug. Rates of abstinence after going through a stop-smoking program have been abysmally low. The nicotine substitution approaches offer some advantage in terms of long-term success at stopping smoking, perhaps mostly by making the withdrawal process easier and less abrupt.

The principal approaches to smoking cessation which have been developed over the last few years rely on substituting alternative forms of nicotine for cigarettes. The first developed is the use of nicotine chewing gum (Nicorette), which is chewed whenever the person feels like having a cigarette and provides approximately the nicotine equivalent of a Marlboro cigarette. By using Nicorette, the individual gets away from the mechanical actions of smoking (the ritual of lighting, holding, sucking, and blowing smoke) and avoids the carcinogens contained in inhaled smoke and yet maintains the addiction to nicotine. Nicotine has a very short duration of action, so the individual who would smoke a cigarette every thirty to sixty minutes typically chews a piece of Nicorette at about the same time intervals and experiences some feeling of the nicotine high with each dose.

Another alternative is the nicotine transdermal skin patch (Habitrol or Nicotrol). These patches provide a very even, smooth blood level of nicotine when they are applied to the skin daily. The skin patches come in different dosage strengths. Each dose is used for about two to four weeks and then a lower dose is used. This provides a very gradual withdrawal from the nicotine over about six to twelve weeks. The major withdrawal problem of most smokers is weight gain. Diet and exercise may prevent this, but even if they do not, the gain in health from stopping smoking is well worth the risk of a few extra pounds of body weight.

Nicorette gum and nicotine patches are available over the counter (without prescription). Nicotine nasal spray (Nicotrol) is another form of nicotine that has been recently marketed.

Zyban (bupropion slow release) is the same as Wellbutrin SR. It was a surprise to find that when Wellbutrin was given to depressed smokers to treat their depression, many of them found their urge to smoke decreased. Subsequent studies have shown that the optimal dose for smoking cessation is 150 mg twice daily, and this is more effective than the nicotine skin patch. The combination of Zyban and a nicotine skin patch can yield a higher abstinence rate than either treatment alone, however. Usually, Zyban is started a week before the planned quit date. On the quit date, the nicotine skin patch is started and all cigarettes and associated equipment (lighters, ashtrays, and so on) are discarded. The well-motivated smoker using this technique may be surprised at how much easier it is to quit using Zyban and the patch than it had been to stop "cold turkey." The urge to resume smoking just isn't nearly as strong as it had been when the smoker tried to quit on his own.

In summary, all forms of drug addiction involve a sensitization to the drug's effect on the body, a craving for the drug, a withdrawal when the drug is no longer present, and a long-term risk of relapse into drug use. Any pharmacologic approach mentioned in this chapter is merely a way to ease the transition from substance abuse to sobriety in the context of what are usually the most effective treatment options, such as a twelve-step program plus individual or family counseling.

FAMILY ISSUES OF SUBSTANCE ABUSE

When one person in the family is abusing substances, the entire family is obviously affected. Whether the person is still using or is in recovery, it is very important for the family to obtain treatment. Family therapy can be utilized to work through dynamics that in essence lock the abuser into her role to get the abuser to accept treatment. For instance, families engage in enabling behaviors that help to keep the addict abusing substances. Enabling includes being in denial of the problem, making excuses for the addict, trying to regulate the amount of intake, obtaining substances for the addict in order to please her or quiet her, joining in abuse of substances, entering control battles with the abuser, taking over the family responsibilities of the addict, and taking on the shame and guilt of the addict. When a family is educated to see in which behaviors they are engaging and they begin to alter these patterns, the addict is more likely to seek treatment and/or to remain in a recovery mode. These patterns are usually so intricately ingrained in the family's mode of operation that they can be tricky to identify and change. A therapist who is outside of the system is often required to effect change.

INTERVENTIONS CAN HELP

Interventions are sometimes necessary in order to get the substance abuser to seek treatment. Often, these take place after the family members have engaged in some family treatment themselves and have learned to identify their roles in the dynamics that foster substance abuse. It is ideal if the family has already become educated about substance abuse and has begun to attend Al-Anon, a self-help support group for the significant others of addicts. There are also groups geared toward children associated with Al-Anon, Ala-Teen and Ala-Tot.

Interventions are often held at home, in the therapist's office, or at the addict's workplace. They involve bringing significant people in the addict's life together and confronting him about his behavior and the effect it is having on their lives as well as the life of the addict. This may include ultimatums; for example, that the person will have to move out unless he ceases drinking. The addict is not allowed to make excuses for his behavior or to blame others. Attendees are straight to the point and speak one at a time. An intervention should also include referral sources for the addict to obtain help, such as Alcoholics Anonymous (AA), Narcotics Anonymous (NA), Cocaine Anonymous (CA), residential treatment programs, and inpatient detox programs. It is important to note that it may not be medically safe for the addict to stop using substances "cold turkey." It is usually important that a medical doctor be consulted regarding the need for detox. If the intervention is not effective in getting the addict to accept treatment, it is imperative that the family follow through with its ultimatums. Otherwise, all will have been a waste. In the future, when the family is forced to do another intervention, it will carry less weight.

Usually, people who are abusing substances are deemed to be untreatable until they are clean. I often engage the addict in family treatment in the beginning stages even if he is still using. I set a rule that he may not come to therapy sessions intoxicated or after using a substance. The reason for this inclusion is the hope that the seriousness of the family seeking treatment will break through the denial of the addict enough to get him started in his own treatment and abstinence. Often, the family hasn't even identified a substance abuse problem, but is seeking treatment for other issues, such as children experiencing difficulties at school, behavior problems, or on referral by some agency. Family therapy is an effective way of identifying the problem of substance abuse. It also provides a neutral environment for an intervention if it becomes apparent that this is necessary.

SECONDARY GAIN AND ENMESHMENT PLAY ROLES IN ISSUES OF SUBSTANCE ABUSE

Secondary gain is a concept that has been discussed throughout this book. It is a critical factor that enables the substance abuser to use. Frequently, on an unconscious basis, families find it advantageous to have the person using. The person may appear less angry, less intrusive, and less aware of other problems that are going on in the household. She may be home less often or more often, whichever is more desired by the family. Fears of her becoming more independent and perhaps leaving home may be lessened. It is not uncommon when the addict decides to stop using that the family consciously or unconsciously pushes her back to using drugs or alcohol. The usual complaint is that the abuser is now more irritable, unpredictable, and overbearing. If these issues are dealt with, the rate of relapse is decreased.

I have written about enmeshment throughout this book and cannot emphasize enough that it needs to be addressed in order to relieve many of the symptoms of the person identified as having the illness. This entanglement is present in some form in all psychiatric disorders. Once the tangles are combed through, all family members can thrive with a new closeness that allows people to grow and develop to their fullest potential. People actually become closer when they encourage each to be who they are at the core of their being, because they will be able to share openly rather than masking feelings with acting out, rage, and substance abuse.

Enmeshment shows up in families where substance abuse is a problem. Often, there is a disturbed parental system in that one parent is teamed with the substance abuser against the other parent; this is usually the opposite-sex parent of the one who is abusing the substance. In other words, the boundaries between the generations are blurred. One parent usually presents herself as the more understanding one or becomes apologetic for the behavior of the other parent, who is deemed as the "bad guy." The parent who plays the role of the "good guy" repeatedly is the enabler.

Sandy and Denny had three children. Denny was a recovering alcoholic and cocaine addict, and at the time of beginning treatment was terminally ill. The twins were teenagers. Tom was addicted to crystal methamphetamine, and Jimmy was addicted to alcohol. Gina was off at college most of the time and drank alcohol on occasion. Rather than being an alcoholic herself, Gina tended to date young men who were fostering an addiction of some sort. There was a clear theme that was expressed throughout the life of this family: Denny was viewed as being mean and withholding, so whenever a child wanted or genuinely needed something he went to Sandy, who would then go to heroic measures to obtain whatever it was for the child. She would most often include a warning to the child to not let Denny know she was giving this because he wouldn't understand and would be angry at her. This set up a coalition between Tom and Sandy and between Jimmy and Sandy from the very beginning. Gina was sometimes included in Sandy's game; however, she was often in a coalition with Denny. As the children grew older and the twins became serious substance abusers, this coalition with Sandy became deadly. The primary way this was enacted was that she would bail them out of financial problems. She was in denial about events that were happening right in the boys' bedrooms. All of this bailing out occurred without Denny's knowledge. The behavior was very difficult for Sandy to break. In fact, when Denny died, the behavior increased, since it was even easier for her to have access to money. The dynamic remained the same and even the warnings to the children were the same when Denny was dead. Both boys became so addicted that each almost died. Tom became so entrenched in the use of crystal meth that he became involved with seriously dangerous characters and, in fact, engaged in criminal behavior himself temporarily while using. It took the near death of both twins to shift this dynamic in the family. The blame is not on Sandy for the boys' addiction; the entire family fit together like the perfect puzzle of addiction. I am simply pointing out the role she played in the dynamic that kept the twins locked into the abuse pattern.

Substance abuse issues are almost always multigenerational. Looking further into the family history of Sandy and Denny would reveal the dynamics that led to this sad scenario. If one drew a family tree and honestly put down traits about each person, one would find drug abuse, alcoholism, gambling, and compulsive overeating dotted throughout each generation. Addictive behaviors run like wildfire throughout families. Children of those who engage in addictive behaviors tend to become addicts themselves or to marry addicts. The family of origin tends to provide a poor environment that is lacking in growth, so that movement through normal stages of development is resisted.

SUBSTANCE ABUSE LEADS TO CHAOS IN RELATIONSHIPS

Substance abuse often leads to primitive conflict which can erupt in violence. At the very least, stormy scenes prevail. Another family I worked with demonstrates just how dangerous this is and how entrenched the family can become in the substance abuser's trap. Helen and Roy were in their eighties. Roy was bedridden and Helen was his primary caregiver. They had a son, Henry, who was fifty years old, was in and out of prison, and was a heroin addict. When Henry was between prison terms, he would come home looking for a place to crash. There was a strong coalition between Helen and Henry, similar to the one described above, with Roy seen as the bad guy. Roy would scream from his bed obscenities at Henry, and Helen would call Henry into the kitchen and say, "You know your father loves you; he doesn't mean what he says." All the while, she would slip a twenty-dollar bill into his hand and kiss him on the cheek as if to say, "This is our little secret." Only this little secret would turn into Henry wanting more and Helen exclaiming they were living on a fixed income with only enough money for food for the month. It was not unusual for these situations to result in Henry threatening to kill his parents and beginning to shove Helen against the wall. As the scene continued, Roy could hear all this from his bed and would begin to yell frantically, begging Helen to give the money to Henry. I was flabbergasted by such stories and, of course, immediately filed an elder abuse report. On further investigation, the scenario had occurred throughout Henry's life. The parents were always advised to not allow Henry into their home, and by the next day, they were welcoming him with open arms. Henry's sister, who had long ago obtained treatment for herself, had to remove herself from the system except on a very limited basis to maintain her own sanity.

Marital relationships that have substance abuse histories in one or both people are often wracked with conflict and power struggles. In the early phases of substance abuse, the spouse usually enables the addict by excusing his behavior problem as due to stress, something that will pass with time. At later stages, the spouse tries to regulate and moderate the using behavior by either engaging in using behaviors herself or by limiting money or supply. The addict resists this, and the more the spouse tries to stop the using behavior, the more the acting out. The spouse may fall into the trap of forgiving the addict when he acts remorseful, which momentarily relieves the addict of his guilt and makes him feel less responsible for his behavior. Another trap is that of becoming critical of the addict, such as Roy did with Henry. This also relieves the addict's shame and guilt because he can now blame the one who is critical for his drinking.

Children of addicts suffer a great deal and often present later in life with post-traumatic stress disorder. As children, they may display a variety of symptoms that are often not addressed: stuttering, excessive fear, tantrums, fighting, school problems, bed-wetting, and so on. They are upset by the parents' unhappiness, fighting, and lack of interest in their needs. Consequences for growing up with an addict seem to depend on the age of the child at the onset of the substance abuse, the child's gender, sibling order, whether physical or sexual abuse was present, and whether the child had significant other relatives or teachers outside the system who provided support. Children have been found to take on the role of the parentified child, family scapegoat, the child who disappears and is unnoticed and neglected, or the family clown who relieves tension by humor and distraction.

Children of addicts are in need of help. They need relief from anxiety or hypervigilance caused by the erratic behavior of the addict. They need to work through their sense of guilt and responsibility for the addict's behavior, for their parents' conflicts, or for not being able to adequately parent their siblings or themselves. They also have to look at their own enabling behavior that is designed to either rescue or persecute the addict. It is crucial that their denial of the problem be challenged. As children, they were unconsciously taught not to talk about things that occur in the family even to each other. Communication skills are greatly affected and these need to be addressed from the very beginning of treatment.

It is crucial that families learn to recognize that these behaviors, patterns, and dynamics have most likely been ingrained for generations. To have the addict simply stop using substances is not enough. Most are familiar with the term *dry drunk*. What this means is that the person is no longer abusing alcohol, but his behavior is still the same as when he was drinking. In fact, at the time the person stops using, his difficult behavior may even become exaggerated, as he no longer has the numbing effect of the substance to act as a barrier. He has lost a major defense for coping with life, so may overcompensate by engaging in more difficult behavior. Again, at the onset of sobriety, the family is often at risk of pushing the addict back to using because of the worsened situation. But if family members are prepared for this, they can learn to address their feelings openly.

It is common that once the addict stops using and tells everyone he is sorry for the pain he has caused them, he is shocked when they are enraged at him. He thinks everyone should be thanking him for becoming clean and should absolve him of any sins he may have committed. The fact is that the family has been abiding by the "don't talk" rule for a very long time. At last, they learn through treatment to express their feelings and commonly start with rage. When the addict finally stops using, family members become outraged, feeling, "If you can stop using so easily, why did you put us through so much hell?" The addict is very vulnerable and, of course, at risk of using at any moment, so it is vital that he have a support system throughout his recovery, and especially during this phase. Participation in Alcoholics Anonymous or other related groups is a must. If family members engage in Al-Anon or one of the children's groups, they too, can be supported in their vulnerability. They may be expressing feelings for the first time in their lives and also can no longer hide their behavior behind the drug use of the addict.

Substance abuse is a family problem. A family that is willing to work together to heal themselves has the most success. Choosing to live in a way that promotes growth is essential.

SUMMARY AND CONCLUSIONS

We have discussed many aspects of psychopharmacology, psychiatric diagnoses, and family dynamics at this point, and it is important to try to summarize these. Our goal is a greater ability to collaborate with a psychiatrist in treatment of a problem, so let's review how you can get this sense of empowerment.

DIAGNOSIS

Psychiatric diagnosis is a complex process. It begins by telling the story of the illness to an expert professional who asks lots of questions to flush out the details. The questions are asked to try to determine if there is a connection between what is happening to you right now and what has happened in your past, what genetic (family) loading may be present, what medical symptoms or illnesses might be contributing to the difficulty, and how relationships at work and home might be aggravating or helping the problem. Are prescription drugs or drugs of abuse getting in the way of recovery? This dialogue is a search for clues as to what medication and/or psychotherapy approaches might be most beneficial.

Additional sources of information can be very helpful in providing a long-term perspective and others' assessments of the problem: records of previous evaluations and treatment, hospital summaries, family history of psychiatric illness and treatment, lab data, psychological testing, and pharmacy records. Talking with an additional informant (spouse or parent) may add an extra perspective on both the illness and what strengths have been helpful in coping with it. Family members are often involved as informants, observers, cotherapists, and helpers in monitoring medication compliance and risk of dangerous behaviors. All of this information is synthesized into a differential diagnosis (list of possibilities) by the psychiatrist, and from this an initial treatment plan follows.

Diagnosis is typically made using the American Psychiatric Association's *Diagnostic and Statistical Manual,* fourth edition. This requires five semi-independent axes of diagnosis, including major psychiatric syndrome, personality disorder or traits, medical problems, stressors, and global assessment of function.

GOAL SETTING

The first part of treatment planning is setting goals. This should be an openly discussed, collaborative effort. At the conclusion of one to three interviews, the doctor-patient dialogue should include such explicit issues as what the diagnosis is; what treatment is supposed to help the patient to do; how long treatment will take; what it will cost in terms of hours working together, dollars, medication trials, and possible side effects, and lab tests; and how doctor and patient will know if treatment is succeeding or failing. The best way to do this is to prepare a set of goals of treatment or target symptoms and an expected approach to dealing with them. Don't be shy! Even if your doctor doesn't explicitly state his or her goals, tell him yours and make sure that you negotiate to the point where you both understand what you're trying to do together. What is expected of the doctor, the therapist (if there is one other than the doctor), and the patient? There are no magical cures, so you'll have to work at developing the goals and plans of treatment together. Examples might be as follows.

For a panic/agoraphobia patient:

1. Stop having panic attacks over the next one to two months. This will involve trying antidepressants and perhaps minor tranquilizers and fine-tuning the dose to make sure they are effective and side effects are tolerable.
2. Resume normal life. Start going to the movies, driving on the freeway, and return to school or work over the next two to four months. This will involve therapist encouragement, spouse or friend accompaniment the first time new things are done, and willingness to practice the exposure.
3. Take an airplane trip over the next three to six months to visit relatives or have a vacation. This will involve getting the panic under control, facing smaller fears repeatedly to build confidence, using medication to cut the acute anticipatory anxiety, going to the airport, and getting onto the airplane.

For a bipolar depressed patient, the goals and plans might be:

1. Get through this depression without trying to hurt myself or going into the hospital over the next few weeks.
2. Get a full family history, compile my medication history, get lab work done, and carefully choose an antidepressant and/or mood stabilizer to try as soon as possible. Discuss side effects and dose of the first-choice medication and alternative medications.
3. Start an antidepressant and/or mood stabilizer and take it for at least four weeks to see if it helps clear the depression.
4. If medicine helps, make a commitment to myself to stay on it for at least six to twelve months, and to stay away from abusable drugs.

5. Start to deal with the contributing factors and consequences of the mood disorder in psychotherapy, perhaps with spouse or other family members.

For a schizophrenic individual, the goals and plans might be:

1. Get the voices in my head to stop yelling nasty, critical things and arguing. Take the dose of medicine up just enough to do this without feeling really drugged. Talk with the doctor and ask for ways to control side effects if they bother me. If side effects get too bad, ask for a change of medicine.
2. Try to get some daily structure in my life. When the voices are controlled, call the local vocational rehabilitation office, community college, or employment office. Start a school or vocational training program or part-time job within the next two to four months.
3. Meet a few new friends. Life is too lonely with no one to talk to, so go to a support group and try to meet some new people. Maybe a few different groups will be worth visiting in order to find one where I'm comfortable.

MEDICINES, PSYCHOTHERAPY, AND SELF-HELP

The goals and plans described here obviously require different facilitators to make them happen. Eliminating symptoms such as panic, depression, or hallucinations usually involves medicines. Taking a good look at life and what's working and what isn't (or worse, may even be causing problems) is best done in psychotherapy. Behavioral changes can be aided by a therapist who has the expertise to translate global wishes into a series of smaller achievable steps. Throughout the case examples, we've seen how psychiatric illness impacts families and sometimes ruins relationships; couple or family therapy can help to deal with these issues. Self-help groups can make a real difference by relieving the loneliness and isolation of an illness, by teaching how others cope with the problems associated with being ill, and by providing educational speakers, books, and referrals to the best health care professionals.

SELF-OBSERVATION

Charting symptoms and the associated factors that made them better or worse is the best long-term habit you can possibly develop. Simply choosing the most bothersome symptoms and graphing them every day on a scale from 0 (awful) to 5 (excellent), and then filling in a few details of situations and medications, can make a world of difference in deciding if medication and psychotherapy are doing what is needed. A graph of depressed mood versus time might show relationships such as heavy drinking, working overtime, missing sleep, arguing with a loved one, or being premenstrual make things worse every time they occur, and taking an antidepressant at a minimum effective dose, exercise, meditation, or a long weekend away from home and work makes things better. The goal here is to look for long-term repetitive patterns of events, automatic thoughts, situations, or actions that make things better or worse, and then to begin making the appropriate corrections in lifestyle to feel better more consistently.

MEDICATION TRIALS

Attempts to treat symptoms with medications are just that. They may be very well informed, expertly planned, and executed, using the very best and newest of medicines and technology, yet still a medication trial might not work. If it doesn't work, ask the following questions: Were the dose and duration of the medication trial enough? Did I take the usual recommended dose, or maximum I could tolerate, or have a therapeutic blood level test, and continue taking the medicine for a full four to six weeks? Did I give it a fair chance by taking the medicine regularly and not abusing substances? If it didn't work, what does that mean? It might mean a missed diagnosis of a psychiatric or medical problem. Is a second opinion necessary? Getting an evaluation from an internist or neurologist or a second opinion from another psychiatrist might be reassuring for both doctor and patient in confirming that no major problem has been overlooked. Nonresponse might mean a correct diagnosis, but the medication just isn't right for the patient. If that is the case, it's not a personal failure. A decent doctor won't give up and neither should you. Most psychiatric illnesses have gone on for months (often years when people take a careful and honest look back at their lives) before I see the patient. I'll often tell people that if we need to try two to four different medications over as many months in order to find the one that works best with the fewest side effects, it is time and effort well spent because that medicine may well impact their quality of life for many years to come.

DURATION OF TREATMENT

Most of the psychiatric illnesses we have discussed are present throughout the life span. They may come and go over fairly long periods of time, or they may be consistent, chronic problems. The duration of treatment is dictated by several factors. A very recurrent or chronic illness is best treated long term. This may mean six to twelve months for some people, with a gradual tapering off of medicine when symptoms are stable for several months and possible retreatment in the future, but it may mean lifetime medication for others. As we begin to acknowledge that some psychiatric problems are biologic, familial, and chronic, and thus bear a remarkable resemblance to medical illnesses such as diabetes and high blood pressure, we can start to think of psychiatric medicines as correcting an underlying brain chemistry problem. Like their medical counterparts, psychiatric illnesses have major stress and lifestyle components, require a commitment to healthy lifestyle for optimal control, and may require lifetime treatment with the support and caring understanding of a good physician and loving family.

APPENDIX 1

COMMON DRUGS: THEIR USES, ADVANTAGES, AND SIDE EFFECTS

Drug Family	Examples	Uses	Advantages	Side Effects
Selective serotonin reuptake inhibitors	Prozac, Zoloft, Paxil, Luvox, Celexa	Major depressive episode, obsessive-compulsive disorder, panic disorder, bulimia, social phobia, premenstrual dysphoric disorder, post-traumatic stress disorder, premature ejaculation	Side effects mild for most people; safe in overdose	Upset stomach, diarrhea, insomnia or tiredness, sexual dysfunction
Tricyclic antidepressants	Elavil, Tofranil, Sinequan, Pamelor, Vivactil, Norpramin, Surmontil	Major depression, panic disorder, obsessive-compulsive disorder (Anafranil only), irritable bowel syndrome, chronic recurrent headaches, chronic pain/fibromyalgia	Generic forms are very inexpensive; blood levels may help dose adjustment	Dry mouth, blurred vision, constipation, dizziness with standing up quickly, weight gain, sexual dysfunction; overdose very dangerous
Atypical antidepressants	Wellbutrin (same as Zyban)	Major depressive episode, smoking cessation	Energizing, no weight gain or sexual dysfunction	Headache, insomnia, dry mouth, 0.1–0.4 percent seizure risk
	Serzone	Major depressive episode	Anxiety relieving, no sleep disruption or sexual dysfunction	Sedation
	Remeron	Major depressive episode	Same as Serzone	Sedation, weight gain
	Effexor	Major depressive episode, generalized anxiety disorder (chronic anxiety)	Effective for treatment of resistant or very severe depression	Nausea, tiredness, sexual dysfunction; stimulating at high dose

Drug Family	Examples	Uses	Advantages	Side Effects
Typical antipsychotics (neuroleptics, major tranquilizers)—oral	Haldol, Prolixin, Stelazine, Navane, Thorazine, Mellaril, Moban, Loxitane	Schizophrenia, severe agitation in mania or major medical illness, psychotic symptoms in severe depression	Inexpensive generics available for most	Muscle stiffness, restlessness, emotional dulling, breast enlargement, irregular menstrual periods, weight gain, very rare neuroleptic malignant syndrome (high fever and muscle breakdown), long-term risk of tardive dyskinesia (involuntary facial movements)
Typical antipsychotics (neuroleptics, major tranquilizers)—injectable long acting	Haldol Decanoate, Prolixin Decanoate	Same as above	Long-acting injection form may last one to four weeks and eliminates daily struggles over medication compliance	Same as above

Drug Family	Examples	Uses	Advantages	Side Effects
Atypical antipsychotic	Clozaril	Schizophrenia or schizoaffective disorder	"Rescue drug" when numerous other antipsychotics have failed or been intolerable. Works on both positive symptoms (hallucinations, delusions, agitation) and negative symptoms; social withdrawal, lack of drive, lack of pleasure, lack of conversation	Rare suppression of bone marrow, leading to inability to fight off infection; requires blood sample every one to two weeks; weight gain, drooling, sedation, seizures at high dose
Atypical antipsychotic	Zyprexa, Risperdal, Seroquel, Zeldox	Same as above	Works well on both positive and negative symptoms; vastly more tolerable than typical oral antipsychotics; people often feel much more normal on them than older drugs	Weight gain (except Zeldox), sedation, rare muscle stiffness or restlessness

Drug Family	Examples	Uses	Advantages	Side Effects
Lithium	Lithobid, Eskalith CR, Lithane	Mood normalization in bipolar affective disorder (antimanic, antidepressant, and cycle prevention effects); augmentation of antidepressant response in major depression, antiaggressive effects	Blood levels well known, inexpensive generics and slow-release forms available	Increased thirst and urination, tremor, upset stomach, diarrhea, sometimes loss of mental acuity (energy and memory), weight gain, occasionally hypothyroidism, rare kidney damage; requires blood testing every one to three months (drug level) and every six to twelve months (thyroid and kidney monitoring)
Anticonvulsant	Depakote, Depakene	Antimanic, cycle prevention	More effective than lithium in rapid cycling bipolar affective disorder, mixed mania with depression symptoms (dysphoric mania), drug-induced mania	Tremor, hair loss, nausea, weight gain; rare hepatitis, pancreatitis; requires blood testing every one to three months for drug level and liver monitoring

Drug Family	Examples	Uses	Advantages	Side Effects
Anticonvulsant	Tegretol	Antimanic, cycle prevention (widely used in the past; not FDA approved except for seizures)	May be more effective than lithium in rapid cycling and mixed mania	Induces enzymes that can make birth control pills ineffective, occasional bone marrow suppression with risk of infection; requires blood testing every one to three months for drug level and white blood cell count, liver monitoring
Anticonvulsant	Lamictal	Antidepressant, cycle prevention, antimanic (not FDA approved except for seizures)	Among mood stabilizers, perhaps the most effective against depression	Rare but potentially serious rash; requires very slow dose increases
Anticonvulsant	Neurontin	Antidepressant, antimanic, cycle prevention, social phobia (not FDA approved except for seizures)	Appears effective in chronic pain and reducing anxiety	No drug interactions or biologic metabolism

Drug Family	Examples	Uses	Advantages	Side Effects
High potency anti-anxiety benzodiazepine	Xanax, Klonopin	Panic disorder, chronic, situational, or medical illness–related anxiety	Able to block panic attacks without being overly sedating for most people, useful on as needed basis; safe in overdose	Physiologic and psychologic dependence with daily use over about one month, abuse in some individuals, difficult to stop using (withdrawal), sedation, incoordination, occasional memory impairment
Low-potency anti-anxiety benzodiazepine	Librium, Valium, Tranxene, Serax	Chronic, situational, or medical illness–related anxiety; alcohol withdrawal	Inexpensive generics available; safe in overdose	Same as above
Short-acting sedative-hypnotics (sleeping pills) benzodiazepine-type drugs	Halcion, Ambien, Sonata	Insomnia, especially problems getting to sleep	Rapid action, no morning hangover	Same as above
Long-acting sedative-hypnotics (sleeping pills) benzodiazepines	Dalmane, Doral	Insomnia, especially problems staying asleep	Longer action, some daytime anti-anxiety effect	Same as above; may accumulate with daily use leading to toxic levels

Drug Family	Examples	Uses	Advantages	Side Effects
Non-benzodiazepine tranquilizer	BuSpar	Useful for chronic generalized anxiety disorder (chronic worriers); ineffective for panic attacks	No sedation, muscle relaxation, withdrawal syndrome, memory effects, but requires daily use for a few weeks to be effective	Dizziness
Barbiturates	Tuinal, Nembutal, Seconal, Phenobarbital	Anticonvulsant and anesthetic uses only; use for anxiety or insomnia is obsolete	None!	Lethal in overdose, high risk of seizures on abrupt withdrawal, induce enzymes that metabolize other drugs faster

APPENDIX 2

Drugs Categorized by Brand and Generic Names

Brand name	Generic name	Primary use
Ambien	zolpidem	Insomnia
Ativan	lorazepam	Panic, Anxiety
Celexa	citalopram	Depression
Clozaril	clozapine	Schizophrenia
Depakote	divalproex sodium	Bipolar
Effexor	venlafaxine	Depression
Elavil	amitriptyline	Depression
Eskalith CR	lithium carbonate controlled release	Bipolar
Halcion	triazolam	Insomnia
Haldol	haloperidol	Schizophrenia
Klonopin	clonazepam	Panic, Anxiety
Lamictal	lamotrigine	Bipolar
Lithane	lithium carbonate	Bipolar
Lithobid	lithium carbonate slow release	Bipolar
Loxitane	loxapine	Schizophrenia
Luvox	fluvoxamine	OCD
Marplan	isocarboxazid	Depression
Mellaril	thioridazine	Schizophrenia
Moban	molindone	Schizophrenia
Nardil	phenelzine	Depression, Panic
Navane	thiothixene	Schizophrenia
Neurontin	gabapentin	Bipolar
Norpramin	desipramine	Depression
Pamelor	nortriptyline	Depression
Parnate	tranylcypromine	Depression, Panic
Paxil	paroxetine	Depression, Panic, OCD
Prolixin	fluphenazine	Schizophrenia
Prozac	fluoxetine	Depression, Bulimia, OCD
Remeron	mirtazapine	Depression
Risperdal	risperidone	Schizophrenia
Serax	oxazepam	Anxiety, Insomnia
Seroquel	quetiapine	Schizophrenia
Serzone	nefazodone	Depression
Sinequan	doxepin	Depression
Stelazine	trifluoperazine	Schizophrenia
Tegretol	carbamazepine	Bipolar
Thorazine	chlorpromazine	Schizophrenia
Tofranil	imipramine	Depression
Tranxene	clorazepate	Anxiety, Insomnia
Valium	diazepam	Anxiety, Insomnia
Vivactil	protriptyline	Depression
Wellbutrin	bupropion	Depression
Xanax	alprazolam	Panic, Anxiety
Zoloft	sertraline	Depression, Panic, OCD
Zyban	bupropion	Smoking cessation (see Wellbutrin)
Zyprexa	olanzepine	Schizophrenia

GLOSSARY

Anhedonia: The inability to experience joy or pleasure in life.

Anticholinergic: Side effects of some drugs that involve dry mouth, blurred vision, and constipation. Often seen with tricyclic antidepressants (especially Elavil), some side-effect medicines used with the major tranquilizers (Cogentin, Artane, Akineton), or major tranquilizers (Thorazine, Mellaril).

Anticonvulsant: A drug usually used to prevent the recurrence of seizures (convulsions). Some anticonvulsants, such as Depakote, Tegretol, Lamictal, and Neurontin, are used "off label" (without FDA approval) as mood stabilizers.

Augmentation: The use of a second drug along with the primary one in an attempt to get a better or more complete response by taking advantage of two different mechanisms of action.

Barbiturate: Sedative-hypnotics characterized by their ability to cause dependence, respiratory depression, withdrawal seizures, and overdose deaths. These drugs are obsolete in psychiatry.

Benzodiazepine: See *minor tranquilizer.*

Cognitive behavioral therapy: Psychotherapy that is structured, short term, involves homework, and is oriented toward discovering and changing maladaptive thoughts (such as childhood scripts imposed by others) and behaviors.

Comorbidity: The existence of two or more distinct psychiatric disorders in the same person.

Day treatment: Often this is a step in between twenty-four-hour-a-day hospitalization and once-a-week outpatient psychotherapy. Typically, the patient spends three to five hours per day several days per week in group therapies designed to help achieve stabilization, socialization, and rehabilitation while still living at home.

Delusions: Firmly held, fixed, false beliefs that are not subject to argument or testing and that are not shared by others in one's culture or religion. Examples may include feelings of jealousy, persecution, people talking about oneself, or thoughts being broadcast out loud or put into one's mind.

Depersonalization: Feeling detached from oneself, as in a dream.

Depot injection: A form of a drug that may be given as a long-acting injection; for example, Haldol Decanoate, which is often given as a monthly injection.

Derealization: Feeling that the world is unfamiliar, strange, or unreal.

Differential diagnosis: This is the list of diagnostic possibilities early in the process of getting to know a patient. For example, a patient with depression might have major depression, bipolar affective disorder, alcohol abuse, or hypothyroidism. This list of possibilities would be further explored (with family history, laboratory studies, and more questioning) to determine which is the most accurate label for the illness.

Diurnal variation: A pattern of mood variation characterized as better at one time of day and worse at another.

Drug metabolism: The body's processing of drugs. This involves absorption (from the gut), distribution to various parts of the body including the active site (the brain for psychiatric drugs), breakdown (usually in the liver), and excretion (in urine or feces).

Dysphoria: Unpleasant, miserable.

Electroconvulsive therapy (ECT): The use of electrically induced seizures to treat psychiatric disorders. Now always done with general anesthesia and muscle paralysis so that the person is not aware of the seizure and the muscle contractions do not cause damage to bones. ECT is usually reserved for cases of severe depression in the United States.

Euthymic: Normal mood, neither depressed nor elated.

Exposure treatment: The treatment of choice for simple phobias as well as obsessive-compulsive disorder; involves actual time being in close contact with the object of the fear or anxiety in order to get used to (habituate) to the anxiety. In OCD, this is often accompanied by response prevention, which involves preventing the person from performing his usual ritual in response to the anxiety.

Grandiosity: An inflated sense of one's worth, power, or sense of being very special.

Half-life: The time it takes the body to eliminate half of a drug dosage. Typically, it takes four to five half-lives to build up to a steady level of a drug when it is started and a similar amount of time to get it out of the body when it is stopped.

Hallucinations: Abnormal sensory experiences that are not apparent to other people, such as hearing voices or seeing visions that seem very real.

Hamilton Anxiety Rating Scale: Similar to the Hamilton Depression Rating Scale but used to measure severity of anxiety.

Hamilton Depression Rating Scale: A series of questions asked by the doctor about depression symptoms, each of which is numerically scored, to get a total score that is a measure of severity of depression. Similar self-rating scales have been developed by Beck and Zung.

"Helper" drug: See *augmentation*.

Hypomanic: Mild manic symptoms, not enough to get a person into serious trouble or hospitalized, often considered a pleasant, energized, very social, and creative state by individuals with bipolar II affective disorder.

Ideas of reference: The thought that others (strangers on the street, radio, or TV) are talking about oneself.

Insight-oriented psychotherapy: Therapy oriented toward deeper understanding of how and why a life problem developed and long-term change or resolution of psychological problems.

Labile: Mood that changes rapidly, often from moment to moment; for example, sudden shifts from normal or good mood to sad or angry.

Major tranquilizer: Drugs used for treatment of psychotic symptoms or severe agitation, especially in schizophrenia, severe mania, or depression. Often called antipsychotics or neuroleptics. Older examples include Haldol, Prolixin, and Thorazine. Newer examples include Clozaril, Risperdal, Zyprexa, and Seroquel. These drugs do not produce dependence and are effective for psychotic symptoms such as hallucinations or delusions.

MAOI: Monoamine oxidase inhibitor, the name of a class of antidepressant/antipanic drugs. These drugs, such as Nardil, Parnate, and Marplan, are seldom used due to their potentially risky interactions with other drugs (cold pills, decongestants, diet pills, Demerol) and aged fermented foods (such as beer, wine, cheese).

MFCC: Marriage Family and Child Counselor, an individual trained at the master's level in psychology to provide psychotherapy to individuals and families

Minor tranquilizer: Drugs used for the treatment of anxiety, also used for alcohol withdrawal; chemically, members of the benzodiazepine family, such as Librium, Valium, Xanax, and Klonopin. These drugs may produce dependence and are not effective for psychotic symptoms such as hallucinations or delusions.

Mixed state (dysphoric) mania: Manic syndrome along with depressive symptoms.

Mood reactivity: The ability to be responsive to the environment, to be cheered up in response to something nice happening.

MSE (mental status exam): The observations and specific questions that are asked to determine how a person is thinking and feeling. This usually includes appearance and behavior, thinking, memory, orientation, mood, affect (expression of feelings), unusual thoughts (delusions) or hallucinations, and evaluation of suicidal, homicidal, and paranoid ideation. It may include tests such as interpreting similarities and proverbs, remembering words, subtracting numbers, naming objects, drawing objects, and reading.

MSW or LCSW: Master's of Social Work or Licensed Clinical Social Worker. An individual trained to work with individuals as well as social systems (such as families and government agencies) to help deal with problems both psychologically (through psychotherapy of the individual or family) and practically (for example, knowing how to get government benefits).

Negative symptoms of schizophrenia: Psychological functions that are missing or blunted, such as lack of willpower (avolition), restricted emotional expression (flat affect), lack of logical thinking, lack of socialization, lack of enjoyment (anhedonia).

Neuroleptic: See *major tranquilizer.*

Neuroleptic malignant syndrome: Sudden development of high fever and muscle breakdown while taking neuroleptic (antipsychotic) medication. This is unpredictable, potentially lethal, and requires intensive monitoring.

Oriented/orientation: Awareness of the date, place, personal identity, and situation in which one finds oneself.

Paranoia: The suspicion that others are plotting against, harassing, or persecuting one.

Partial hospitalization: See *day treatment.*

Pathologic gambler: One who gambles compulsively and excessively, to the point where it interferes with normal budgeting and paying bills such as rent and groceries.

Personality disorder: Long-standing ways of thinking about and relating to oneself and others that may cause problems in relationships, often without a sense of insight, and with a sense of disappointment that others do not respond as the person wants and expects them to respond.

Positive symptoms of schizophrenia: Symptoms that are present and should not be, such as hallucinations, delusions, or bizarre behavior.

Pressured speech: Rapid, often nonstop speech.

Prodromal: An early sign or symptom of a disorder, which may be nonspecific discomfort such as social withdrawal, anxiety, or insomnia before a fully developed episode of illness occurs.

Psychiatrist: An individual who first trained as a medical doctor and then specialized in diagnosing and treating mental disorders with both medications and psychotherapy.

Psychoanalytic therapy: Therapy oriented toward deeper understanding of how and why a life problem developed and long-term change or resolution of psychological problems. This usually involves interpretation of transference (feelings toward the therapist who is generally a quiet listener) and resistance to change. Psychoanalysis involves three to five sessions per week, lying on a couch so that there is no eye contact with the therapist. Both psychoanalytic therapy and psychoanalysis are usually long-term treatments.

Psychologist: An individual trained at the master's or Ph.D. level to provide diagnostic assessments (by interviews and specialized tests) and psychotherapy to an individual or family.

Psychomotor agitation: Restlessness, inability to sit still, pacing, hand-wringing, a driven energy without a clear goal.

Psychomotor retardation: Slowed thinking, moving, and speech, appearing to lack energy or movement.

Psychosis: Delusions or prominent hallucinations, usually with a loss of sense of reality and impaired ability to function in everyday life.

Rapid cycling affective disorder: More than four episodes per year of major depression or mania.

Residual: A late remaining sign or symptom of an illness after it has been partially controlled and started to improve.

SSRI: Selective serotonin reuptake inhibitors, a group of antidepressants used also for panic, obsessive-compulsive disorder, bulimia, and sometimes for premenstrual syndrome, post-traumatic stress disorder, and other problems. They share a common mechanism of action, blocking presynaptic neurons from taking serotonin back up into the neuron that released them. Examples include Celexa, Luvox, Paxil, Zoloft, and Prozac.

Suicidal ideation: Thoughts about one's own death, which may vary from passive (it's okay if I get run over) to active (such as plans to buy a gun and bullets).

Supportive psychotherapy: Therapy geared to enhancing coping skills and problem solving during a period where the patient's usual coping strategies may be overwhelmed.

Taper: Gradually decreasing the dose of a medicine in order to see if it is no longer needed, to see if side effects will decrease, or to see if symptoms will return.

Tardive dyskinesia: Late-onset movement disorder in an individual taking neuroleptic drugs, usually involving mostly facial muscles and the tongue, predominantly occurring after several years of use of typical antipsychotics. New atypical antipsychotics may have substantially lower risk of this problem.

TCA: Tricyclic antidepressants, a group of antidepressants used for depression and sometimes for panic disorder, obsessive-compulsive disorder (Anafranil only), and chronic headaches or pain. They share a common three-ring structure. They are relatively old and available as inexpensive generic forms.

Titrate: Adjusting the dose of a medicine gradually, over time, to get the maximal benefit with minimal side effects.

SUGGESTED READING

Books for the general reader who wants to become familiar with psychiatry and psychopharmacology, written in a way that makes them very readable and generally understandable to the nonphysician:

Gitlin, Michael J. *The Psychotherapist's Guide to Psychopharmacology,* 2d edition. New York: The Free Press, 1996.

Gorman, Jack M. *The Essential Guide to Psychiatric Drugs,* 3d edition. New York: St. Martin's Griffin, 1997.

Julien, Robert M. *A Primer of Drug Action: A Concise, Nontechnical Guide to the Actions, Uses, and Side Effects of Psychoactive Drugs,* 8th edition. New York: W. H. Freeman and Company, 1998.

Nathan, Peter E. and Jack M. Gorman. *A Guide to Treatments That Work.* New York: Oxford University Press, 1998.

Stahl, Stephen M. *Essential Psychopharmacology: Neuroscientific Basis and Practical Applications.* New York: Cambridge University Press, 1996.

Comprehensive psychiatric textbooks that are more technical and detailed include the following:

American Psychiatric Association (Task Force on DSM-IV, Allen Frances Chairperson). *Diagnostic and Statistical Manual of Mental Disorders,* 4th edition. Washington, D.C.: American Psychiatric Association, 1994. (Note: this is referred to as *DSM-IV* throughout our book and by most mental health professionals.)

Bezchlibnyk-Butler, Z. Kalyna, and J. Joel Jeffries. *Clinical Handbook of Psychotropic Drugs,* 9th edition. Seattle: Hogrefe & Huber Publishers, 1999.

Dunner, David L. *Current Psychiatric Therapy,* 2d edition. Philadelphia: W.B. Saunders Company, 1997.

Hales, Robert E., Stuart C. Yudofsky, and John A. Talbott. *The American Psychiatric Press Textbook of Psychiatry*, 3d edition. Washington, D.C.: American Psychiatric Press, 1999.

Janicak, Philip G., John M. Davis, Sheldon H. Preskorn, and Frank J. Ayd, Jr. *Principles and Practice of Psychopharmacotherapy*, 2d edition. Baltimore: Williams & Wilkins, 1997.

Kaplan, Harold I., and Benjamin J. Sadock. *Comprehensive Textbook of Psychiatry/VI*. Baltimore: Williams & Wilkins, 1996.

Schatzberg, Alan F., and Charles B. Nemeroff. *The American Psychiatric Press Textbook of Psychopharmacology*, 2d edition. Washington, D.C.: American Psychiatric Press, 1998.

Tasman, Allan, Jerald Kay, and Jeffrey A. Lieberman. *Psychiatry*. Philadelphia: W. B. Saunders Company, 1997.

INDEX

acute mania
  Klonopin (clonazepam), 246
  lithium used for treatment, 245–46
agoraphobia, 21–22
  panic disorder with, 22
alcohol and drug abuse
  family issues, 325
  interventions can help, 326–27
  nicotine addiction, 323–25
  opiate abuse, 322–23
  secondary gain, 327–29
  stimulant abuse, 321–22
  substance abuse and chaos in relationships, 329–32
  tranquilizer abuse, 320–21
alcoholism, 317–18
  complications of, 318
  older approach of prevention, 320
  pharmacologic treatment, 319–20
  significant genetic component, 318
  treatment by psychiatrists, options for, 318–19
Anafranil, 66
  long-term use, 67
  side effects, 66–67
antidepressant(s)
  new generation of, 153–54
  that should not be used for panic disorder, 24
  useful in treating panic disorder, 24
antidepressant treatment of panic order, process of
  MAO inhibitors, 26
  SSRIs, 25–26
  tricyclic, 24–25

anxiety, 18
anxiety, medical causes of, 19
Anxiety Disease, The (Sheehan), 37
anxiety disorder, generalized, 113
  benzodiazepine, 114–15
  BuSpar (buspirone), 116
  other anxiety disorders, 122
  symptoms, 113
anxiety disorders, drugs to avoid when treating
  antipsychotic drugs (Haldol and Stelazine), 122
  barbiturates and meprobamate (Miltown), 122
anxiety disorders: panic and phobias
  anxiety, medical causes of, 19
  epidemiology, 19–20
  family issues in panic disorder and anxiety disorders, 57–60
  panic attacks, 20–23
  panic disorder, medical treatment of, 23–29
  psychotherapeutic treatment of panic disorder, 29
  social phobia, 30–32
  specific phobias, 30
assertiveness training, 31–32

benzodiazepine, 114
  with driving and alcohol, 114
  half-life, 115
  minor tranquilizers, 115
  short-acting, 115
benzodiazepine anxiolytics for treating panic disorder
  Klonopin (clonazepam), advantages of, 26, 27–28

Xanax (alprazolam), doses, side effects and advantages of, 26–27
benzodiazepine treatment issues, 132–134
bipolar affective disorder (manic depressive illness), 243–45
   acute bipolar depression, 247
   acute mania, 245–47
   cyclothymic, 244
   diagnostic criteria for, 243–44
   hypomania, 243
   long-term maintenance treatment, 248–51
   natural history of, 244–45
   seasonal subtype, 244
body dysmorphic disorder, 62–63
BuSpar (buspirone), 68, 116, 164–65

catatonic symptoms in depression, 141
codependency, 111–12
cognitive behavioral therapy, 29

Dalmane (flurazepam), 125
depression
   antidepressants, new generation of, 153–54
   BuSpar, 164–65
   drug dosing, 160–63
   drugs, unresponsive to, 143–44
   drugs that cause depression, 138–39
   electroconvulsive therapy (ECT), 168
   family issues in depression, 230–41
   psychiatric diagnosis, 137–38
   illness and depression, 142–43
   MAO inhibitors, 163–64
   medication for, 148–53
   medication trials, 154–55
   primary depression, 137
   psychotherapy or medications?, 144–46
   refractory depression, 165–68
   response lag, 158–59
   safety and overdose risk, 154
   seasonal affective disorder, 165
   secondary depression, 137–38
   subtypes of depression, 140–42
   suicide, 146–47
   treatment, duration of, 159–60
   unpolar and bipolar mood disorders, 139–40
depression, acute bipolar
   antidepressants, 247
   cycling, 247
depression, proper medication for treatment, 148–49
   side effects: helpful or harmful?, 149–53
depression, family issues in
   depression among elderly or terminally ill, 238–39
   enmeshment, 232–36
   family depression, dynamics of, 230–31
   suicide threats and attempts, coping with, 239–41
depression, laboratory evaluation of
   biologic markers, 148
   physical causes of, 147–48
depression, refractory, 165–18
depression, subtypes
   atypical depression, 140–41
   catatonic symptoms, 141
   melancholic subtype, 140
   psychotic, 141
   seasonal depression, 141–42
Desyrel (trazodone), 149–50
diagnosis, psychiatric, 1
   chief complaint, 4–5
   data, identifying, 4
   medical, 3–4
   nonmedical, 2–3

Diagnostic and Statistical Manual,
 fourth edition (American
 Psychiatric Association), 1
Doral, 125
dosages for anxiety disorders, 28–29
drug dosing
 Celexa, 161
 Effexor (venlafaxine), 162–63
 Paxil, 161
 Prozac, 160, 161
 Wellbutrin, 161–62
 Zoloft, 160–61
drug half-life, 125
drug treatments for OCD, 66
 Anafranil (clomipramine), 66–67
DSM-IV, 122
dysthymia, 143–44

Elavil (amitriptyline), 150
electroconvulsive therapy
 (ECT)(shock treatment), 168
emotional aloofness, 312–13
enmeshment in families with bipolar
 affective disorder, 271–73
epidemiology
 diagnosis of anxiety disorders, 20
 onset of anxiety disorders, 19–20
 percentage of adult population
  with symptoms, 19
exam(s)
 mental status, 9
 physical, 9–10

family dynamics and insomnia
 double bind, 131
 good sleep hygiene, 131
 secondary gain, 130–31
family dynamics in bipolar disorder,
 271
family issues
 with OCD, how obsessive-compulsive disorder affects families, 91–92

 in panic disorder and anxiety disorders, 57–60
 in schizophrenia, entire family is
  affected, 308–9
Feighner, 162–63

generalized anxiety disorder
 benzodiazepine, 114–15
 BuSpar, 116
 characteristics of, 113

habits of patient, 8
Halcion (triazolam), 126
history (of patient)
 developmental, 8
 family, 7–8
 medical, 7
history of present illness, 5
hypnosis or relaxation training, 29
hypothyroidism and anxiety, 19

illness, 5–6
 denial of, 274
 and depression, 142–43
impairment in relationships
 (insomnia)
 described, 129–30
 marital discord, 130
insomnia, family issues with,
 129–130
insomnia and minor tranquilizers,
 123–27
 acute situational insomnia, 123
 acute stress-related insomnia, 123
 anticholinergic, 125
 antihistamines, 125
 behavioral approaches to, 124
 benzodiazepine treatment issues,
  132–34
 chronic insomnia, 123–24
 circadian rhythm disturbance, 124
 major sleep disorders, 123–24
 periodic leg movements, 124

rapid eye movement (REM), 124
sleeping pills, 125–27
interventions, 326–27

Janicak, Phillip, 28, 125

Klonopin, 115, 120, 121, 122
Kupfer, 159

Librium, 114, 115
life situation, current, 8–9
Luvox (fluvoxamine) for treating OCD, 68

maintenance treatment, long-term, 248
  Lithium, 248–250
  psychotherapy and depression, 250–51
MAO inhibitors
  Nardil (phenelzine), 163–64
  Parnate (tranylcypromine), 164
  for treating OCD, 69
medical diagnosis, medical model, 3–4
medication not working, what happens
  additional data, 156
  augmentation strategies, 156–57
  charting moods and depression ratings, 155–56
medication trials, how to best utilize
  adequate antidepressant trial, 155
  flexibility, 155
melancholic subtype (of depression), 140
mitral valve prolapse and panic attacks, 19
monoamine oxidase inhibitors, MAOIs (Nardil)
  restrictions and drugs to avoid, 24, 26
multiple disorders and obsessive-compulsive personality

acknowledgments before treatment can begin, 65
average age of onset, 64
follow-up studies, long-term, 64–65
obsessive-compulsive personality disorder, 64
OCD and simple phobias, differences in, 64
treatment, 65

nicotine addiction, 323–25
Nierenberg, 162–63
nonmedical diagnosis, 2–3

obsessive-compulsive disorder (OCD), 61
  body dysmorphic disorder, 62–63
  disorders, multiple, 64–65
  drug treatments for OCD, 66–69
  hoarding, 62
  multiple disorders, 64–65
  other disorders with OCD, 63
  symptoms among adults, 61–62
  Tourette's disorder, 63
  trichotillomania, 63
OCD, drug treatments for, 66
  Anafranil (clomipramine), 66–67
  BuSpar (buspirone), 68
  Luvox (fluvoxamine), 68
  MAO inhbitors, 69
  Prozac (fluoxetine), 67
OCD, family issues with, 91–96
  how OCD affects families, 91–92
  symptoms, families encouraging, 92
  when a family member refuses to admit there is a problem, 94–95
  when the family member agrees to accept help, 96
opiate abuse, 322–23

panic attack(s), 20–21
  agoraphobia, 21–22
  characteristics of, 20
  first person scenario, 34
  full-blown and small, 21
  onset and situations that trigger, 20
  situational or unexpected, 20–21
  symptoms, 21
panic disorder, 22–23
  complication of, 23
  onset of, 22
panic disorder, medical treatment, 23–28
panic disorder, psychotherapeutic treatment of
  cognitive behavioral therapy, 29
  hypnosis or relaxation training, 29
panic disorder and anxiety disorders, family issues in, 57–58
  examples, 58–59
  managing, 60
  power boss role, 60
  separation from primary caregiver, 57–58
performance anxiety, 31
phobia, social
  assertiveness training, 31–32
  characteristics of, 30
  and depression, 31–32
  drugs for treating, 31
  performance anxiety, 31
  population affected, 31
  underdiagnosed, reasons for, 31
phobias (specific), of anxiety disorders, 30
post-traumatic stress disorder (PTSD), 99
  acute stress disorder, 99–100
  codependency, 111–12
  comorbidity, 100
  drugs used in treating, 101
  education about PTSD and its effects, 105–6
  emotional responses to trauma, 100
  epidemiological studies, 100
  family history, importance of, 109–10
  how PTSD affects families, 104–5
  primary treatment, 100–1
  substance abuse and alcoholic family, 110–11
  triggers, 107–9
Prozac (fluoxetine), 67
psychiatric diagnosis
  current life situation, 8–9
  defining target symptoms, 12–13
  developmental history, 8
  diagnosis, 1–5
  evaluating an illness (symptom description), 5
  family history, 7–8
  habits, 8
  history of present illness, 5
  how to help your doctor, 11–12
  laboratory examinations, 10–11
  medical history, 7
  mental status exam, 9
  physical exam, 9–10
  psychiatric treatment, past, 6–7
  review of systems, 9
psychiatric treatment, past, 6–7
psychotherapeutic treatment of panic disorder, 29
psychotherapy or medications?, 144–46
psychotic (subtype of depression), 141
PTSD: family history, importance of, 109–10
PTSD and how it affects families, 104
  family participation in treatment, 105
  traumatic events that affect families, 104–5
PTSD and its effects, education, 105–6

refractory, 165–66
response lag, 158–59
risk factors with benzoiazepine treatment
   medical benefits, 134
   rebound or withdrawal symptoms, 132–33
   seizures, 133

safety and overdose risk, 154
schizophrenia, 279–81
   antipsychotic selection, 283–86
   communication, 309–11
   delusions, 279–80
   development of, 281–82
   emotional aloofness (requires patience), 312–13
   family issues in, 308–9, 314–316
   hallucinations, 279
   helpful hints for, 313–14
   negative effects of criticism, 311–12
   neuroleptic malignant syndrome, 287
   psychosis, 279
   psychosocial treatments, 287
   symptoms, 280–281
   tranquilizers, minor, 283
   tranquilizers (major), neuroleptic and antipsychotic, 282–83
   treatments, alternatives and adjunctive, 286–87
seasonal affective disorder, 165
seasonal depression (subtype of depression), 141–42
secondary gain and enmeshment, 327–29
selective serotonin reuptake inhibitors (Prozac, Zoloft, and Paxil), 24, 25–26

Serzone (nefazodone), 149–50
side effects (of medication)
   anticholinergic, 150
   sedating antidepressants, 149–50
   weight loss, 150
sleeping pills
   classes of, 125–27
   long-half-life, implications of, 125–26
stimulant abuse, 321–22
Stop Obsessing (Foa), 87
stress, chronic, 8–9
substance abuse. *See* alcohol and drug abuse.
suicide, 146–47
   risk factors, 147
systems, review of, 9

target symptoms, 12–13
thyroid disease and anxiety, 19
Tourette's disorder, 63–64
tranquilizer abuse, 320–321
trichotillomania (compulsive hair pulling), 63
tricyclic antidepressants (imipramine and desipramine)
   doses, side effects, anticholinergic effects and availability, 24–25
triggers (PTSD), 107
   examples, 107–9

unipolar and bipolar mood disorders
   major depression, symptoms of, 139–40
   primary mood disorders, 139

Valium, 114

Xanax, 114, 115, 132–33